Half a Century of Medical Research

Volume One

Medical Research Council

Half a Century of Medical Research

Volume One: Origins and Policy of the Medical Research Council (UK)

A. Landsborough Thomson
(late Second Secretary of the Council)

London Her Majesty's Stationery Office
1973

SBN 11 450025 8 *

Author's Preface

The subject of this work is a British agency created to promote research in the biomedical field, namely the Medical Research Council. The first volume deals with the history of this body, particularly in its constitutional and administrative aspects. The second volume will deal with the development of its scientific programme.

The period covered is the first half-century of the Council's existence as such, 1920–70, plus the seven years of the predecessor Medical Research Committee, 1913–20. The steps taken to establish that Committee, in 1911–13, are also described, with some retrospect upon still earlier events in the United Kingdom leading up to the recognition of a public responsibility for medical research. Some points relating to 1971 (or even early 1972) that it would have been pedantic to ignore have been inserted during the final stages of preparation for press.

The first six chapters present a continuous chronicle, but limited to the constitutional aspect; otherwise the approach has been analytical, the method being to treat different facets of the subject separately, each for the whole period. No attempt has been made to build the story round outstanding personalities, which would have been invidious and lacking in proper balance. An institution is an organism of which the whole is greater than the sum of its parts; it has a corporate existence to which very many people contribute in different ways and degrees, and it acquires a continuing momentum of its own which transcends individual lives. It is an ideal that anyone may well be proud to serve during his time, but that nobody can claim as his own.

It is a fundamental tenet that science is international and that its advance cannot be described in terms of the contribution made by one country or a particular organisation. A new line of investigation may be opened up here or there, or in different parts of the world simultaneously, when the general state of knowledge is ripe for the particular development. These beginnings depend, firstly, on the ideas of workers in the front line of scientific advance. They depend, secondly, on opportunity—the earlier training of these workers, their material support and intellectual freedom as investigators, and their provision with appropriate technical resources. It is in the creation of such opportunities that promotion consists. The primary concern in these pages thus lies with the origins of policy, such as the reasons why particular methods of promotion were adopted, the considerations governing the relation between administration and science, and the circumstances in which certain subjects of research were selected for special support. The subsequent advance of research soon becomes part of the general history of scientific progress.

The writer has accordingly been primarily concerned to describe the beginnings of what later became major developments in the Council's scientific programme, and the early formulation of administrative principles that are now either accepted as axiomatic or have been overlaid by subsequent amendment or retrospective rationalisation. This has involved checking with contemporary records, of which the long series of published annual reports provides a rich source that is still far from exhaustion. Unpublished minutes, memoranda and letters filed in the Council's office have added further information on many points. Personal recollection of events over the greater part of the period covered has been of much help in guiding the search, but it has not by itself been relied upon unduly.

It has been necessary to keep in view the requirements of several kinds of possible readers—those who have been directly involved in the Council's work; those who are concerned with the promotion of research in other contexts; and those with a general interest in the subject. For these last some explanations have been given that must seem elementary to the scientifically informed.

Acknowledgements

Personally, I am grateful to the Council for the opportunity to write this history, which has been for me a task of absorbing interest in my retirement; and also to the successive Secretaries, Sir Harold Himsworth and Sir John Gray, for encouragement of the enterprise and for the provision of facilities and assistance in the headquarters office. I am indebted to many other members of the staff, at all levels, for help as occasion has required.

Two former colleagues, the late Sir Charles Harington and Dr F. H. K. Green, have critically read the whole account in draft; I have had much benefit from their comments, which were in both cases based on long association with the Council. Others have critically read one or two chapters referred to them because of their special concern with the subjects covered.

Still others, in the office, have helped me in different ways. I particularly mention Mr D. J. Cawthron, himself trained as a historian, who has pursued many inquiries on my behalf and has also brought a variety of relevant biographical and other matters to my notice. Mrs Norma Morris (followed by Mrs Anne Sanderson for a shorter period) gave part of her time to assisting me in the search for information (with the cooperation of the staff of the office registry), in critically checking my drafts, and in controlling the typing operations. Miss Daphne Gloag, head of the publications group in the office Secretariat, has given invaluable help in the final editing for press. My need for day-to-day secretarial assistance in this work has over the years been well met by, in turn, Mrs Heather Stephenson and Mrs Julia Smith.

A final acknowledgement, not for help in writing history but for their part in making it, is to the research workers and particularly those who have been my colleagues in the service of the Council. It is for what they achieve that the organisation exists. The administrator may do much to create opportunities and he may help to tend the growing tree; but it is they who plant it and they who bring it to fruition. Space has allowed me to name only a minority, and seldom to say more, but here I greet them all—whether still working or retired. Some pioneers to whom I have been able to make fuller reference were my seniors or contemporaries, and most of them have gone; they also were my friends, and I salute their memory.

L. T.
April 1972

Medical Research Council Headquarters Office
20 Park Crescent
London WiN 4AL

Contents of Volume One

APPENDICES

INDEXES

Illustrations in Volume One

Introduction

by

Sir Harold Himsworth, KCB, MD, FRCP, FRS
late Secretary and Deputy Chairman, Medical Research Council

To those who have been part of an institution, to those who have been involved in its development and to those who have depended upon it for their support, the history of its origins, growth and difficulties cannot fail to have a special and intimate interest. If, in addition, the institution in question has stood as a prototype in a continuing field of human activity, interest passes beyond the special to become of wider relevance. When, therefore, the Medical Research Council reached the half-century of its existence, it was decided, for both these reasons, to take advantage of the availability of Sir Landsborough Thomson after his retirement and to ask him to put together an account of the Council's evolution in the developing context of the growing needs of this country for ever more scientific knowledge.

For this task Sir Landsborough was uniquely equipped. It was in October 1919, after a distinguished academic career in zoology at Aberdeen, and an equally distinguished military career in the First World War, that he joined the staff of the old Medical Research Committee, which preceded the setting up of the Council itself. From then, until his retirement thirty-eight years later, he was second-in-command at the Council's headquarters to three successive Secretaries. During this period, he saw the Council grow from its embryonic form to become a pervading national influence in the development of biomedical knowledge. Sir Landsborough is thus in an exceptional position to give an account of the developments during the last fifty years and, more important, to put on record the significance of the considerations that underlay these.

The Research Councils, in the form we know them, are a peculiarly British institution and, although they have been copied to a greater or lesser extent elsewhere, it is questionable whether they could have arisen save in the context of the ethos of this country. The idea that it is in the best interests of a country that research (as distinct from development) should be established independently of political interest or administrative commitment is not one that would normally occur to those concerned with the machinery of government, even though it is but the translation into the scientific sphere of the time-honoured caution that no man should be judge of his own case. That a committee including men as able as Haldane and Morant, in consultation with so far-seeing a Minister as Addison, could conceive such a scheme may occasion no surprise. It is doubtful, however, if even they could have ensured its acceptance but for the general climate of self-confidence and assurance that had carried over into the public life of this country from a century of unchallenged authority and power. Be that as it may, the pattern proposed by the Haldane Committee in 1918 was adopted in place of the traditional arrangement of putting research under the control of an administrative department with a particular interest in its findings. That the research council scheme has in principle been a success, that it is economic, that it has been, and is, a material factor in promoting public and scientific confidence, was shown by the conclusions reached by the Trend Committee, appointed more than forty years after its inception, when reviewing its performance.

It has been said that the greatest problem facing modern society is that of incorporating expert knowledge into government. It may well be, therefore, that now we have clearly entered an age when policy, not only at the departmental but also at the national level, is coming to depend increasingly upon the objective quality of the scientific knowledge available, the organizational pattern of which the research councils are the prototype might find increasing application. In any event, an informed account of the evolution and problems of one such council should be invaluable in promoting a more informed appreciation of the points at issue and the bearing of these on the public interest. It has been provided by Sir Landsborough Thomson in this book.

London, April 1971

Part I
Origin and Status: Constitutional History

Chapter 1
Predecessors in Great Britain (before 1911)

General retrospect—Early state-aided researches—Research under the Privy
Council—Research under the Local Government Board—Research in the
Services—The Lister Institute—The twentieth century—The Royal
Commission on Tuberculosis

General retrospect

The conception that the promotion of medical research is a responsibility of the State is almost wholly a growth of the twentieth century
so far as concerns the United Kingdom, which lagged in this respect
somewhat behind France and Germany. Nevertheless, there were in
the nineteenth century certain sporadic and partial incursions of the
British Government into this field, presently to be mentioned. In
earlier centuries the advancement of medical knowledge depended
on the spontaneous enterprise of men engaged in professional practice and working either in the hospitals or in the general community.
The advances mostly took the form of improvements in methods
evolved in the course of practical experience. On the other hand,
there were outstanding examples of results obtained from deliberate
research in anatomy and physiology and into the nature and causes
of disease. One need only recall such illustrious names as those of
William Harvey (1578–1657) for the experimental demonstration of
the circulation of the blood, of Thomas Sydenham (1624–89) for the
clinical description of diseases as such and for studies of epidemiology,
of John Hunter (1728–93) for work in comparative anatomy and
physiology and for the foundation of scientific surgery, and of
Edward Jenner (1749–1823) for inoculation with vaccinia against
smallpox. One may also mention James Lind (1716–94), an Edinburgh graduate and "founder of naval hygiene", who among other
things made a controlled clinical trial to prove the value of citrus
juice against scurvy. There followed in the nineteenth century such
events as the discovery of the anaesthetic properties of chloroform
and its use in midwifery by James Young Simpson (1811–70) and the
introduction of antiseptic surgery by Joseph Lister (1827–1912); and
the latter part of that century was marked by many discoveries
which laid the foundations of modern medical science.

The pioneer discoveries stand out against the relatively undeveloped state of knowledge in their times; they were made under
social conditions and in scientific circumstances immensely different
from those of today. The Industrial Revolution in the middle of the

eighteenth century initiated a drastic change in the whole structure of society; the population vastly increased, the balance between rural and urban communities was radically altered, and the pattern of existence acquired new aspects for many people. More recent times have seen further growth in the complexity of life and in the sheer pace of living.

In parallel with these vast social changes there was, and continues to be, an immense development of science over the whole field of discovery and invention. Growing knowledge in different branches, both physical and biological, has many potential applications to the problems of human health; and thus a great responsibility has been placed on the medical research worker to see that they are in fact applied. New techniques of investigation of great refinement have been introduced, calling for higher standards of training in their use. A tendency towards specialisation, if sometimes overdone, has been inevitable. The time has long passed when medical research could progress solely as a by-product of the work of exceptional men in professional practice—itself much affected by the wider extent of knowledge and the need for more highly specialised skills of its own. No longer, indeed, is it the prerogative of the medical profession, for other disciplines have necessarily been brought to bear upon its problems.

The implications were beginning to be appreciated in the closing years of the nineteenth century. In America, Frederick T. Gates, the far-seeing lay adviser to John D. Rockefeller on his philanthropic expenditure, wrote in a memorandum of 1897:

> Medicine can hardly hope to become a science until it can be endowed, and qualified men enabled to give themselves to uninterrupted study and investigation, on ample salary, entirely independent of practice. (Quoted by Fosdick, 1956.)

The twentieth century has seen great developments in Britain, especially that with which the present work is concerned. First, however, it is of interest to look back more closely at earlier events, using Sir Arthur MacNalty's Fitzpatrick Lectures (published in 1948) as the main source of the next three sections of this chapter; the Heath Clark Lectures by Sir John Charles (1961) are also relevant.

Early state-aided researches

It is not surprising that the beginnings of State medicine, and with it the early forerunners of state-aided medical research, took place in the preventive field. Curative medicine was until the present century financed by the fees paid privately to general and specialist practitioners, by charity through the voluntary hospitals, and only at the lowest economic level by the Poor Law administration. Measures of public health, on the other hand, had of necessity to be supported by the community, from the funds of central or local government. Public hygiene is indeed a subject of great antiquity, traceable from prehistoric times through such ancient civilisations as those of Egypt, Assyria, Israel (Mosaic law), Greece, and Rome. In England the first sanitary act was passed in 1388; for long, however, hygiene was a matter for legislation rather than administration, and enforcement lay with local rather than central authority.

The first essays in state-aided medical research arose as a by-product of administrative measures taken in the interests of the public health. Thus, in the period 1833–54 Dr Thomas Southwood Smith (1788–1881) was intermittently employed on inquiries for official commissions and, latterly, for the General Board of Health; he published reports on the causes of sickness and mortality, on the results of sanitary improvement, on quarantine, and on outbreaks of cholera and yellow fever. Inquiries for the Poor Law Commission, at the instigation of Edwin Chadwick (the salaried member), were likewise made by Dr Southwood Smith, and also by Dr Neil Arnott (1788–1874) and by Dr James Phillips Kay (later Sir James Kay-Shuttleworth—1804–77); in particular, they reported on fevers in London, and Kay later reported on fevers in Edinburgh and Glasgow.

A General Board of Health for England and Wales was set up as part of the machinery of central government in 1848; and although it did not last for long it had successors. Dr J. Simon, to be mentioned later, was Medical Officer of the Board and had a definite policy as regards research. Although he had no staff to assist him, he was able to employ specialists on a temporary basis to report on particular matters. Thus, in addition to Dr Southwood Smith, Dr E. H. Greenhow (1814–88) was employed to inquire into the proportion of deaths from different diseases in different districts; and at the same time Dr William Farr (1807–83), compiler of statistics in the General Register Office, was making his great contribution.

Research under the Privy Council
The General Board of Health was abolished in 1858, when its functions were transferred to the Privy Council—strangely fore-shadowing a much later event (Chapter 5). Sir John Simon (1816–1904) was transferred from the Board as first Medical Officer of this new central health authority and played the outstanding part in the events that followed. The surname was pronounced in accord with his French ancestry; there is a recent biography (Lambert, 1963). Those were the days of the great all-rounders in the medical field, and Simon was a pre-eminent example: he was a pathologist who had been elected a Fellow of the Royal Society at an early age for his work on the thyroid, and a surgeon who was later President of the Royal College of Surgeons of England; he had also been Medical Officer of Health of the City of London. He was not deterred by the fact that the administrative scope of his office was limited to public vaccination, the Quarantine Act, and certain special powers (during epidemic emergencies) under the Disease-Prevention Act.

Otherwise the Privy Council, in matters of health, had only the functions of inquiry and report: the Privy Council were "to cause to be made from time to time such inquiries as they may see fit in any matters relating to the Public Health in any place or places". In Simon's view, this power should be used to "develop a scientific basis for the progress of sanitary law and administration and to aim at stamping on public hygiene a greater exactitude than it had hitherto had".

During the Privy Council regime, 1858–71, Simon promoted careful inquiries into outbreaks of disease and many new facts of epidemiology were established. Among the investigations were those of Dr Greenhow and Dr (later Sir) John Burdon-Sanderson (1829–1905) into diphtheria, and of Dr Edward Smith (1818–74) into the nutrition of the populace on a basis of sample dietaries. In 1865 Simon sent investigators to report on typhus in Russia and on cerebrospinal meningitis in Germany. The great cholera epidemic of 1865–66 was made the subject of epidemiological and pathological studies. Other inquiries ranged over a wide field, including social and industrial medicine and touching on such varied subjects as infant mortality, tuberculosis, food, housing, parasites, and hospital hygiene.

Simon was indeed the first State organiser of medical research. As a pathologist, he had followed the work of Pasteur with much interest; and in 1864 he obtained authority from the Privy Council to promote laboratory investigations:

> Investigations, not necessarily connected with our practical business at the moment, but tending to be of powerful indirect influence on our practical business as a whole; investigations, which we knew could be of no rapid effect, but which we hoped would by degrees—even if only by the slow degrees of exact science—surely lead us to more precise and intimate knowledge of the causes and processes of important diseases, and would thus eventually augment more and more the vital resources of Preventive Medicine.

Of special interest, as a pioneer effort in biochemical study, was Simon's employment of Dr John Lewis William Thudichum (1829–1901) for research work intended "to promote an improved chemical identification of diseases". The great interest of the various organic substances which Thudichum isolated from the body, particularly from the brain, was not fully recognised at the time; his findings indeed provoked a storm of hostile criticism, but they were later fully confirmed by others—including Dr Otto Rosenheim, working at the National Institute for Medical Research. In 1929, as a gift from his daughters, a valuable collection of chemical preparations made by Thudichum passed into the keeping of the Medical Research Council, as recorded in its Report for 1928–29. This remarkable man, born in the Grand Duchy of Hesse and originally named Ludwig Johann Wilhelm Thudichum, has been the subject of a biography by Drabkin (1958) and more recent annotations by Debuch and Dawson (1965) and reference by Charles (1961).

Nearly thirty years after Thudichum's death, his four by then aged daughters were found by Dr Rosenheim to be living in dire poverty in what had been their father's house; the Council was glad to be instrumental in obtaining for them a pension from the Civil List.

In 1870 Parliament approved a special item of £2000 per annum for "Auxiliary Scientific Investigations" in the estimates of the Privy Council, and this must be reckoned as a landmark in State provision for medical research. As MacNalty wrote:

> The great value of these scientific investigations under the Privy Council lay not so much in the results achieved, although these were considerable, as in the principles won. State grants were made to workers in medical research, and the laboratory work was closely associated with epidemiological field inquiries. For the first time the State had officially recognised the importance of research into health and disease.

At this time, and until 1883, Burdon-Sanderson continued to receive grants—latterly at the Brown Institution for the Study of Animal Diseases—for work on such subjects as cattle plague, tuberculosis, the nature of contagion, wound infection, and the pathology of blood poisoning. Other grant-aided investigators had been paying special attention to cholera, and their reports to the Privy Council indicate a growing belief in the spread of this and other diseases by living organisms; they were also influenced by the classical demonstration in 1854 by Dr John Snow (1813–58), a general practitioner in London, that cholera infection was spread in drinking water.

To quote MacNalty again:

> With the aid of the novelists [notably Charles Dickens] and his classical reports, Simon educated public opinion in the importance of public health and built up the great edifice of English State Medicine with sound scientific knowledge and with the active support of the medical profession. Much of the success of the Medical Department of the Privy Council was due to the fact that its work was scientific and unaffected by political considerations to which National Health should never be subordinated.

Research under the Local Government Board
Simon's administration led to the great Sanitary Act of 1866. This was followed by the Royal Commission of 1869–71, from which resulted the establishment in 1871 of the Local Government Board, forerunner of the Ministry of Health—the Local Government Board for Scotland was set up in 1894—and in the consolidated Public Health Act of 1875. Simon passed from the service of the Privy Council to that of the new Board. So did (as he became) Sir George Buchanan (1831–95), a scientifically distinguished successor as Principal Medical Officer of the Board; he was a Fellow of the Royal Society, which once in every five years awards a Buchanan Medal instituted in his honour.

The policy of promoting special investigations and research was continued by the Local Government Board, although without any noteworthy increase in the scale of effort. The latter part of the nineteenth century was the period during which the causal organisms of many infective diseases were discovered, and this new knowledge had obviously great importance for public health. On the basis of earlier findings, the threat of further invasions of this country by epidemic cholera was repulsed. Investigations on similar lines were now directed towards typhus, plague, and food poisoning.

Some of the investigations were made by members of the Board's medical staff, and others through the agency of research grants; as MacNalty has said, "the financial grants were meagre, the recipients distinguished, industrious and enthusiastic". It was a method whereby men specially skilled in research could be brought, as a rule temporarily and partly, into the service of the Board. As a result, many papers advancing knowledge of bacteriology and chemical pathology were published in the reports of the Board's Medical Officer. Particular mention may be made of the experiments on rabies performed by Mr (later Sir) Victor Horsley (1857–1916), pathologist and surgeon, as secretary of a Commission appointed by the Board to inquire into Pasteur's method of dealing with the infection. Dr E. E. Klein (1844–1925), an Austrian by birth, made many investigations for the Board—mainly into infections—while director of the Brown Institution (see Chapter 12). Pioneer work in the chemical pathology of infectious diseases was done for the Board by Dr Sidney Martin (1860–1924); and on the purity of water supplies by Dr (later Sir) Alexander Houston (1865–1933). Many other eminent pathologists contributed in like manner, including Professor F. W. (later Sir Frederick) Andrewes (1858–1932), who became a member of the Medical Research Council, and Dr M. H. Gordon (1872–1953), who became a member of the Council's scientific staff. An eminent physiologist, Dr J. S. Haldane (1860–1936), did work for the Board on the use of carbon monoxide for the destruction of rats in ships infected with plague. Dr S. A. Monckton Copeman (1862–1947) spent most of his working life in the service of the Local Government Board (and latterly in that of the Ministry of Health), doing research work on smallpox vaccine in particular.

In 1910 the Board established a laboratory in London for bacteriological investigations related to its work, and the staff undertook research on food-poisoning, streptococcal infections, and other subjects. This laboratory was later continued by the Ministry of Health until 1939, when on the outbreak of the Second World War it became the nucleus of an Emergency Public Health Laboratory Service organised by the Medical Research Council—but that is looking ahead (see Volume Two).

Research in the Services
Medical research, particularly on tropical diseases, was incidentally supported by the State through the work of medical officers in the various Services of the Crown; a few outstanding examples must suffice. David Bruce of the Royal Army Medical Corps (later

Major-General Sir David Bruce; 1855–1931) discovered the causative organism of 'Malta' fever in 1887; and in 1895 he showed that the 'nagana' of domestic animals in Africa was due to a trypanosome carried by species of tsetse fly (*Glossina*), and subsequently that human sleeping-sickness was likewise due to trypanosomes similarly carried and that wild animals acted as carriers of trypanosome infections. Ronald Ross of the Indian Medical Service (later Colonel Sir Ronald Ross; 1855–1932) elucidated in 1895–97 the life-history of the malaria parasite in its transmission from man to anopheline mosquito, and back to man; in so doing he confirmed (in parallel with independent Italian investigators) a hypothesis of Dr (later Sir) Patrick Manson(1844–1922), the acknowledged 'father of tropical medicine' but himself at that time working in the service of the Chinese Imperial Maritime Customs and in the University of Hong Kong.

William Boog Leishman of the RAMC (later Lieut.-General Sir William Leishman; 1856–1926) discovered the parasite causing kala-azar and also did important work on African tick fever. He was later a member of the Medical Research Council; and he had the unusual distinction for a pathologist of becoming Director-General of Army Medical Services. Leonard Rogers of the Indian Medical Service (later Major-General Sir Leonard Rogers; 1868–1962) made numerous researches into leprosy, cholera, and other tropical diseases. Some of his later work was published by the Medical Research Council, of which he was also a benefactor (Chapter 16).

Although it is not possible to rival the record of the Indian and armed services, officers of the Colonial Medical Service also contributed an impressive total to medical knowledge in the tropical field.

The Lister Institute
An event in the final decade of the nineteenth century, although involving no use of public funds, was of much significance in the development of the general situation. This was the establishment in London, in 1891, of 'The British Institute of Preventive Medicine'. In 1898, on the receipt of funds commemorating the centenary (in 1896) of Edward Jenner's discovery of vaccination, the title was changed to 'Jenner Institute of Preventive Medicine'; but later a commercial organisation was found to have prior claim to a similar name. The title was accordingly changed again in 1903 to 'The Lister Institute of Preventive Medicine'. And in 1966 the Lister Institute celebrated its 75th anniversary, with a great record of scientific achievement to its credit. Its history has been briefly related by two of its Directors (Drury, 1948; Miles, 1966) and more fully by three former members of its staff (Chick, Hume and Macfarlane, 1971).

Some quarter of a century later, the Lister Institute—with greatly increased endowments and a high scientific reputation—was to be involved in the plans for a medical research organisation under Government (Chapter 10). In the event, no constitutional involvement materialised; but many instances of close scientific cooperation with the Medical Research Committee, and its successor Council, are mentioned in the present work.

The twentieth century

Some of the examples already quoted overlap into the twentieth century, at the beginning of which the general position remained very much the same as during the preceding few decades. The only medical research that was deliberately state-aided consisted of some special investigations promoted by the Local Government Board; incidental support continued to be given through research work undertaken by whole-time medical officers in the public service.

Certain research projects overseas did receive official support. Thus, in 1905 the Secretary of State for India, together with the Royal Society and the Lister Institute, appointed an Advisory Committee to direct inquiries into problems of plague and to administer an annual grant provided for the purpose. The Advisory Committee in turn appointed a working Commission to make investigations in India; the results were published in a series of reports from 1906 onwards.

Otherwise, the advancement of knowledge was mainly the responsibility of the universities, at that time largely self-supporting, and of the associated teaching hospitals maintained by charity. On the clinical side, however, progress in research was handicapped by the fact that the professors in such subjects were part-time teachers engaged in practice. Nevertheless, there were exceptional men in the medical profession who were able to undertake important research work while in specialist or general practice—Dr (later Sir) James Mackenzie (1853–1925), for instance.

Around the turn of the century also, privately financed institutes for medical research were beginning to appear. The outstanding example of the Lister Institute has already been mentioned. The Imperial Cancer Research Fund was established in 1902, and from funds raised by subscription maintained its own research laboratory and other projects. Research was also done in the laboratories of some of the drug manufacturers, notably in the Wellcome Physiological Research Laboratories; the latter had begun work in 1894, but it was not until some ten years afterwards that they undertook important researches in physiology and pharmacology in addition to the main original function of producing antitoxins.

In 1909, Sir Otto Beit founded and permanently endowed—in memory of his brother Alfred—the Beit Memorial Fellowships for Medical Research. They were intended "to promote the advancement by research of medicine and the allied sciences in their relation to medicine". These highly competitive awards have enabled a series of young men and women to devote a few years wholly to research work and by so doing, apart from the immediate value of their results, to equip themselves for careers in which research would at least play an important part. The list of former Beit Fellows shows how many who began in this way subsequently became leaders of research in medical science. The list includes a good number who became members of the Medical Research Council or directors of its establishments or (in two instances) its Secretary.

The Royal Commission on Tuberculosis
The true predecessor of the Medical Research Committee (later Council) was the Royal Commission Appointed to Inquire into the Relations of Human and Animal Tuberculosis. This was set up by an Order in Council of 31 August 1901, under the chairmanship of Sir Michael Foster, Professor of Physiology in the University of Cambridge. Its remit was to inquire whether the disease in animals and man was one and the same; whether animals and man could be reciprocally infected with it, and under what conditions, if at all, the transmission of the disease from animals to man took place, and what were the circumstances favourable or unfavourable to such transmission. So great an authority as Robert Koch had stated publicly, at a meeting in London, that the bovine bacillus was so different from the human bacillus that there was virtually no danger of its causing tuberculosis in man. The truth or falsity of this was a matter of vital importance in preventive medicine.

The Commission's brief first Interim Report, published in 1904, contains the following highly significant sentence: "After duly considering the matter, we came to the conclusion that it would be desirable not to begin the inquiry by taking evidence, that is to say, by collecting the opinions of others (though this might be desirable at a later stage), but to attack the problem laid before us by conducting experimental investigations of our own." The Royal Commission on Tuberculosis thus became a research body, eschewing mere opinions and seeking to establish facts by promoting scientific investigation. To this end it was provided with money from public funds for the employment of a scientific staff and for the cost of experiments. The 'observers', so called, were Dr Louis Cobbett, Dr A. Stanley Griffith, Dr Arthur Eastwood, Dr H. J. Hutchens, and later Dr F. Griffith. Dr E. J. Steegmann was Secretary of the Commission.

The main purpose of the Commission's first publication was to announce the finding that "tubercle of human origin can give rise in the bovine animal to tuberculosis identical with ordinary bovine tuberculosis". The converse, not being a matter suitable for direct experiment, took longer to prove, but meanwhile the Commission urged that it would be most unwise to base legislative measures on the view that the disease caused by the one bacillus was wholly different from that caused by the other. The Commission remained active for 10 years in all, and during the greater part of that time its scientific staff was engaged in bacteriological researches in the Royalcot Laboratory at Stansted, Essex. The results were published in the Commission's reports, the last of which appeared in 1911 (with subsequent appendices), and constituted an important addition to knowledge of the disease. One of the Commission's staff, Dr A. Stanley Griffith, moved to Cambridge and after three years as a Research Scholar of the Grocers' Company passed to the service of the Medical Research Committee, in which (and in that of the successor Council) he long continued his work on tuberculosis (Volume Two).

The problem of tuberculosis, however, still remained one of the gravest in the field of health. It appears to have been in some measure the need for research on the subject that led—in the same year, 1911—to the legislative provision from which the Medical Research Committee originated (Chapter 2).

Chapter 2
Construction Period (1911-1913)

The National Insurance Act 1911—Origin of the provision for research—
Interpretation of the provision—The Departmental Committee on Tuberculosis—The views of witnesses—Implementation of the provision

The National Insurance Act 1911
In 1911, the year in which the Royal Commission on Tuberculosis
issued its Final Report (Chapter 1), Parliament passed the National
Insurance Act—a measure, introduced by Mr David Lloyd George
(later Earl Lloyd George of Dwyfor) as Chancellor of the Exchequer,
which took a pioneer step towards what later became known as the
Welfare State. It established schemes for health and unemployment
insurance, based on contributions from employees, employers, and
the State. Among other works, the scholarly history of national
insurance in Great Britain by Professor Bentley B. Gilbert (1966) is
especially worth consulting.

One of the provisions, that of sanatorium treatment for cases of
tuberculosis, has particular significance for this history. Subsection
(2) of Section 16 of the Act laid down that one penny in respect of
each insured person should be contributed annually to the expenses
of sanatorium benefit out of moneys provided by Parliament; but
that the Insurance Commissioners might retain the whole or any
part of that contribution "for the purposes of research" (see
Appendix B). In this rather indirect way a national fund for medical
research was created. The yield was in due course estimated as
being of the order of £57 000 per annum (Chapter 15).

This first National Insurance Act was epoch-making from several
points of view, and in the promotion of medical research it was an
authentic landmark. Sir Walter Fletcher used to say that the three
British statesmen who had notably furthered the cause of medical
science were King Henry VIII, who founded the regius chairs of
'physic' at Oxford and Cambridge (although in fact the regius chair
of medicine at Aberdeen is the oldest foundation of its kind in what
is now Great Britain); King Charles II, who gave the Royal Society
its Charter; and Mr Lloyd George with his Act.

Origin of the provision for research
It would be of much interest to know whose idea it was to include
provision for research in the Bill—if indeed it was not Lloyd George

himself, and it has been suggested that his mind did not run in that sort of direction. There was for long a tradition, and there have been published statements up to recent dates, ascribing the idea to Dr Christopher (later Viscount) Addison; but his own memoirs state that he had never met Lloyd George until after the Bill was before the House of Commons, although he was a valiant supporter from the Second Reading onwards. Nor afterwards did Addison ever claim the credit in this particular matter; and the only evidence for it is a press report of a far from explicit compliment paid by Lloyd George in an after-dinner speech in 1914.

There have also been public statements attributing not only this provision but much, if not the whole, of the Act to Sir Robert Morant, the Permanent Secretary of the Board of Education. There is no foundation for this; Morant did not come into the picture until he was appointed Chairman of the National Health Insurance Commission (England) when the Bill was almost law; that he later played the biggest part in implementing the Act is a different matter.

Another name suggested is that of Sir George Newman, then Chief Medical Officer of the Board of Education, but virtually all the evidence is against his having been involved; the only apparent exception is a remark, again far from explicit, made by Lloyd George in conversation as long afterwards as 1937 and quoted by Newman in his personal diary without comment. In the course of much writing about the research provision and its outcome, Newman never himself claimed credit in the matter. A name that has also been suggested is that of Sir Arthur Newsholme, then Principal Medical Officer of the Local Government Board, but this is solely on the ground that he was the only medical man regularly consulted during the drafting period; in fact, none of his minutes among the Bill papers mentions research. The whole question has been discussed elsewhere by the present writer (Thomson, 1973) in more detail and with full references.

Another tradition was that originally the draft Bill limited the research to tuberculosis, as inclusion of the provision in a clause dealing with sanatorium benefit might suggest. This was probably a subsequent attempt to rationalise the contextual position, and there is no evidence that there was anything more in the latter than a matter of drafting convenience. It might well be, nevertheless, that the originator of the provision had research on tuberculosis particularly in mind; this would not have been surprising, with the background supplied by the recent Royal Commission (Chapter 1) and the disease being in any event singled out in the Act for special attention. (The terms of the Financial Resolution related to the Bill are even more suggestive, referring to "sanatorium benefit, including research work in connection therewith".) The context did afterwards raise a question of legal interpretation, as noted below.

The only contemporary evidence on record appears to be that of William John Braithwaite (1876–1936), the civil servant who chiefly helped Lloyd George in the preparation of the Bill. His memoirs, based largely on his diary, were edited after his death by another civil servant, Sir Henry Bunbury, and published only in 1957. In these, Braithwaite names those who were associated with him, notably John S. (later Lord) Bradbury of the Treasury; and he makes it plain that Lloyd George himself was the principal architect of the measure, framing it without having the resources of a major administrative department behind him.

In his diary for 8 May 1911, the day on which the draft was delivered to the Bill Office at 10.30 p.m., Braithwaite recorded:

> Meeting in the Chancellor's room, many persons, to finish up the bill. Many points decided of a smaller kind. The three days' newspaper criticism has not added a single point, but the Chancellor is setting aside a small sum for research.

To this extract he appended, in his memoirs, the following comment:

> The "small sum set aside for research" was the 1d a member, to which the Medical Research Council is due—a great contribution. I do not know who deserves the credit for thinking of it.

What Braithwaite did not know on such a matter is probably now beyond discovery; search of the Bill files in the Public Records Office, and of the Lloyd George papers in the Beaverbrook Library, has yielded no clue. During the passage of the measure through Parliament, the provision attracted little attention amid the highly controversial social and financial issues. Even Dr Addison, in a long speech on the Second Reading on 24 May 1911, made no reference to it; and at the committee stage in the House of Commons, on 2 August 1911, the entire sub-section was passed without debate (*Hansard*).

Although Clause 16 (originally numbered 15) went through the Committee stage in the House of Commons unchallenged, there had been a debate on 12 July 1911 over Clause 8, which set forth the rates and conditions of the benefits to be provided. Mr (later Sir) Austen Chamberlain moved an amendment to omit Sub-Section (1)(b), relating to sanatorium benefit, on the ground that it was inappropriate to single out one disease, tuberculosis, for special provision in a measure of otherwise general scope. This evoked a long and reasonable debate, resulting in withdrawal of the motion for amendment. In the course of this there were several sympathetic references to research, in relation to tuberculosis, although the subject was not explicit in the wording currently under discussion. In particular, Dr Arthur Lynch (representing an Irish constituency) urged that more emphasis should be laid on the research aspect; he went so far as to say that sanatorium treatment, about which much was still uncertain, would be of no value without provision for further research.

In the House of Lords two amendments were moved to Clause 16(2). One, by Lord Tenterden, was to delete (b) of the sub-section, including the proviso; this was frankly an anti-vivisectionist objection to research and, on being opposed by Lord Haldane, the motion was negatived without division. The second, moved by Lord Balfour of Burleigh (10th Baron), was to add the words 'and education' after 'research' at the end of the proviso; on its being pointed out by Lord Haldane that education was covered in a later section, the motion was withdrawn.

Interpretation of the provision

It may seem somewhat tortuous to have provided the money as a discrete item towards "defraying the cost of sanatorium benefit" and in the next breath to have given power to retain it for research; the formula does indeed appear to have involved some risk that the provision would be interpreted in a restricted sense by reason of its immediate context. Certainly, the National Health Insurance Commissioners almost at once thought it advisable to obtain a legal opinion on the point. The opinion given by the Law Officers on 22 January 1913 is preserved in the files of what is now the Department of Health and Social Security and is in the following terms:

> The Insurance Commissioners may frame their regulations under the proviso to section 16(2) so as to enable the monies therein referred to to be applied for purposes of research in connexion with any disease to which insured persons may be liable.

This was paraphrased by the Commissioners, with a slight change of emphasis, in their Report on National Health Insurance in 1913–14, as follows:

> Advice has been obtained to the effect that the application of the Research Fund is not limited to research in tuberculosis, but that the money may be expended on research into any disease to which insured persons are subject.

The opinion was never tested in the courts, during the few years that this part of the Act remained operative, and so did not acquire the force of a judgement. The terms of the opinion—especially in the paraphrased version—were actually not wholly meaningful in a scientific sense, as medical research cannot properly be regarded as consisting solely of the direct investigation of diseases, especially if limited to particular diseases within some administrative category.

In practice, the purported limitation of subject matter was interpreted so widely as to impose no restriction at all. For instance, the earliest research schemes under the Act included work specifically directed to conditions found only in children, who were not at that time covered by insurance benefits. A few years later, on 29 December 1919, Sir Robert Morant, by then at the Ministry of Health, said in a semi-official letter to the Treasury (about research in tropical medicine):

> Legal advice was taken at the outset, to support us in holding that there was no sort of limitation, under the Act, upon the spending of the money in the interests of insured persons in particular; the money was to be available for

spending upon all forms of medical research. This, after all, was only rational, since the employed population of this country cannot but be benefited by any form of investigation that could conceivably come within the phrase 'medical research'.

This seems to go somewhat beyond the official statement quoted earlier. By an extension of the argument, to which further reference is made in Volume Two, there was not even thought to be any geographical limitation on the places where research could be undertaken.

A further point is that the power to retain money for research was permissive and not mandatory; but there was clearly an intention to provide funds for research, and when the measure became law nobody doubted that the permissive power would be exercised. Formally at least, the discretion rested with the Insurance Commissioners appointed for the purposes of Part I (National Health Insurance) of the Act, and of these there were four bodies—respectively for England, Scotland, Ireland, and Wales. There was, however, to be "a joint committee of the several bodies of Commissioners"; and, although its stated function was to make interterritorial adjustments of a financial nature, it later came to have important significance for the promotion of research, which clearly called for an undivided administration. This Joint Committee was incorporated under a later Act (Appendix B).

The Departmental Committee on Tuberculosis
The Act itself gave no guidance as to how this money, if retained for research, was to be applied or administered. Much of the public thinking on the subject was done by the Departmental Committee on Tuberculosis appointed by the Treasury on 22 February 1912, under the chairmanship of Mr Waldorf (later Lord) Astor, MP— and with the recurring name of Dr Christopher Addison, MP, in the list of distinguished medical and other members. The remit was: "To report at an early date upon the consideration of general policy in respect of the problem of tuberculosis in the United Kingdom, in its preventive, curative, and other aspects, which should guide the Government and local bodies in making or aiding provision for the treatment of tuberculosis in sanatoria or other institutions or otherwise."

Although these terms of reference made no explicit reference to the National Insurance Act, its provisions relating to tuberculosis and the associated provision relating to research were very much in the Committee's minds.

In its Final Report, published in 1913, the Committee made the following comment on the provision for research contained in the Act:

This provision marks a most important development in the attitude of the State towards scientific research into the causes, treatment and prevention of disease. Hitherto, apart from a small annual sum expended by the Local Government

Board and occasional grants for particular objects, the State has, in the main, left research to voluntary agencies. The Committee welcome the fact that by the National Insurance Act a considerable sum of money is now permanently available for the purpose of research. . . . [It is] their opinion that research under the National Insurance Act should be organised in such a way as not to discourage either voluntary contributions or voluntary research towards the same ends. The aim should rather be to stimulate and cooperate with voluntary agencies.

It was natural that a Committee specifically concerned with tuberculosis should, having regard to the origin of the provision, consider that research on that subject should have a predominant claim; but it was aware that the claim would probably not be exclusive. The view on this aspect is stated as follows:

The Committee are of opinion that the whole of the moneys made available by the National Insurance Act could usefully be spent on research in connection with tuberculosis. They understand, however, that the Insurance Commissioners have been advised that the moneys in question may properly be applied to research in connection with any disease which may affect insured persons. The Committee anticipate that for the present, at any rate, the moneys will be applied mainly to research in connection with tuberculosis and its allied problems, but, in view of the possibility of extension of research to other diseases, they consider that any scheme for dealing with these moneys, and any machinery which may be established for that purpose, should, as far as possible, be on lines which will be applicable to and facilitate such an extension.

It may be doubted, however, whether any sum approaching the total available for research could at that time have been effectively spent on tuberculosis alone.

The Committee appreciated the need for promoting research work on the widest possible geographical basis:

The boundaries between the different parts of the U.K. which it may be necessary or desirable to observe for political or administrative reasons are not necessarily applicable to a scheme for scientific investigation. The work of research should be carried on in places having the best facilities for the particular investigation contemplated without being limited by consideration of geographical situation, provided that every part of the U.K. has the advantage of close association with the work of the scientific investigators.

The Report then proceeded to recommend a research organisation consisting of an Advisory Council and an Executive Committee:

The Advisory Council should include representatives from different parts of the U.K. of the various Government Departments concerned, of medical, scientific and teaching bodies interested in the question of research, together with scientific persons of distinction, and men of business capacity and proved ability with, in most cases, experience of public work. The representatives of Government Departments should be in a minority and should be members *ex officio*. The Executive Committee should consist of not fewer than five nor more than ten members. The majority, but not all of these members, should be experts.

Further recommendations followed on the duties of the two bodies:

The duties of the Advisory Council should be to advise, make suggestions and submit the Executive Committee's budget to the Government, and to advise, criticise and make suggestions to the Executive Committee. The duties of the Executive Committee should be to frame a budget which should be discussed and considered with the Advisory Council before being submitted by the Council to the Government; to determine, after consultation with the Advisory Council, the scheme of research work; to make periodic reports to be transmitted by the Advisory Council to the Government; and generally to organise and supervise the research work wherever carried on.

It will be seen later that the respective duties and the relationship of the two bodies were in the event, and fortunately, defined in rather different terms. Further:

It is obvious that the Executive Committee will need a permanent whole-time Secretary in order to assist them in carrying out their duties. In view of the character and importance of these duties, he should be an expert of high standing in research, possess administrative capacity, and be paid a salary of 1,200 *l.* to 1,500 *l.* per annum. If practicable, he should also act as Secretary to the Advisory Council.

The mention of "high standing in research" as a qualification is interesting; later this essential requirement was for a time in danger of being overlooked, although it was eventually fulfilled (Chapter 3).

Other recommendations on administrative matters included this far-sighted comment on financial arrangements:

It is impossible to forecast accurately whether research work will produce positive or negative results, the exact length of time required to carry out a particular piece of work, the amount of money required to complete it, or what further work the results obtained may necessitate. Accordingly the Executive Committee will find it difficult to frame any hard and fast estimates of expenditure, or lay down with accuracy what sum of money will need to be spent in a given year. The balance unexpended in a given year should, therefore, be carried forward to the next.

The Committee expressed the opinion that the methods of expending money on research should include:

(a) The establishment of a central bureau at the headquarters of the Advisory Council and the Executive Committee; this should have "a statistical and sociological department", and also "a library and publishing department".

(b) Clinical, pathological, bacteriological, chemical and other scientific researches carried out by competent investigators employed by the Executive Committee in institutions approved by them.

(c) Researches of the same nature in an institution or institutions (including laboratories and hospital wards) which should be under the immediate control of the Executive Committee to the extent and for the purpose in question.

(d) Special inquiries, e.g. of a statistical and sociological nature, carried out by the Executive Committee independently of any particular institution.

The question was also raised whether a sum of money, not exceeding £1000 per annum, should be available as a prize or prizes for the best original research work done, but to be awarded only if the discovery was of sufficient importance and utility (see Chapter 9).

Finally, and again far-sightedly, the Committee was "of opinion that some workers of proved and exceptional ability should be enabled to devote their whole time to research work, and should be given a definite and adequate salary and be entitled to a pension. Efforts should also be made to retain for research work young and talented investigators who would otherwise tend to drift into other lines".

The views of witnesses

The Committee expressed, as above, a clear concept of how the money for research should be used. Going behind this, it is of some historical interest to review the varying opinions contained in the memoranda submitted for the Committee's consideration and published in an appendix constituting the second volume of the Final Report. In general, considering that the Committee was dealing with tuberculosis in all its aspects, a remarkable degree of interest was shown in the provision for research.

Some of the memoranda submitted to the Committee were not concerned with the research aspect at all. Others dealt with research in part or even exclusively. Among these, some writers assumed that research would necessarily, or even desirably, be restricted to tuberculosis; their proposals have therefore only a limited interest, although they include expression of general principles having wider application. Some, on the other hand, assumed that the money would be available for a more comprehensive scheme of research, although perhaps not in the first instance; and a few strongly urged the desirability of this. Of those who examined the financial implications most formed low estimates, relatively to the total available, of the cost of a research scheme limited to tuberculosis; one spoke of the need to avoid suddenly placing a large sum in 'the pathological market', where there was already a dearth of experienced workers.

The extreme views on this question were voiced, on the one hand, by Professor Sheridan Delépine, who propounded a budget of £60 000 per annum for research on tuberculosis alone; and, on the other hand, by Sir James Kingston Fowler, who wrote:

Nothing would afford me greater pleasure than to hear that a sum of 60,000 *l.* a year was to be devoted to research in pathology, yet, notwithstanding that tuberculosis is a subject in which I am deeply interested, I should regard it as little short of a calamity if that, or any such sum of money, were to be allocated to research in tuberculosis alone.

Although I recognise that when it is only possible to obtain money from private sources for research in connection with a special subject, such as cancer or tubercle, it is better to accept than refuse it, yet I believe that advances in our knowledge of the pathology of those diseases is more likely to follow upon increased support being given to general pathological research in an Institute, similar to the Institut Pasteur, where many workers are engaged upon a variety of researches, under the guidance and inspiring influence of men like Roux and Metschnikoff, than by devoting large sums annually to research in a given subject.

Dr James Ritchie of Edinburgh wrote that "the problems of tuberculosis cannot be fruitfully considered apart from those of infections generally". Professor Matthew Hay of Aberdeen proposed that additional funds should be provided, independently of the National Insurance Act, to permit of extension of the research to infectious diseases other than tuberculosis.

It is implicit in most of the memoranda dealing with research (and explicit in Dr Ritchie's) that there should be a unified scheme and a single controlling authority for the United Kingdom as a whole.

A few writers apparently regarded 'laboratory work' and 'research' as synonymous terms, urging the need for a chain of pathological laboratories for diagnostic work. Most of those who concerned themselves at all with research naturally did not fall into this error. Some wished to see different laboratories set up for the two purposes; thus, Professor Matthew Hay proposed local laboratories for routine purposes and a central institute for research. Dr A. Eastwood went further; drawing a clear distinction between routine diagnosis and research (although they might sometimes be related), he stated that there was no justification for defraying the cost of routine work out of research funds.

Many of the writers, whether considering research on tuberculosis alone or on a wider basis, discussed the relative merits of a central institute and of a system of subsidies or grants for work in the universities and other existing agencies. Dr Simon Flexner wrote from America, with experience of the Rockefeller Institute in mind, to stress the essential role of a central research institution; some of the others did not attach importance to this. A fairly general view favoured a balanced research scheme which would include central and peripheral elements. Dr W. S. Lazarus-Barlow of the Middlesex Hospital and Professor E. J. McWeeney of Dublin favoured the idea of a special research hospital. Dr A. Eastwood, Dr A. C. Inman of the Brompton Hospital, and Professor (later Sir) Robert Muir of Glasgow recommended that the research institute should have a farm for experimental work with large animals. Some mentioned the desirability of provision to enable research workers to visit foreign countries.

Some of the writers who were themselves highly experienced in research had cogent things to say about the recruitment and employment of scientific staff. Thus Professor Muir stressed that for work aiming at new discoveries "men of the highest qualifications are necessary; they must possess originality and breadth of outlook, and must have had the most complete scientific training possible in their particular department". Sir Ronald Ross, then of Liverpool, proposed subsidies to private research workers, part-time grants to laboratory workers throughout the country, and the employment of whole-time workers—some temporary and others permanent. He also thought that there should be money prizes to be awarded in retrospect for the best work done.

Sir Almroth Wright of St Mary's Hospital urged the need for creating a medical research service, to which suitable men would be attracted by prospects of whole-time careers and eventual pensions. For the education of recruits to the service he envisaged the central institute as a kind of college with five departmental heads of professorial status. Dr Eastwood pointed to the importance of avoiding a commitment of funds by apportioning lump sums to existing external institutions in accordance with the strength of their claims. Such payments would be difficult to terminate and the central authority would lose control of expenditure.

A few of the writers discussed the nature of the central authority which should be set up to administer the funds for research. Dr E. J. Steegman, who had been Secretary of the Royal Commission on Tuberculosis, mentioned that it had already in 1908 recommended to the Local Government Board that a permanent research body should be created. Dr (later Sir) Charles Martin actually used the title 'National Medical-research Committee'. Professor Muir stressed that the controlling body should consist of experts. Dr Eastwood pointed out that there was no guiding precedent, as the research project was envisaged as continuous and it would be impossible to lay down a complete scheme for it at the outset. Sir Ronald Ross said that in the past research workers had been inadequately remunerated, and "the direction of the work is put under men who have not themselves been greatly distinguished in the line, and, in fact, there is not a great show of intelligence in the organisations, even where funds are available". Sir Almroth Wright considered that, after the first appointments had been made, his proposed collegiate central institute should achieve autonomy under its own senate—a contention to which he was to return at a later date.

Finally, it is interesting to note that, of those who submitted memoranda, the following later served as members of the Medical Research Committee or Council (see Appendix H): Clifford Allbutt, F. W. Andrewes, W. Bulloch, A. K. Chalmers, Matthew Hay, C. J. Martin, and R. Muir—while some of the others became closely associated with the project in different ways.

Implementation of the provision
The Report of the Departmental Committee gave a firm lead for implementation of the Act's provision for research, as the Insurance Commissioners acknowledged in their own Report for 1913–14. Administrative action certainly followed without any substantial delay; but there must have been some hard in-fighting behind the scenes, possibly while the Committee was still sitting, as Addison later recorded (1924) that there had been "a long battle between those who wanted to departmentalise the scheme by appropriating

the money for the Local Government Board, and those of us who were determined to secure the utmost possible freedom for whatever body had to administer it".

The Committee's Report is a document of great historical interest, in the particular field, because it presents the first formulation of a number of ideas that were not only translated into action at the time but have remained effective to the present day. An account of the original implementation follows immediately (Chapter 3).

(A statement that has been repeated several times in print, once quite recently, must here be discounted in order to clear a misconception from the record. It was to the effect that in 1913 "the Government" approached the Lister Institute of Preventive Medicine with a suggestion that the latter might agree to become "the nucleus" of a new "Medical Research Department" to be set up under the Act; that after much debate the proposal was rejected by the Institute; and that the Government then proceded to set up the Medical Research Committee. This account seems to have arisen from misunderstanding of an episode of narrower significance and later date that is hereafter recounted, from original sources, in its proper context (Chapter 10). In short, the approach was made by the Lister Institute to the already established Medical Research Committee in 1914; and it referred to a possible use of the Institute as the Committee's central establishment.)

A vital decision was that there should be a single research organisation for the United Kingdom, and not one under each of the four Commissions. These had first, however, to pass separate resolutions formally 'retaining' the penny per person for research; this is recorded in the Report for 1913–14 of the English Commission.

The credit for this unity was claimed, no doubt justly, by Sir Robert Morant, in a personal letter to Mr A. J. (later Earl of) Balfour on 22 October 1919 (with copy to Fletcher):

This Medical Research Committee has been a particularly favourite child of mine since the beginning of 1912, when I was able to prevent the small sum of money then made available for Medical Research from being broken up into four parts for the four divisions of the United Kingdom; and we managed to get a Committee set up for the Kingdom as a whole, which has done quite magnificent work, and particularly so during the war.

The eventual formal step implementing this decision, by placing the responsibility on the National Health Insurance Joint Committee, is mentioned later (Chapter 3).

Chapter 3

The Medical Research Committee (1913-1920)

Appointment of the Medical Research Committee and the Advisory Council
—Statutory regulations—The first Chairman—Early proceedings of the
Committee—'Central Institute'—Scientific staff—First scheme of research—
Appointment of a Secretary—The First World War—Constitutional changes—
End of the Advisory Council

Appointment of the Medical Research Committee and the Advisory Council
It was implicit in the action taken to set up an organisation for
promoting medical research, with the funds to be provided under the
National Insurance Act 1911, that the research was not to be limited
to tuberculosis, and also that the organisation was to be a single one
for the whole United Kingdom (Chapter 2). The action, in the first
instance, consisted in the signature by Mr Lloyd George, as
"Minister responsible to Parliament for National Health Insurance"
(Chancellor of the Exchequer), of two Minutes of Appointment
dated 20 June 1913.

One Minute appointed nine persons to be "a Committee with
executive functions, to be known as the Medical Research Committee, for the purpose of dealing with the money made available for
research under the proviso to Sub-Section (2) of Section 16 of the
National Insurance Act 1911". Lord Moulton, a law lord who was
also a Fellow of the Royal Society, was named as chairman; the
others were two Members of Parliament and six persons appointed in
respect of their scientific qualifications (Appendix H). From 1916
three members were to retire at intervals of two years, their places
being filled (by reappointment or otherwise) by the Minister. The
terms of reference were as follows:

> The duties of the Committee will be to formulate the general plan of research
> and enquiry at the outset, and for each year to make arrangements for carrying
> it out, and to supervise its conduct so far as may be necessary, and in particular to
> secure adequate coordination of the various parts of the scheme. It will also deal
> with the collection and publication of information and of the results of statistical
> and other enquiries so far as suitable or necessary. For this purpose it will deter-
> mine, subject to the assent of the Minister responsible for National Health
> Insurance, the expenditure of the money available each year; the total of the sums
> available under paragraph (b) of subsection (2) of section 16 being about
> £57 000 per annum. Before the Minister responsible for National Health
> Insurance gives his final assent to the scheme of the Medical Research Com-
> mittee for any year, he will receive criticisms and suggestions in regard to it
> from the Advisory Council for Research, which is being appointed for this
> purpose.

The second Minute appointed an "Advisory Council for Research". Lord Moulton, again, was named as Chairman; and there were 40 other members. The list included the names of two Members of Parliament and one veterinary surgeon (Appendix C); the others, including two women, were all members of the medical profession; several held positions in the public service and five were Fellows of the Royal Society. The Minute stated that the expenditure of the money annually available for research would be directed by the Medical Research Committee appointed for the purpose, subject to the assent of the Minister responsible for National Health Insurance; and that the Scheme drawn up by the Committee would, before ministerial assent, be referred to the Advisory Council,

whose duty it will be to consider the Scheme when referred to them and to afford to the Minister all such criticisms and suggestions in regard to it as they may think desirable to submit to him from the point of view of securing that adequate consideration is given to the different problems arising and the various kinds of research work going on in the different parts of the United Kingdom, and in other portions of the Empire, in America, and in foreign countries, and also to the general scope of the research work to be undertaken under the Committee's Scheme.

The two Minutes were printed, and the substance of both was also published in a circular. According to the circular, the members of the Advisory Council were appointed by the Minister "after receiving suggestions for suitable names from each of the universities of the United Kingdom, from the Royal Colleges of Physicians and of Surgeons, from the Royal Society, and from other important public bodies interested in the question". It also included "medical representatives of the four National Health Insurance Commissions, and the other principal Government Departments concerned in medical work". It said, further, that in and after 1916 one-third of the members should retire, their places being filled (whether by reappointment or otherwise) by the Minister; but this provision was varied in the subsequent Regulations.

Statutory regulations
It may be, however, that the whole of the procedure by Minutes of Appointment was in the nature of an administrative short-cut and did not satisfy the requirements of the Act, in that the latter empowered, not "the Minister responsible for National Health Insurance" (Chancellor of the Exchequer), but the Insurance Commissioners. Whatever the reason, the appointment of the two bodies was re-enacted two months later, without reference to the foregoing and with some amplification of detail, as described below.

Meanwhile, the National Insurance (Joint Committee) Amendment Regulations made by the Treasury on 7 August 1913 had dealt further with the question of the moneys provided by Parliament which might be retained for research under the Act. These Regulations were originally provisional but, needing no amendment, eventually became definitive in effect. They vested solely in the National Health Insurance Joint Committee the power (so far as the terms of the grant by Parliament might permit) of retaining the monies in whole or part for research, and the power to make regulations about the manner in which any sums so retained should be applied for the purpose.

The Provisional National Health Insurance (Medical Research Fund) Regulations were issued by the Joint Committee on 20 August 1913, appointing the Medical Research Committee and the Advisory Council; the latter included one member who had not been named in the earlier Minute. These Provisional Regulations prescribed the periods of office of members of the Medical Research Committee and the Advisory Council, and the method of appointing or reappointing persons into the vacancies. They required the Committee to appoint a Treasurer from among its members, and empowered the Committee to appoint "officers and servants". They required the Committee to prepare schemes of research from time to time, with estimates of expenditure, and on such schemes the Advisory Council was to be consulted. They authorised expenditure for various purposes, including honoraria of approved amounts to members of the Committee other than the Chairman and any who were Members of the House of Commons. They dealt with points of accounting and audit, and with the investment of any sums standing to the credit of the Medical Research Fund. They provided that balances unexpended at the end of the financial year should be carried forward "if the terms of the Parliamentary grant so provide". They prohibited payments to members of the Committee or Advisory Council, other than the honoraria already mentioned and travelling and subsistence expenses incurred in attending meetings. Wherever higher approval was required the power was vested in the Chairman of the Joint Committee; the latter, the Rt Hon. C. F. G. Masterman, MP, was a member of the Government as Financial Secretary of the Treasury and had become "the Minister responsible for National Health Insurance".

On 21 March 1914, the Provisional Regulations were replaced by the National Health Insurance (Medical Research Fund) Regulations 1914. These differed in having two additional clauses enabling the Medical Research Committee to acquire real property (such as the site and building of the 'Central Institute') and providing for the appointment of two members as Trustees to hold such property, the Committee not being a body corporate. These Regulations may be said to be the definitive constitution of the Medical Research Committee, although the latter had already been operating for several months, and for that reason they are recorded in full (Appendix C).

The first Chairman

A remarkable man was Chairman of the Committee, and of the Advisory Council, for the first three years—and during one of them, before a Secretary took office, performed the executive function as well. John Fletcher Moulton was born in 1844. At Cambridge he was Senior Wrangler in 1868 and became a Fellow of Christ's College. In 1874 he was called to the bar; but he still found time to collaborate with William Spottiswoode in studies of electrical phenomena, and he was elected a Fellow of the Royal Society in 1880. Later he became a Queen's Counsel; he specialised in cases of patent law, where his grasp of technical issues was outstanding. For three short periods he was also a Member of Parliament in the Liberal interest. In due course he became a judge and was knighted; and from 1912 he was a Lord of Appeal in Ordinary, with a life peerage. Lord Moulton was chairman of several official bodies; and in 1914 he was appointed Director-General of Explosive Supplies at the Ministry of Munitions of War. He died in 1921. There is a biography by H. Fletcher Moulton (1922), in a preface to which the first Earl of Birkenhead wrote:

> I was never myself brought into contact with a mind which impressed me more by its brilliancy, scope and power . . . no man since the great Bacon has brought to the Bench so consummate a scientific equipment.

After Lord Moulton's retirement from the Committee, the latter paid tribute to him in its Report for 1915–16:

> His unrivalled powers of apprehending the true lines of development in the natural sciences enabled him to give invaluable guidance to the Committee in essential matters from the beginning of their work. . . . The Committee recognise gratefully that they were able to receive this help at the time when it was most needed.

Early proceedings of the Committee
The Medical Research Committee came into being, without waiting for completion of the formal stages described above, and met for the first time on 24 July 1913. In addition to the Chairman, the two parliamentary members were Dr Christopher Addison, MP, and Major Waldorf (later Lord) Astor, MP. The others were Sir Clifford Allbutt, Regius Professor of Physic in the University of Cambridge; Mr C. J. Bond, a Leicester surgeon with wide scientific interests; Professor William Bulloch, who held the University of London Chair of Bacteriology at The London Hospital; Professor Matthew Hay, of the Chair of Forensic Medicine in the University of Aberdeen (and Medical Officer of Health, City of Aberdeen); Professor (later Sir) Frederick Gowland Hopkins, of the Chair of Biochemistry in the University of Cambridge; and Colonel (later Lieut.-General) Sir William Leishman, of the Army Medical Service. (The last named has already been mentioned in Chapter 1, and several of the others in Chapter 2.)

All the members were present at the first meeting; they had already sent in suggestions, which the Chairman had embodied in a memorandum as a basis for discussion. They met again on the next day,

B*—M.R.

when a broad scheme of research was accepted. Organisation was discussed; and the research field was divided among the six scientific members with a view to their framing proposals.

At this stage the Committee had no premises and no Secretary or other staff. All the earlier meetings were held at the Chairman's house, 57 Onslow Square, South Kensington. The minutes were written by hand (by the Chairman's secretary, it is believed) in a large notebook, which was properly bound at a much later date. The Chairman apparently conducted such correspondence as there was, but little of this survives.

The Committee resumed its meetings on 22 and 23 October 1913, when important decisions were taken. It was agreed that a 'central institute' in London under the Committee's own control was essential; and thought was given to the choice of senior staff to head its departments. The need for a statistical department, and for hospital beds for clinical research, was also noted. Thereafter, meetings were held at weekly intervals and the projects were rapidly developed; these were of course still all in the planning stage, and there was nothing in being which called for administration. By the end of 1913 the Committee had obtained ministerial approval for its initial research programme; and arrangements had been made for members to make individual visits to centres of research throughout the British Isles.

'Central institute'

On 30 October the view that the then so-called 'central institute' must be in London was reaffirmed; the purchase of a house in the country, with grounds in which further buildings could be erected, was considered as a possibility for a later date. At the same meeting it was made known that a building at Hampstead, hitherto used as a hospital, would be available; an option on the property was secured, and within a few months the purchase was completed (Chapter 10). There was some discussion, inconclusive at that stage, on the question of whether part of the building should be used as a research hospital.

Early in 1914 overtures were made by the authorities of the Lister Institute of Preventive Medicine proposing an arrangement whereby it would be taken over by the Committee as the latter's central institute; the negotiations continued for a further nine months before they fell through. Details of this episode are given later as part of a fuller history of what eventually became the National Institute for Medical Research (Chapter 10).

Scientific staff

On 22 October 1913, the question of staff for the central institute was considered and the relevant minute of the meeting reads as follows:

A staff of skilled observers must be obtained and a careful review made of possible men. At the head of all these should be a Chief Director who should be the best man obtainable at any price. He should have the cooperation of other Heads who should again be men of the highest standing, and all these directors should be given efficient assistants with adequate help.

After the meeting had been adjourned to the following day, it was considered, after some discussion, that Sir Almroth Wright was "the only man satisfying the requirements of such a post" as that of Chief Director. It was also agreed that, in addition to a bacteriologist, the heads of departments should be a biochemist and a physiologist. Names of possible men to fill these posts, including several foreign workers, were mentioned.

On 11 December 1913, it was decided that Sir Almroth Wright was the only possible person for the chief post in the Department of Pathology, and that Dr H. H. Dale and Dr G. Barger would form a good combination to lead the Department of Biochemistry. At subsequent meetings Dr J. Brownlee as Statistician and Dr Leonard Hill as Applied Physiologist were added. Thereafter Dr Benjamin Moore and Captain S. R. Douglas were added as colleagues of Dr Hill and Sir Almroth Wright respectively. A fuller account is given later (Chapter 10). The salaries offered were well above the absurdly low current level for academic posts.

On 30 October 1913, it was agreed that it was also essential that the Committee should have staff available for work in other institutions, and this was apparently with research in clinical medicine particularly in mind. On 5 March 1914, the names of Dr T. R. Elliott and Dr Thomas Lewis were mentioned in this regard (Chapter 11).

After various preliminary approaches and further negotiations, all those proposed for posts in the central institute were in fact appointed to the staff early in 1914. That this did not happen earlier was, at least in some cases, partly due (*fide* Sir Henry Dale) to a reluctance of the scientific men to commit themselves until they knew who was to be appointed as Secretary of the Committee. Other reasons were the difficulty in assessing appropriate salaries in an organisation of a completely new type, and the fact that there was as yet no definite provision for pensions or even for security of tenure. The solution of this last problem was contained in a document of some constitutional importance. A letter (of which copies were printed, but marked 'Confidential') was sent on 15 December 1913 by the Chairman of the National Health Insurance Joint Committee to the Chairman of the Medical Research Committee in the following terms:

> You are aware that, technically, the money for Medical Research under the Insurance Act and the Regulations thereunder has to be reserved for that purpose by Resolution of the Joint Committee, and therefore that, strictly speaking, the only money actually available is the money for the first year. But it is, of course, obvious that no scheme of research to be on sound lines and productive of lasting value could be undertaken on a basis rendering the whole thing liable to cessation at the end of any year. And it is clear that your Committee must feel assured of adequate permanence as regards monies devoted either to capital expenditure, spread over a period of years, for the purposes of

Central Laboratories and Offices and so forth, or to the remuneration of a suitable staff without which such buildings would clearly be useless; an expert staff requiring, it is plain, a reasonable permanence of employment, for such work to be effectually undertaken.

Hence, in proceeding to carry out the scheme which I have today approved, you may rest assured that such expenditure as you find it necessary to incur upon what I may call a continuing basis, for a reasonable period of years, will be regarded by me, as Chairman of the Joint Committee, and I am sure by the Chancellor of the Exchequer also, as properly incurred, in spite of the technical difficulty to which I have referred above. And, in such circumstances as these, you need, I am sure, feel no doubt that this view would be upheld and the necessary provision made in any future year, should other Ministers be in our places—i.e., that all reasonable commitments would be continued.

First scheme of research

In November 1913 the Medical Research Committee submitted its first 'Scheme of Research' for ministerial approval. This was done in a minute from the Chairman of that Committee to the Chairman of the National Health Insurance Joint Committee. The scheme, unlike those for later years (Volume Two), was in very general terms and is quoted here in full except for a brief section on immediate requirements:

THE SCHEME OF RESEARCH

Type of Research   The object of the research is the extension of medical knowledge with the view of increasing our powers of preserving health and preventing or combating disease. But otherwise than that this is to be the guiding aim, the actual field of research is not limited and is to be wide enough to include, so far as may from time to time be found desirable, all researches bearing on health and disease, whether or not such researches have any direct or immediate bearing on any particular disease or class of diseases, provided that they are judged to be useful in promoting the attainment of the above object.

Method of Conducting the Research   The organisation by which this research will be carried out should consist of the following departments:
(1) A competent body of investigators of the highest class in the permanent employ of the scheme and devoting their whole time to research under it. They would be supplied with proper laboratories, duly qualified assistants, etc., and would ordinarily carry on their researches in such laboratories.

(2) Skilled investigators in the permanent or temporary employment of the scheme who would be engaged in procuring their material clinically or otherwise in connection with hospitals or other institutions furnishing the requisite opportunities for so doing. This material would in some cases be worked upon in local laboratories and in some cases at laboratories provided for them elsewhere under the scheme, and sometimes by a combination of both methods.

(3) Individual investigators not in the employment of the scheme who are carrying on independent investigations of a kind which are suitable to form

part of or to be coordinated with the research under the scheme, and to whom it is desirable to give help either in money or otherwise to enable them better to carry on their researches.

(4) *Statistical Department* This will mainly consist of persons in the permanent employment of the scheme who will be engaged in enquiries relating to diet, occupation, habits of life and other matters bearing upon the incidence of disease, and who will collect and deal with all types of vital statistics including the distribution of disease, the relative frequency of special types of lesions in diseases such as Tuberculosis, and in general with all statistical investigations useful either as preliminary to research or confirmatory of its results. It will possibly have to consider and advise how the statistical material provided for under the Insurance Act should be dealt with.

It is hoped that when the scheme is in actual work there may become associated herewith a Bureau through which those engaged in research unconnected with the scheme or otherwise working on kindred questions may be able to obtain information, references to special publications and other help of a like nature.

All these four departments are essential to the success of the organisation and are intended to co-operate with one another and will be used separately or together according to the nature of the work in hand. It is neither possible nor desirable to lay down any hard and fast lines of demarcation of their spheres of action.

Thus was the field of operation broadly defined, in terms which could still serve today although they might be amplified in detail. Thus, also, were four methods of promoting research proposed: (1) by maintaining a permanent staff in the Committee's own laboratories; (2) by maintaining permanent and temporary staff for work wholly or largely in hospitals and other institutions not under the Committee's control; (3) by making grants to investigators not in the Committee's employ; and (4) by maintaining a Statistical Department. Except that the fourth is no longer regarded as a separate administrative category, these remain at the present time the principal ways in which research work is supported (Chapter 9).

On 4 December 1913, the Advisory Council met and duly endorsed the Committee's proposals. On 15 December the Chairman of the National Health Insurance Joint Committee signified his approval.

Appointment of a Secretary

At the Committee's meeting on 30 October 1913, consideration was given to the need for an 'Organising Medical Secretary'. By this date spontaneous applications for such a post—which was an obvious necessity—had already been received, but none of the correspondents appears to have been thought worthy of serious consideration; their names are not on record. The contemporary minutes suggest that the future scope and importance of the position had not yet been clearly envisaged. It was usually, but not invariably, thought that the Secretary must be a medical man; but the idea that he must also be a man of experience, and indeed eminence, in research had not yet been assimilated. Hopkins later recounted that someone had suggested a part-time appointment.

A proposal to advertise the post was not pursued. During the next three months two people were tentatively proposed—Dr (later Sir) Andrew Balfour and Sir George Newman—but, on being sounded, these did not wish to be considered for the post; and one member of the Committee, Professor Matthew Hay, was definitely offered the appointment but declined. One may say frankly now that, in the light of later experience, it may be greatly doubted whether any of these three distinguished persons could have brought to the post the appropriate scientific attainments.

On 19 February 1914, it was decided to approach two people, one being Dr Walter Morley Fletcher, a physiologist working at Cambridge, and the other a man who was a non-medical hospital administrator of repute; but this second possibility was never followed up. It is a matter of record that Fletcher's name was put forward in Committee by Professor Hopkins; but Hopkins later made it known that the suggestion was first made informally to him by Dr T. R. Elliott, although he had then immediately recognised how appropriate it was. Dr Fletcher proved to be interested, and within a very short time a definite offer of appointment had been made to him and he had accepted it. He could not take up full duty until 1 July 1914, but he gave such time as he could during the interval; he was in attendance at meetings of the Committee from 19 March 1914 onwards. The minutes of the Committee from those of the meeting on 2 July 1914 (and for some time afterwards) are in his hand. Soon after he took up whole-time duties an office was obtained in St Stephen's House, Westminster, at a rent of £25 per annum.

The history of the Committee during the first few months of its existence shows how much can be accomplished by a small group of talented men, ably led, willing to meet together as often as once a week and to take individual action at other times. Clearly, however, it was neither an economical arrangement in its use of manpower nor one which could be indefinitely maintained. It may well have had its advantages during the planning stage, when a combination of abilities and a diversity of views would have an especial value. It would inevitably have proved inadequate when the stage of active operation commenced, as it was about to do, calling for decisions from day to day and requiring both a sharp focus for corporate policy and a consistent level of administrative action.

It was indeed high time that the Committee had headquarters of its own, with a permanent official handling its affairs. Not only was there now an undeniable demand for regular administration, but there had already been some disquiet among the members that business was concentrated in the hands of a rather autocratic Chairman—however brilliantly capable—and recorded mainly in his personal papers. The minutes of meetings were merely read out on the next occasion, no copies being provided to members, and this almost clandestine procedure gave rise to misunderstandings. There was even an unhealthy feeling that a few people who knew him best had readier access to the Chairman than had others. Indications of this situation exist in surviving correspondence of only slightly later date (and in an oral tradition within the writer's memory); a letter of Fletcher's mentions that Lord Moulton was very angry about not being offered reappointment in 1916.

The potentiality of the Committee as an instrument of Government must have radically changed when Fletcher assumed whole-time duty as its Secretary. In such circumstances the initiative must pass to the man, assuming him to have the requisite qualities, who is devoting his main energies to the task and keeping its problems always in the forefront of his mind. The role of the councillor, with primary obligations elsewhere, remains of great importance; but it becomes consultative and critical. More and more, as he gains experience of the special function, must the permanent officer be not only the executant of policy but the main source or medium of new proposals. And as the staff organisation grows he, as its official leader, becomes also the representative of its views to the governing body. That body is no longer alone but forms the apex of a larger entity—a research service—which develops certain corporate characteristics; and in this the Secretary is naturally the focal point.

That Dr Fletcher—Sir Walter as he became in 1918—had the requisite qualities can never have been in doubt, and was later amply proved by his achievement. He was a man of outstanding personality, about which more is said later (Chapter 17). He had an established reputation as a research worker in physiology; and he quickly displayed a talent for administration, a type of work which he enjoyed.

Yet it was a special type of administration that he developed—and later handed on; a type which was based on an understanding of the peculiar conditions required for successful research work and on sympathy with scientific men. Its means were always subordinated to the end; its methods were adapted to the special type of people with whom it had to deal. It was essentially flexible (Chapter 17).

When Fletcher was absent through illness for some months in 1916, Dr H. H. Dale of the scientific staff and Mr C. J. Bond, a member of the Committee, kept his work going.

The First World War

For an organisation so planned and so served, everything seemed propitious. But, as was said, "the lamps are going out all over Europe". The outbreak of war on 4 August 1914 created an entirely new set of circumstances, and to these the infant organisation had to adapt itself as best it could. In short, the Committee's main task for the next four years was to mobilise the aid of medical science for the national war effort; some account of this is given in Volume Two.

Nevertheless, the normal programme was never wholly submerged; plans already made were put into operation, and indeed often further developed, so far as conditions permitted. The establishment of the central institute had to be deferred, to allow the building to be used for hospital purposes, but the several departments were constituted in borrowed accommodation in other institutions (Chapter 10).

Constitutional changes

On 22 October 1913, the Committee appointed Major Astor, from among its members, to be Treasurer. On 5 March 1914 the Chairman and Treasurer were appointed as Trustees.

On 20 August 1916, the Chairman and two other members of the Committee retired, in fulfilment of the Regulations, and were replaced by others (Appendix H). Major Astor became Chairman and the Viscount Goschen, one of the new members, succeeded him as Treasurer. Two further retirements and replacements occurred in 1918.

Final changes were made in February 1920, with a view to coming events. Two members resigned and three new members were appointed, increasing the total to ten. And on the resignation of Major (by then Viscount) Astor, he was followed in the chairmanship by the Viscount Goschen, and the latter in the treasurership by a new member, the Hon. Edward Wood (later Lord Irwin, eventually Earl of Halifax).

By this latter date, however, a major constitutional change was impending, an account of which will be found in the next two chapters. On 31 March 1920 the Medical Research Committee, as such, ceased to exist. Before then, from 1 July 1919, there had been a transitional period in respect of ministerial responsibility for the Committee's activities (Chapter 4).

End of the Advisory Council

In retrospect it is difficult to be sure what effective function this large and mainly professional body was originally intended to perform, if indeed this was ever clearly envisaged. As already mentioned, it was appointed on a representational basis, whereas the members of the Medical Research Committee (and successor Council) were expressly chosen as individuals. It may have been considered politic to provide a dignified role for representatives of professional, institutional, and departmental interests in the medical field, in order more easily to limit membership of the executive body to persons with special qualifications for controlling scientific work. Or there may have been a reluctance to give too much independence to a small expert body, as yet untried; or perhaps it was thought that an imposing façade was a necessity for maintaining public confidence in the new organisation. Whatever may have been in the minds of the framers of the original constitution, it is clear that at a later date the interposition of such an assemblage between the active body and the responsible ministers would have been regarded as not only superfluous but intolerable.

The history of the Advisory Council—domestically known by the cheerful sobriquet of 'the forty thieves'— is soon told. It met on 4 December 1913, as already mentioned, to approve the first research schemes of the Medical Research Committee; it met again on 17 November 1914, to approve those for the second year. It performed its function of benediction faultlessly on both occasions; it may well have been aided in doing so by the fact that it had the same Chairman as the Medical Research Committee itself, and this was indeed the saving grace of a potentially awkward constitutional arrangement.

On 26 May 1915, the members of the Advisory Council received a letter from Fletcher, under direction by the Chairman of the National Health Insurance Joint Committee, forwarding a White Paper on work being done by the Medical Research Committee in connection with the war, and explaining that for the time being the annual submission of schemes of research was thought to be unnecessary. There followed this paragraph:

> Upon the question whether the Medical Research Committee should place their services, together with all the resources under their direction, freely at the disposal of the National Executive in the existing circumstances, Mr Montagu feels assured that there will be no difference of opinion among the members of the Advisory Council, and accordingly he does not propose at this time of strain to summon a special meeting of the Advisory Council, for consultation with regard to the emergency activities of the Committee connected with the war.

Thereafter the body passed into oblivion, apart from the somewhat equivocal memorial given to it in this chapter, and apparently no steps were taken to reappoint or replace the members in 1916 as the Regulations required. On 31 March 1920 it ceased to have even a notional existence. No question of replacing it seems ever to have been raised in discussion of the reconstruction next to be considered (Chapter 4).

Chapter 4
Reconstruction Period (1918-1920)

General situation—Proposed Ministry of Health—The Department of Scientific and Industrial Research—The Machinery of Government Committee—Ministry of Health Act 1919—The scientific independence of medical research—Some founding fathers

General situation

The approaching end of the First World War (1914–18) was the signal for replanning in many branches of public activity. Some things had disappeared and others were recognised as obsolescent; new needs had become apparent and a spirit of change was in the air. 'Reconstruction' was the slogan.

It might have been thought unnecessary to make any change in respect of a body so new as the Medical Research Committee, and as yet so untried under the normal conditions of peace. On the other hand it might in any event have been considered desirable to take the opportunity of providing a more appropriate link with the Government than through the organisation dealing with National Health Insurance, an arrangement derived from the manner in which the Committee came to be established (Chapter 2)—an accident of birth, so to speak—rather than from any fundamental rationalisation. The question in fact arose inevitably as a side-issue of proposals of wider import.

Proposed Ministry of Health

A major item in the proposals for reconstruction was the creation, unsuccessfully mooted on previous occasions, of a Ministry of Health in place of the old Local Government Board—this was for England and Wales, but with a corresponding change for Scotland. Among other things, it was proposed that the new Ministry should take over, from Commissioners under the Treasury, responsibility for National Health Insurance in England and Wales. In the absence of special provision to the contrary, therefore, the Medical Research Committee would have found itself automatically transferred to the jurisdiction of the Ministry.

To some this appeared to be a logical and obviously proper arrangement—such is the compelling power of names! There were, however, some very serious objections. Firstly, the powers of the Ministry were limited to England and Wales, whereas the Committee's functions related to the whole of the British Isles; and it had

34

indeed already operated overseas during the war. Secondly, the Ministry had functions covering only a part of the medical field. For example, health in industry was the responsibility of the Home Office; and until a much later date the Ministry had little direct concern with curative, as distinct from preventive, medicine. The Committee, on the contrary, was charged with the promotion of research relating to all aspects of health and disease. Thirdly, a large administrative department necessarily has certain declared policies and urgent day-to-day requirements, both tending to create pressures of a kind inimical to the initiative and perspective essential for long-term research. In contrast, the Committee had already achieved independent power, in its scientific discretion, to frame and execute its programme for the advancement of knowledge; even a suspicion of bureaucratic control or political expediency would have destroyed the Committee's authority and have lost it the sympathetic co-operation of scientific men.

The Department of Scientific and Industrial Research
Another factor in the situation was that by an Order in Council of 28 July 1915, two years after the original appointment of the Medical Research Committee, there had been established a Committee of Privy Council for Scientific and Industrial Research; and this provided a precedent for an appropriate form of ministerial control over a research organisation expending public funds. After a few months during which administrative action was taken within the Board of Education, a separate Department of Scientific and Industrial Research was established in 1916. It was soon given charge of two organisations of earlier date: the Geological Survey, founded in 1835, was transferred from the care of the Board of Education to that of the Department, on the recommendation of the Reconstruction Committee; the National Physical Laboratory, founded in 1899, was placed under the financial control of the Department, although the Royal Society continued to be closely associated with its scientific administration.

The Department, although separate from any other, had no Minister entirely its own. Ministerial responsibility was in commission, so to speak, in the hands of the Committee of Privy Council. The members of this body were ministers serving *ex officiis*; the Lord President of the Council was Chairman, and the others were the heads of the departments chiefly concerned with science and industry. Such a committee—the device was an old one—was not designed to hold meetings; in practice the Lord President, as chairman, became the minister responsible to Parliament, consulting his colleagues as he thought necessary.

The internal constitution of the Department, brought into being in 1916, was less happily conceived. Its scientific body was an Advisory Council, with no formal authority over the executive; all action was taken in the name of the Committee of Privy Council.

Moreover, the Department was staffed by administrative civil servants, of whom—at least at the senior level—few had a scientific background and none had research experience. It is significant that subsequent reforms were in the direction of assimilation to the pattern adopted for medical research (and later for agricultural research). It was, however, not until 1927 that a man of science became Secretary of the Department, although he had been deputy for some years, and not until the passage of the Department of Scientific and Industrial Research Act 1956 that the former Advisory Council became a Scientific and Industrial Research Council with executive control. Further changes are mentioned later (Chapter 8). The origins of the Department have recently been discussed by McLeod and Andrews (1970).

The Machinery of Government Committee
In July 1917, a Machinery of Government Committee was appointed by Lloyd George as a subcommittee of the Reconstruction Committee; both it and the parent body were very shortly afterwards transferred to the jurisdiction of Addison on his appointment as Minister of Reconstruction. It was a small body of distinguished membership, under the chairmanship of Viscount Haldane, and its terms of reference were "To enquire into the responsibilities of the various Departments of the central executive Government, and to advise in what manner the exercise and distribution by the Government of its functions should be improved". The members included Morant, Sir George Murray of the Treasury, Mrs Sidney (Beatrice) Webb and three Members of Parliament, with Michael Heseltine as secretary. The proposal to set up this body was initiated by Mr E. S. Montagu, Financial Secretary to the Treasury, in a memorandum of 30 April 1917, presented in circumstances discussed by Daalder (1963); but Haldane, in his autobiography, claims to have prompted it. According to Lord Bridges (1959), referring to the memorandum just mentioned:

> Montagu seems first to have suggested that the Privy Council should be the centre for all research activities of Government. Haldane disagreed. He thought that the Lord President would be too busy with other things.

This Committee reported in 1918, devoting a chapter to "Research and Information". In this it recommended "that increased importance should be attached to the organisation of enquiry and research, and that the activities of the central Government in this direction should be extended". It proceeded to consider intelligence work in, and research work supervised by, administrative departments, contrasting these particular functions with intelligence and research work for general use. For the latter it held that special arrangements were essential, and it found that those already made for the Department of Scientific and Industrial Research were appropriate:

> The establishment in 1915, under the Lord President of the Council, of a new Department to develop and organise the knowledge required for the application

of Science to Industry, to keep in close touch with all Departments concerned with scientific research, to undertake researches on behalf of Departments, and to stimulate the supply of research workers, marked a stage in the recognition of a need which is not merely local or departmental, but national, and there is in our opinion good reason for extending what has been done here to other fields in which thinking is required in aid of administration.

A Cabinet with such knowledge at its disposal would, we believe, be in a position to devolve, with greater freedom and confidence than is at present the case, the duties of administration, and even of legislation. . . . We may here add that the gradual introduction of the co-operation of the Ministers of the Dominions in affairs which belong to a Cabinet now charged with the interests of the Empire as a whole, points to the probability that the organisation of the kind of knowledge we have in view is likely to become requisite in new directions.

Citing as a model the direction of the Department of Scientific and Industrial Research by its own Committee of Privy Council, the report states:

As regards the methods to be adopted for conducting enquiry and research in any branch of knowledge, so far as it is determined that the work should be carried out under supervision of a general organisation, and not under that of an administrative Department, we think that a form of organisation on the lines already laid down for Scientific and Industrial Research will prove most suitable.

It is therefore not surprising that a similar constitutional position was thought desirable for the organisation concerned with medical research. Speaking of the Medical Research Committee, as it existed, the report says:

It is important, also, to observe that, although the Minister in charge of an administrative Department is answerable to Parliament for the work of the Committee, we have of set purpose, and for two clear reasons, classified the Committee as a service of a general character, and not as a body engaged upon research for the immediate purposes of a single administrative Department.

The first reason is that, although the operations of the Medical Research Committee are within the province of the Minister responsible for Health Insurance, so that he would defend the proceedings of the Committee if they were criticised in Parliament, in practice, as we understand, the Minister relies, under the arrangements described in paragraph 37, upon the Medical Research Committee to select the objects upon which they will spend their income, and to frame schemes for the efficient and economical performance of their work. The Minister has, of course, always received a full explanation of their schemes from the Committee before giving his approval, but he has never sought to control their work, or to suggest to them that they should follow one line of enquiry rather than another.

There is, therefore, an important distinction to be drawn between this research work and all other work within the sphere of the Department; and the judgement of the scientists who form the majority of the members of the Medical Research Committee as to the value of this understanding is clear. In their first Annual Report (1914–15, Cd. 8101, page 48) the Committee say that they 'venture to acknowledge their indebtedness to the three successive Chairmen of the National Health Insurance Joint Committee under whom they have worked, for having allowed them the most complete freedom, within their constitution, to bring flexible and rapid assistance to the national need on occasions of emergency with the least possible delay in the motion of constitutional machinery'.

The second reason is that the Committee had not long been established before the outbreak of war in 1914; and that, as their four Annual Reports clearly indicate, they have, in consequence, from the first devoted almost the whole of their energies to the investigation of problems arising out of war conditions, and referred to them by administrative Departments, including the Admiralty, War Office, Air Ministry, Home Office and Ministry of Munitions, for the purpose of concentrating the whole of the scientific forces available in the country upon the search for a solution.

The actual recommendation in respect of the Medical Research Committee, after agreement that all the other powers and duties of the English and Welsh Insurance Commissions should pass to the proposed Ministry of Health, was:

The operations of this Committee have never been limited, as would presumably be the case with the new Ministry of Health, to England and Wales, but have extended over the whole United Kingdom. We think that it is essential to make provision for enabling the work to be continued on the same lines, so as to secure the fullest dissemination of its results, and the best use of the limited funds available for it.

For these reasons, and on the grounds which are set out in the Chapter of this part of our Report dealing with Research and Information, we recommend that, on the establishment of the Ministry of Health, the Medical Research Committee should be reconstituted so as to enable it to act under the direction of a Committee of the Privy Council on the lines already followed in the case of the Committee of Council for Scientific and Industrial Research.

While stressing the advantage of the Privy Council formula, the report ends the particular chapter on a warning note. It was envisaged that a multiplication of research organisations on this footing might place too heavy a burden on the Lord President, whose other duties often included the leadership of the House of Lords. The eventual formation of a number of such organisations was thought to be not unlikely:

It may, therefore, not be premature to anticipate that the distinctive character of the organisation of Intelligence and Research for general use; the proper scope of such an organisation; and its potential relations with analogous organisations throughout the Empire, could thenceforth all be maintained by a Minister specifically appointed on the ground of his suitability to preside over a separate Department of Intelligence and Research, which would no longer act under a Committee of the Privy Council, and would take its place among the most important Departments of Government.

The extent to which these words proved to have been prophetic will be seen later (Chapters 6, 8).

Ministry of Health Act 1919
The recommendation was accepted and the necessary legislative provision inserted in the Ministry of Health Bill. The reasons given in the Report of the Machinery of Government Committee were elaborated—although some paragraphs are identical—in a memorandum prepared by, or under the direction of, Addison in his capacity as Minister of Reconstruction. This memorandum was apparently available in 1918 to those who were then drafting the Bill, and also to the professional bodies consulted about it, although it does not seem to have been made public at that date.

The paragraph emphasising the dangers inherent in control of the research organisation is notably frank and cogent:

> A progressive Ministry of Health must necessarily become deeply committed from time to time to particular systems of health administration. The Minister of Health at any moment may be appointed by the Government on the ground that he is something of a scientist or takes a special interest in health matters. One does not wish to attach too much importance to the possibility that a particular Minister may hold strong personal views on particular questions of medical science or of its application in practice; but, even apart from special difficulties of this kind, which cannot be left out of account, a keen and energetic Minister will quite properly do his best to maintain the administrative policy which he finds existing in his Department, or imposes upon his Department during his term of office. He would, therefore, be constantly tempted to endeavour in various ways to secure that the conclusions reached by organised work under any scientific body, such as the Medical Research Committee, which was substantially under his control, should not suggest that his administrative policy might require alteration. The more active the administration of his Department the greater this danger becomes. It is essential that such a situation should not be allowed to arise, for it is the first object of scientific research of all kinds to make new discoveries, and these discoveries are bound to correct the conclusions based upon the knowledge which was previously available, and, therefore, in the long run to make it right to alter administrative policy.

Nevertheless, during the debate on the Second Reading of the Bill in the House of Commons on 25 February 1919, there were Members who suggested that it would be preferable to place the Medical Research Committee under the direct control of the Minister of Health rather than, as implied in the Bill, to reconstitute it so as to enable it to act under the direction of a Committee of Privy Council. The reasons for the proposal in the Bill were explained by Astor, in his capacity as Parliamentary Secretary to the Local Government Board; and the President of the Board, Addison again, circulated a White Paper giving the text of the memorandum mentioned above. This important historical document was later reproduced in the Report of the Medical Research Council for 1950–51, as an appendix to an obituary appreciation of Addison.

The Government view prevailed, and the Ministry of Health Act 1919 became law with the particular provision included; and the provision came into operation on 1 April 1920, by virtue of an Order in Council of 9 February 1920 (Appendix D). There had, however, been an anomalous transitional period in respect of ministerial control, owing to the fact that related provisions of the Act had been brought into operation on 1 July 1919, by an Order of 25 June 1919. The effect was that the powers of the Insurance Commissioners were transferred to the Minister of Health as from 1 July 1919, but that the proviso excluding the power to retain sums for medical research remained in abeyance; and also that the provision of the National Insurance Act 1911 creating that power was not yet repealed. As a result, the Minister of Health replaced the Chairman of the National Health Insurance Joint Committee as the responsible minister during the nine months from 1 July 1919 to 31 March 1920.

The scientific independence of medical research
Before the new constitutional position had been achieved, there had been other threats to the independence of medical research than that of attachment of the agency to a large administrative department. The existence of the Department of Scientific and Industrial Research created the hazard that empire-building or uninformed logic might exert pressure for the creation of a single research organisation in which that for medical research would be merged; some such moves were indeed tentatively made behind the scenes. Amalgamation would have meant subordination for the smaller body, and this would have been disastrous. Not only did the Department, in those days, suffer from the disabilities mentioned above, but these and associated factors seriously delayed the time when it could command the full confidence of the scientific world. Moreover, it was especially concerned with 'applied' research directly bearing on industrial needs; and the nature of this work involved a high level of expenditure and the establishment of large research stations, which were staffed by scientific civil servants and not associated with universities. The needs of research aimed at medical discovery were quite different. Close consultation and collaboration between separate organisations was another matter, and this was in due course amicably and fruitfully achieved (Chapter 7).

There was, alternatively, a proposal to bring both research councils, and probably other agencies, into juxtaposition under a single Committee of Privy Council, with the Lord President as its Chairman. This Committee was to have a central secretariat for finance, which would undoubtedly have been the embryo of a 'Department for Research', a term which was actually used in contemporary discussion. There was also some talk in the Treasury of a 'Ministry of Research', and it has been noted above that the Report of the Machinery of Government Committee did indeed provide some basis for this. There was, however, strong objection on the part of the Ministry of Agriculture and Fisheries to yielding its control of research in these two fields, and this may have had force against the idea of a unified research organisation.

Looking back, one finds it hard to believe that the Medical

Research Council could have built up its present reputation and strength of position had it not enjoyed the fullest measure of independence during its formative period.

Some founding fathers

It has been seen that David Lloyd George (1863–1945) can be acclaimed as the father of the Medical Research Committee, whether the original idea was his own or that of some unsung hero among his parliamentary and official helpers (Chapter 2). Two statesmen, Haldane and Addison, and one outstanding official, Morant, may be named as the godfathers who particularly sponsored the Committee's reincarnation as the Medical Research Council. There are, of course, biographies of these men, but none is satisfactory from the angle of the present work ("Addison did nothing to deserve so bad a biography", as Gilbert has said).

First was Lord Haldane, who presided over the Machinery of Government Committee ('Haldane Committee') and claimed to have drawn up its report himself (in a letter to Mr Ramsay Macdonald, cited by Gilbert). To him, therefore, the Council was in large measure indebted for its extra-departmental status and for the attachment to the Privy Council that fostered its independence of action during the formative years. The career of one so well known as Richard Burdon Haldane (1856–1928) needs only the briefest mention here—graduate of Edinburgh and Göttingen, philosopher, lawyer, parliamentarian, eventually an outstanding Secretary of State for War and finally Lord Chancellor. It was said of him by Sir Henry Tizard: "He was the kind of Minister under whom scientists rejoice to serve; constant in support, imaginative and helpful in his understanding". On the same authority, he was the "consultant and strong supporter" of the President and Parliamentary Secretary of the Board of Education when they were launching the Department of Scientific and Industrial Research in 1915. Tizard also records that when Haldane went up in a military dirigible balloon, quite a risky thing in those days, he declined to exchange his top hat for the indignity of a flying helmet.

Then there was Christopher Addison (1869–1951), who played a number of roles in the early days of the Committee and Council—and again much later. He was a Doctor of Medicine of London University and a Fellow of the Royal College of Surgeons of England; he became Professor of Anatomy at Sheffield and later held teaching posts in London medical schools. He then turned to political life, and from 1910 was intermittently a Member of Parliament, first in the Liberal and later in the Labour interest. There is no good evidence to support statements that he had a hand in drafting the research provision in the National Insurance Act 1911 (Chapter 2); but he was a member of the Departmental Committee on Tuberculosis (Chapter 3), and thereafter an original member of the Medical Research Committee. In 1914 he became Parliamentary Secretary of the Board of Education and was concerned in the establishment of the Department of Scientific and Industrial Research. In 1915 he became Parliamentary Secretary of the Office of Munitions, and in 1916 Minister of Munitions of War; there he was concerned with setting up the Health of Munition Workers Committee, which was a precursor of the part of the Council's organisation dealing with problems of industrial medicine.

In 1917 Addison was appointed Minister in charge of Reconstruction; the Committee on the Machinery of Government came within his sphere, and likewise the first move towards implementing its recommendations on the future of the organisation for medical research. That question fell even more directly within his responsibility from 1919, when he became President of the Local Government Board for its closing days and then the first Minister of Health. He wrote in his memoirs (1924) that "it was tempting, and it would have been easy, to have brought the Research Committee wholly under the Ministry of Health . . . but it would have been a narrow and mistaken course". That view he actively supported, both in the memorandum already mentioned and in piloting the Ministry of Health Bill through Parliament. He became Lord Addison in 1937 (Viscount in 1945), and when his party later came into power he held various high offices, including that of Lord President. Of his impact on the Council when he returned to it as Chairman in 1948, and was afterwards also its minister, something is said later (Chapter 17).

Sir Robert Morant was described by Addison as "a magnificent and ruthless hustler . . . great in mind as well as in body", and by Sir Harold Nicolson as a "supreme Civil Servant". Sir Laurence Brock, who had served under him, said that "Morant was a great man, the only great man in the Civil Service in our lifetime". Beatrice Webb wrote that he was "the one man of genius in the Civil Service . . . a strange mortal, not altogether sane". He also had some detractors, colleagues with whom he had violently differed and writers taking views from them; Violet Markham wrote in measured rebuttal of their denigrations. Morant was described by Lord Salter (1961) as:

Perhaps the most remarkable civil servant of his day. . . . A man of magnetic presence, tall and with a great leonine head of white hair, he combined dynamic energy with an excitable and nervous temperament. He pursued an undeviating purpose through perplexing and subtle methods, due partly perhaps to the fact that as a young man he had tutored the sons of the King of Siam and absorbed some of the traditions of court intrigue in Bangkok.

Sir Lewis Selby-Bigge, another colleague, wrote in the *Dictionary of National Biography*:

His premature death, in London, 13 March 1920, left the Civil Service with the feeling that it had lost one of the greatest figures it had ever produced— great by both character and achievment.

Robert Laurie Morant (1868–1920) entered the Civil Service at a later age than was usual, having—after leaving Oxford (New College)—spent some years in various forms of educational work at home and abroad. By 1903, at the age of thirty-five, he had become Permanent Secretary of the Board of Education; and he exercised more than the usual influence of an official in moulding the reforms then being undertaken by the department, notably with regard to the medical inspection and treatment of school children. Despite statements to the contrary, he was not concerned with the National Insurance Act 1911 before it became law (Chapter 2); but in 1912 he was appointed Chairman of the new National Health Insurance Commission (England), and he also became Deputy Chairman (to a minister) of the National Health Insurance Joint Committee. He served as a member of the Machinery of Government Committee. In 1919 he became the first Permanent Secretary of the Ministry of Health. In these capacities he played a great part in shaping the Medical Research Committee and its successor.

Sir George Newman, who was his medical colleague at the Ministry of Health, wrote in 1939 of Morant: "It is safe to say that no Civil Servant in our national history has made a more permanent or constructive contribution to the administration of Public Medicine and its application to the well-being of the Nation." Newman seems to give more credit to Morant than to Haldane (see above) for the report of the Machinery of Government Committee, saying that it enshrines "many Benthamite and Morantian views" and "was the last but one of Morant's constructive efforts". He also refers to Morant's work in implementation of the National Insurance Act 1911 "and its medical research clauses and their administration" (there was only one such clause); and in this regard, Newman remarks on Morant's ability to get much action out of little legislative sanction:

> He made the fabric of the school medical service grow out of half a dozen lines in a second class measure, which passed Parliament in the late summer of 1907; and out of an obscure clause in the National Insurance Bill he drew forth the fertile inspiration of the Medical Research Committee. [And on this latter point Selby-Bigge may again be quoted: "Morant had more at heart the wide potentialities, realised in the European War, of the system of national aid for medical research, founded in 1913 on principles which he elaborated . . ."]

The Council paid a tribute to Morant in its Report for 1919–20, after his untimely death on the eve of its own reconstitution:

> To him in great part was due the original constitution of the Medical Research Committee . . . and the formation of the Medical Research Fund for the United Kingdom as a whole, and . . . in these he used all his powers of constructive wisdom to secure the best intellectual freedom for the Committee.

At the Ministry of Health he was directly concerned with the establishment of the Committee of Privy Council for Medical Research, and for constituting the Medical Research Council under its direction; the Report continues:

In this again he showed his concern for the best interests of medical research and for the promotion of the service it has to give to the State. . . . The Council will meet the new responsibilities and opportunities that lie before them in the future fittingly indeed if they can bring to their work a conception of public duty as high as his, and some measure of the eagerness and breadth of his intellectual vision.

That last sentence reflects the sincere esteem in which Morant was held by Fletcher as a staunch ally in the pursuit of ideals that they had in common; the regard was undoubtedly reciprocated. Although this section deals with people who helped from outside, it is well to remember how much Fletcher himself contributed from within to the reconstruction; but of him much is said later (Chapter 17).

Chapter 5
Establishment of the Medical Research Council (1920)

Provisions of the Ministry of Health Act—Appointment of the Committee of
the Privy Council for Medical Research—Incorporation of the Medical
Research Council—Provisions of the Royal Charter—Replacement of
Trustees—The constitution in practice—Membership of the Council—Functions
of the Chairman and Treasurer—Secretary and staff—Financial control

Provisions of the Ministry of Health Act
As has been seen, the Ministry of Health Act 1919 provided the
statutory basis of a reconstituted agency for medical research
(Chapter 4). Under this measure a Ministry of Health replaced the
Local Government Board in England and Wales, corresponding
changes being made in Ireland by the same Act and in Scotland by
the Scottish Board of Health Act 1919. The four bodies of Insurance
Commissioners ceased to exist, and most of the powers of those for
England and for Wales were transferred to the new Ministry by
Section 3(1)(b) of the Act.

Proviso (i) to that Section, however, excluded from the transfer
"the power conferred on the Insurance Commissioners by the
proviso to Sub-Section (2) of Section 16 of the National Insurance
Act 1911, of retaining and applying for the purposes of research
such sums as are therein mentioned". It went on to enact that "the
duties heretofore performed by the Medical Research Committee
. . . shall be carried on by or under the direction of a Committee of
the Privy Council appointed by his Majesty for that purpose".
Section 11(2) and the Second Schedule repealed the above cited
provision of the earlier Act, thus divorcing the finance of medical
research from the National Insurance scheme.

The proviso also enacted that "any property held for the purpose
of the former Committee shall . . . be transferred to and vested in
such persons as the body by whom such duties as aforesaid are
carried on may appoint, and be held by them for the purposes of that
body"; but in the event the Council became a corporation capable
of holding property. The reference to a body which would carry on
the duties is curiously oblique; relegation to an expert executive body
was, in fact, the only practicable formula. In effect there was complete continuity and the Medical Research Committee was *de facto*
succeeded by the Medical Research Council.

The implementation of the Act required certain further instruments—namely, a series of Orders in Council and a Royal Charter,
and in the first place an Order in Council of 9 February 1920

45

appointed 1 April 1920 as the date of the commencement of the Act
for the particular purpose, in circumstances already detailed
(Chapter 4).

Appointment of the Committee of the Privy Council for Medical Research
The Committee of the Privy Council was appointed by an Order in
Council of 11 March 1920 (Appendix D), naming as members: the
Lord President of the Council, the Minister of Health, the Secretary
for Scotland and the Chief Secretary for Ireland. The Minister of
Health was to preside over the Committee in the absence of the
Lord President; the latter was, by implication, to be Chairman. It
was also ordered that the Secretary of the Medical Research Council
for the time being was to be the Secretary of the Committee of the
Privy Council.

Further provisions of the Order were that the Committee of the
Privy Council "may out of moneys provided by Parliament or otherwise available, and subject to such conditions as the Treasury may
prescribe, furnish the Medical Research Council with such funds as
may be necessary"; that the Committee "shall in every year cause
to be laid before both houses of Parliament a report of their proceedings and of the proceedings of the Medical Research Council during
the preceding year"; and that the Committee "shall exercise and
perform in relation to the [Medical Research] Council such powers
and duties as in the Charter aforesaid they shall be authorised and
empowered to exercise and perform" (see next page).

Incorporation of the Medical Research Council
Throughout the reconstruction discussions it was assumed that there
was to be such a body as the Medical Research Council, whatever its
point of attachment to the machinery of state. The first essential was
clearly to create a body that could carry on the work of the Medical
Research Committee. The change of title from 'Committee' to
'Council' was of secondary significance.

The Medical Research Council was first named, so far as formal
instruments are concerned, in the Order in Council of 11 March
1920 appointing the Committee of the Privy Council (see preceding
section). In its preamble the relevant passage reads:

> And whereas for the purpose of securing the continued performance of the
> duties heretofore performed by the Medical Research Committee a Petition has
> been presented to His Majesty in Council by the Minister of Health praying for
> the grant of a Charter of Incorporation to the present members of the Medical
> Research Committee, under the style and title of the Medical Research Council,
> to act under the direction of the Committee of the Privy Council to be appointed
> by His Majesty for that purpose.

An Order in Council of 25 March 1920 (Appendix D) approved the
draft of a Charter "for creating the Members of the Medical
Research Committee a Body Corporate under the style and title of

'The Medical Research Council'." The draft was appended, and the Charter was granted in terms of it on 1 April 1920 (see next section and Appendix E).

So, on the latter date, the Medical Research Council came into being with the same members as the predecessor Medical Research Committee, sitting round the same table and performing the same functions. Its title had changed; it had become a corporation; and there was a new formula for its direction at ministerial level. Although it followed the model of the Department of Scientific and Industrial Research in coming under the jurisdiction of a special Committee of the Privy Council, the Medical Research Council differed from the Advisory Council of that Department in having executive powers and controlling its own administration; therein lay the novelty, and as the Council said in its Report for 1919–20, "the privileges and responsibilities with which the terms of their Charter have endowed them . . . are such as they think have not been given before to any body of scientific men".

Provisions of the Royal Charter

From what has been said, it will be clear that the new double-tiered organisation had no statutory terms of reference except of the most general kind. Its function, as stated in the Ministry of Health Act 1919, was to carry on "the duties heretofore performed by the Medical Research Committee". As the money simultaneously ceased to be retained in accordance with the original formula, the statutory basis for which was in fact repealed, the Act of 1919 apparently implied that the duties covered the expenditure of money to be provided by Parliament in some other way; and, further, that the field of research was no longer even theoretically subject to definition in the context of the Act of 1911.

As has been seen, the Order in Council of 11 March 1920 determined the membership of the Committee of the Privy Council, who was to preside, and who was to be its Secretary. It also implicitly approved delegation to the Medical Research Council, which it mentioned by that name. The Order, further, empowered the Committee to 'furnish' the Council with funds, and instructed it to lay a report annually before Parliament. All the other specific powers and duties of both bodies are derived from the Charter of 1 April 1920, incorporating the Council. This instrument is therefore of chief importance, and its provisions must be summarised here although the full text is given later (Appendix E). For the purposes of the present chapter the original form is followed, subsequent changes being left for separate consideration (Chapter 6 and Appendix E).

The preamble states that the instrument of incorporation was "for the purpose of securing the continued performance of the duties heretofore performed by the Medical Research Committee and with a view to facilitating the holding of, and dealing with, any money provided by Parliament for medical research, and any other property, real or personal, otherwise available for that object, and with a view to encouraging the making of gifts and bequests in aid of the said object". This is the nearest approach to terms of reference that the Medical Research Council has.

The ten members of the Medical Research Committee, listed by name, were to "be one Body Corporate under the name of 'The Medical Research Council', having a perpetual succession and a Common Seal". The general powers granted were those usual for a corporate body of the kind: the Council was empowered to sue and be sued; to enter into contracts or agreements (subject to the direction of the Committee of the Privy Council); to accept, hold, and dispose of, money and other personal property; to accept trusts; and "to do all other lawful acts whatsoever that may be conducive to or incidental to the attainment of the objects for which the said Committee of Our Privy Council has been appointed, and the said Medical Research Council is hereby established". The Council was empowered to acquire and hold real property in the United Kingdom "not exceeding in the whole the annual value of £50 000" (amount subsequently increased); and other persons or bodies were authorized to transfer real property to the Council within the stated limits of value.

It was implicit that the number of members of the Council should remain at ten, as there was provision only for replacements. Three members of the Council were to retire on 30 September 1921, and at intervals of two years thereafter; but they were to be eligible for reappointment. Vacancies were to be filled by appointment by the Committee of the Privy Council, but any appointment to fill a casual vacancy was to be only for the remainder of the period of office of the member replaced. Two members were at all times to be members of the House of Lords and of the House of Commons respectively; and the other members were to be appointed after consultation with the President of the Royal Society and with the Medical Research Council—implying that they were to be chosen in respect of their personal scientific qualifications but in fact two of those named as original members were members of the House of Commons and only seven were scientific. Members of the Council who were not members of either House of Parliament might be paid such honoraria as the Committee of the Privy Council directed. The Council was to appoint one of its members to be its Chairman and one to be its Treasurer, subject to the approval of the Committee of the Privy Council.

The Council was to appoint a Secretary; and it was empowered to appoint "other officers and servants", and to expend money for its administrative purposes, provided that the number of such staff, their rates of remuneration, rates of allowances, and the amount of money expended were approved by the Committee of the Privy Council. More generally, in expending moneys provided by Parliament the Council was to act in accordance with directions given from time to time by the Committee of the Privy Council. Property vested in the Council, or the proceeds of sale of such property, was to be held in such manner as the Committee of the Privy Council might approve, subject to the conditions of the Charter and of any relevant trust. The Council's accounts were to be made up for each financial year ending on 31 March and were to be audited in such manner as the Treasury might direct.

The Council was empowered to amend the Charter by Special Resolution, for which the procedure was prescribed, subject to the amendments being allowed by the Committee of the Privy Council.

Articles 2, 3, 6, 7, 11 and 12 (see Appendix E) of the Charter closely followed, *mutatis mutandis*, the corresponding provisions made for the Medical Research Committee in the Regulations governing its constitution. The points of similarity relate to the retirement of members in rotation, the filling of vacancies in membership, the appointment and duties of a Treasurer, the power to appoint officers and servants, the payment of honoraria to scientific members, the payment of allowances and expenses, the keeping of accounts and the manner of audit.

Replacement of Trustees

One formal step was still required to complete the new constitutional arrangements. The property of the Medical Research Committee, which was not a body corporate, had been held by two Trustees (Chapter 3); but the Act of 1919 had provided for its transfer. Accordingly, an Order of the Committee of the Privy Council, dated 5 July 1920, ordered "that the Medical Research Council be the body of persons to and in whom the property formerly held for the purposes of the Medical Research Committee is transferred and vested in pursuance of the said proviso".

The constitution in practice

The whole implication of the formal constitution just described—and of the discussions leading up to it, and the precedent provided by the earlier arrangement—was that the Medical Research Council should be a mainly expert body with the greatest possible freedom, in the exercise of its scientific discretion, to promote research for the improvement of human health. Its activities were not to be restricted by territorial or departmental limitations of function, and its policy was not to be subject to the pressures of day-to-day expediency. It was to be under ministerial direction only of the most general kind, relating mainly to matters of its own administration and of the financial provision which Parliament would be asked to make.

The Council's point of attachment to the machinery of state, and the form of this attachment, were designed to provide these conditions. A Committee of the Privy Council is a convenient formula for representing a wide field of governmental interest. At the same time, such a body tends to meet rarely, if ever: there was in fact only one meeting of the Committee of the Privy Council for Medical Research in all the years of its existence, and there is no formal record of the proceedings on that occasion. The extent to which the other members of the Committee were consulted depended largely on its Chairman; it was commonly restricted to matters requiring formal Orders of the Committee, and to the annual report for presentation to Parliament.

For the rest, ministerial responsibility devolved on the Lord President of the Council as Chairman of the Committee. That he was likewise Chairman of the other Committee of the Privy Council

C—M.R.

exercising similar jurisdiction in a different scientific field (further bodies being added later) had the advantage of bringing analogous activities into the same focus at ministerial level. The interests of research were thus represented in the Cabinet by an important minister, and one who was not involved in the particular policies of any large administrative department. The Lord President was likewise the minister responsible to Parliament, with the minor disadvantage that he was usually in the House of Lords and therefore not personally available to answer questions in the House of Commons. As he had not a junior minister specially allotted to him, this function was apt to fall to some other minister, often a Government Whip; eventually the duty was assigned, as a standing procedure, to the Minister of Health—an arrangement not wholly free from ambiguity as between his departmental function and his membership of the Committee of the Privy Council for Medical Research. (For the change in these arrangements made in 1961, see Chapter 6.)

A significant item in the formula was that the Secretary of the Medical Research Council, appointed as such by the Council itself, was Secretary of the Committee of the Privy Council. This meant that, for the particular purpose, he was the senior permanent official of the responsible minister; he thus formed the link between the two tiers of the organisation, with a constitutional role in each. It meant, further, that any correspondence of the Committee of the Privy Council, unless conducted at ministerial level, would emanate from the address of the Medical Research Council. In consequence, although the minister naturally had the assistance of his personal staff, these officials could not act in the name of the Committee of the Privy Council; nor had they any jurisdiction over the Medical Research Council or its staff. In practice, most of the external relations of the Medical Research Council were conducted in its own name, that of the Committee of the Privy Council being seldom invoked.

Membership of the Council
The appointment of members of the Medical Research Council was a function of the Committee of the Privy Council, and it was effected on each occasion by a formal Order of the Committee. Appointment of members other than those to be drawn from Parliament had to be made after consultation with the President of the Royal Society and with the Medical Research Council itself. In practice the consultations were usually made by the Secretary of the Committee of the Privy Council before submission of names to the minister, and the Council was consulted first. The initiative in proposing names lay with the Council, and this ensured that the choice would be made on scientific grounds and without the embarrassment of nominations resulting from pressure by professional, institutional or departmental interests. The required concurrence of the President of the Royal

Society ensured that the appointments would be agreeable to independent scientific opinion, and the proposals thus doubly supported were always accepted. This principle and practice were of the highest constitutional importance for preserving not only the Council's status as an independent scientific body but also its general acceptability in that role.

The Council's choice of new members has been based on the principle that members serve as individual scientific counsellors and not as representatives of the institutions to which they belong. Among those serving at any time, a certain geographical spread within the United Kingdom is considered to be expedient; it is convenient to have several London members but undesirable that this element should unduly predominate. In particular, the aim has always been to have at least one member from Scotland, and there have sometimes been more. As the Council's constitution has sometimes been taken as a model for use elsewhere, it has to be remarked that the principle on which members are chosen is not readily applicable in a country with a very small number of universities; the demand for institutional representation, and on a basis of equality, may be irresistible.

The considerations already mentioned have to be reconciled with the need for permanently covering the main branches of medical science (Chapter 17). Obviously, not all branches can be represented continuously, but expert advice in disciplines not covered by Council membership is always obtainable from the special committees appointed for the purpose (Chapter 9). In any event, the role of a Council member is not merely, or even primarily, to represent his particular subject but to participate in a broad consideration of the whole field. A body representing all branches would be too large; and if it were to consist entirely of specialists the effect would be to place many decisions virtually in the hands of a single member. Changes in the number of members, and in their selection for retirement, are mentioned later (Chapter 6).

The honorarium paid to a scientific member of the Council was originally £100 per annum, and it remained at this figure for many years (see Chapter 6).

Functions of the Chairman and Treasurer
In spite of a technical ambiguity, there was never any practical difficulty over the appointment of members to the offices of Chairman and Treasurer. Appointment to membership lay with the Committee of the Privy Council, but appointment to office was made by the Council (subject to the approval of the Committee). The custom was, however, to appoint the Chairman and Treasurer from among those members appointed otherwise than in respect of scientific qualifications—that is, without consultation—and the Committee of the Privy Council was thus able to approach possible new members on the basis that appointment to office would follow. In other words,

appointment to office by the Council became purely formal.

The functions of the Chairman of such a body as the Council are in the main obvious. He presides over its meetings, and between these he is available for consultation by the Secretary and may be asked to approve emergency action in the Council's name. He may, of course, also take the initiative in raising questions with the Secretary. He may likewise represent the Council on special occasions.

On the other hand, the Chairman was not ordinarily called upon to act as the Council's spokesman in representing its view to higher authority. This inhibition was due to the constitutional position of the Council as part of a double-tiered organisation and the consequent dual role of the Secretary as mentioned above. In these circumstances the Secretary was naturally the link between the two tiers, putting forward submissions by the Council on matters requiring ministerial approval. It was therefore only on rare occasions (sometimes in questions affecting the Secretary's personal position) that the Chairman made any representations of an official kind on the Council's behalf.

The functions of the Treasurer were much less obvious. The Charter stated that it was his duty "to receive on behalf of the Council all sums payable to the Council for the purposes of medical research". This was clearly impossible in practice; it could not be a realistic duty unless the financial side of the headquarters office were made directly responsible to the Treasurer and not to the Secretary, an arrangement which would have been in the highest degree inconvenient. Moreover, it was naturally to a permanent official that the Treasury looked in any matter concerning the Council's finances; for long, a senior official of the Treasury was 'accounting officer' for the Council's grant-in-aid, since it was being borne on a vote made to the Treasury by the House of Commons (Chapters 6, 15).

Nevertheless, it was useful to the Council to have among its members one with special qualifications and experience in financial affairs. The Treasurer was indeed expected by his colleagues to take a lead in their deliberations when matters of this kind came before them. He was also available for consultation by the Secretary or his appropriate deputy; his advice was valued by the headquarters staff and was commonly sought at an early stage in framing any major proposals of a financial nature. The Treasurer also, as a matter of custom, came to be regarded as having a special function in respect of the Council's capital funds (of non-official origin), although in practice his role might be confined to approving action on recommendations made by the Council's professional advisers on investments.

Secretary and staff

The Council appointed its own Secretary, and the appointment was not subject to ministerial approval (although the responsible minister might nevertheless expect to be kept informed of the

Council's intentions). The principle was important, because the appointment was obviously a key one in the whole organisation and had to be made largely on scientific grounds. The chief qualification was first-hand knowledge of the aims, methods and current content of medical research, coupled with high standing gained by personal achievement in that field. A new Secretary was therefore usually sought outside the existing headquarters staff, and indeed outside all administrative employment. It was taken for granted that he must be a member of the medical profession. Clearly he had also to have aptitude for administrative work, in addition to exceptional personal qualities of a nature less easily defined.

The Council was also empowered to appoint other staff, both for the purpose of its headquarters administration and for such part of the research programme as it might wish to have carried out under its direct control. For the number and remuneration of staff the approval of the Committee of the Privy Council was required—in effect the approval of the Treasury, which was usually consulted by the ministerial Chairman of that Committee. In practice, specific approval had rarely to be sought; the number of staff was for long governed by the funds made available, and except for a very few of the most senior posts the other condition was regarded as satisfied by conformity with scales of pay authorised for general application to particular categories of staff (see Chapter 15).

Financial control

A primary function of the Committee of the Privy Council was to furnish the Medical Research Council with funds for its work (Chapter 15). In practice this meant that the Chairman of the Committee of the Privy Council approved the estimate submitted annually to the Treasury. In the expenditure of its funds, so far as these were provided by Parliament, the Medical Research Council had to act in accordance with any directions given by the Committee of the Privy Council; and the same applied to the manner of holding property. In effect this meant that the Council was subject to Treasury control, but in practice the requirements of that department were met by a broad conformity with the principles governing the expenditure of public funds. The Council's accounts have, by direction of the Treasury as provided by the Charter, been audited by HM Exchequer and Audit Department.

Article 8 of the Charter implied that the Medical Research Council was not subject to direction by the Committee of the Privy Council in respect of expenditure of moneys provided otherwise than by Parliament. Although this gave the Council some independence in the use of funds of non-official origin, it did not follow that the Treasury could disinterest itself completely—having regard to the total position of the Council as a body financed mainly from public funds. In any event the Council remained subject to the obligations of trusteeship, whether or not the particular funds were received under express conditions of trust. It would therefore not be permissible to use such funds for any purpose which the Treasury would regard as improper (as distinct from abnormal in the practice of Government departments), or for any purpose outside the scope of the Council's appropriate functions.

Chapter 6
Later Constitutional Developments
(1920-1971)

Changes in membership of the Committee of the Privy Council—The Minister for Science—Amendments to the Royal Charter—Assessors to the Council—The National Health Service Acts—Statutory responsibilities—The Council's jubilee—Implications of the Trend Report—Dissolution of the Committee of the Privy Council—The new Charter—Criticisms and new proposals

Changes in membership of the Committee of the Privy Council
As recounted in Chapter 5, the Committee of Privy Council for Medical Research originally consisted of the Lord President of the Council, as chairman, and the three 'health ministers'—the Minister of Health, the Secretary for Scotland and the Chief Secretary for Ireland. The last named office ceased to exist in 1922.

By an Order in Council of 26 July 1926 (Appendix D), the Committee was reconstituted with the addition of three further ministers, the respective Secretaries of State for the Home Department (incorrectly styled in the Order), for Dominion Affairs, and for the Colonies. (Almost immediately afterwards the Secretary for Scotland became a Secretary of State; in 1947 Dominion Affairs became Commonwealth Relations.) The Home Secretary was added, partly on general grounds, partly because he had responsibility for relations with the Government of Northern Ireland, and partly because the Home Office at that time included the Factory Department and had thus a special interest in industrial health. The other two appointments recognised, respectively, that the Council had scientific relations with analogous bodies and other institutions in the self-governing dominions and had concern in promoting research into problems of tropical medicine which were of importance in colonial territories. The Council's Report for 1919–20 refers to the value of a constitutional link with the Dominions, but in practice relations have been maintained at a scientific rather than a political level.

The Committee was again reconstituted by an Order in Council of 28 October 1955 (Appendix D), this time with the addition of the Minister of Labour and National Service (styled Minister of Labour from 1959). The chief reason for this new appointment was that the Factory Department, and with it the interest in industrial health, had meanwhile been transferred from the Home Office to the Ministry of Labour.

Changes affecting the chairmanship of the Committee were made in 1959 and 1964, as related below; and the eventual dissolution of the Committee, in 1966, is mentioned later.

The Minister for Science

In 1918, as already recounted, the Machinery of Government Committee had extolled the virtues of constitutional arrangements whereby Government research organisations came under the direction of special Committees of the Privy Council (Chapter 4). At the same time it expressed misgivings lest multiplication of such organisations should place too heavy a burden on the Lord President of the Council, as chairman of the several committees concerned, in view of the parliamentary duties which he was commonly called upon to undertake. It accordingly concluded its remarks on this subject with a passage, quoted in the earlier chapter, which envisaged the possible formation of, in effect, a Ministry of Science.

A Ministry of Science was more positively mooted at various later dates, but the idea found little favour. The objection was not to the appointment of a special Minister, but to the implied creation of an official hierarchy under him which might seek to have close administrative control over the expert bodies in their conduct of scientific affairs. The compromise formula was apparently not then considered, namely that of retaining the Committees of the Privy Council but transferring their chairmanship from the Lord President to a Minister appointed specially for the purpose but not provided with a large administrative department. That, however, was the solution adopted when, by an Order in Council of 30 October 1959, the Government appointed a Minister *for* Science. He was provided with a personal staff, but his relation to the research organisations remained that of chairman of their respective Committees of the Privy Council.

The first Minister for Science was simultaneously Lord Privy Seal, and a year afterwards Lord President. Although this double role involved heavy parliamentary duties, the responsibility for scientific affairs was emphasised by the additional title and there was a special staff to assist in its discharge; and it remained open to the Prime Minister to separate the appointments at any time if it seemed expedient. In 1961 a Parliamentary Secretary was appointed to assist the Minister for Science; this provided the Minister—usually a peer—with a deputy to answer for him in the House of Commons, obviating the earlier need for makeshift or ambiguous arrangements (Chapter 5).

Amendments to the Royal Charter

The constitution of the Council stood the test of time, and experience demonstrated the far-seeing wisdom of those who proposed its main principles. For forty-five years it was only in matters of secondary importance that the provisions of the Charter required amendment. For this purpose the powers of amendment given by Article 9 of the Charter were invoked on three occasions, amendments having been made by the Council in accordance with the specified procedure and given effect on being allowed by the Committee of the Privy Council.

On one other occasion an amendment, proposed by the Council in like manner, was made by the grant of a Supplemental Charter (on account of the nature of the change rather than of its importance).

The amendments are shown in Appendix E. In brief, amendments allowed on 1 March 1926 increased the number of members of the Council from ten to eleven, making it explicit that eight of them were to be scientific; modified the provisions relating to the retirement of members and their eligibility for reappointment; and made a purely formal change in another respect. Amendments allowed on 1 November 1943 increased the number of members to twelve (including nine scientific) and further modified the provisions relating to retirement and reappointment.

By an amendment allowed on 15 May 1957 a member of the House of Lords ceased to be disqualified from receiving an honorarium as a member of the Council; shortly before this the honorarium, hitherto paid only to scientific members, had been increased from its original £100 per annum to £500, and to £750 in the case of the Chairman, and it was thenceforth paid to every member who was not a Member of the House of Commons.

On 27 July 1949 a Supplemental Charter (Appendix E) was granted, a draft having been approved by an Order in Council of 30 June 1949 (Appendix D). This increased to £100 000 the limit of £50 000 placed by the Original Charter on the annual value of real property that could be held by the Council, a small formal change in wording being made at the same time. The growth of the Council's holdings, at that time including property held for the Public Health Laboratory Service, involved a risk that the original figure might become inadequate.

Assessors to the Council

The constitution made no provision for the appointment of assessors to the Council, but it is clearly inherent in the powers of such a body to invite other persons to attend its meetings, either on occasion or regularly; members of the Council's staff, in addition to the Secretary, in fact attend on this basis. It is understood that persons so attending do not have votes and cannot propose or second formal resolutions—but resolutions and voting play little part in the Council's ordinary proceedings.

In 1935 the respective Secretaries of the Department of Scientific and Industrial Research and of the Agricultural Research Council were appointed as assessors *ex officiis*; this was a reciprocal arrangement. These assessors, however, were not expected to attend meetings of the Council unless by arrangement on some special occasion. On the other hand, they received copies of the papers (other than particularly confidential or purely domestic ones) for meetings of the Council and were expressly at liberty to discuss with the Secretary beforehand any point which might seem to affect their interests.

In 1949 the Council agreed to invite the respective Chief Medical Officers of the Ministry of Health and of the Department of Health for Scotland to become assessors *ex officiis*, and this invitation was officially accepted. These appointments were on a different footing

C*—M.R.

and the two Chief Medical Officers have attended meetings of the Council with regularity and have taken an appropriate and useful part in discussions. This form of liaison with the two health departments, in addition to frequent consultations on particular matters, has proved to be invaluable.

In 1953 it was decided that the Chairman of the Council's Clinical Research Board should also be an assessor if he did not happen to be a member of the Council. He, likewise, has attended regularly and taken a full part in discussions. It was clearly important for the Council to maintain the closest possible touch with this important advisory body, to which a good deal of detailed decision was in effect delegated.

In 1960 the Chairman of the University Grants Committee—the body advising the Treasury on block grants to the universities—was appointed to be an assessor, on the same footing as the Chief Medical Officers. This marked a stage at which direct provision for research projects was increasingly made to the universities, a demarcation of function between them and the central research organisations thus being involved. In 1961 the Royal Society accepted an invitation to nominate an assessor who would attend meetings; and the Biological Secretary of the Society at that time was the first nominee.

The National Health Service Acts
The National Health Service Act 1946 (Appendix B) involved no change in the Council's constitution but had important practical effects on its work in the clinical field. This measure related to England and Wales and *inter alia* empowered the Minister of Health to conduct research or to assist others to conduct research—Section 16(1), and likewise empowered hospital boards and management committees to conduct research—Section 16(2). The earlier of these sub-sections includes the reservation that the power was given "without prejudice to . . . the duties imposed on the Committee of the Privy Council for Medical Research" under the Act of 1919. Incidentally, the reference to the Committee in Section 16(1) apparently represents the first use of its full title in a statutory instrument.

The reservation was included in the Bill only after considerable official argument while the measure was in draft. The principle was not in dispute, but lawyers took the view that there was nothing in the Bill which could in any way detract from the functions of the Committee of the Privy Council (and thus of the Medical Research Council), and that there was therefore no need for explicit protection of these functions. The contrary view was based on mainly psychological grounds, it being feared that the impression on the public mind would be that the Ministry was in future to be the Government agency for medical research, to the exclusion of others. As it was, the Act did indeed create an impression that the Ministry was assuming some new function of a major kind in respect of research, although in fact it already possessed general powers in the matter. (Section 2 of the Ministry of Health Act 1919 included measures for "the initiation and direction of research" among the general powers and duties of the Minister; the words quoted were not in the original draft of the Bill, but were inserted by an amendment, moved by Addison, which the Government accepted. The same words were used in Section 2 of the Scottish Board of Health Act 1919.) In the event, the proposed reservation was included in the Bill and was accepted by Parliament. The point having been made, it was considered unnecessary to ask for any similar reservation in the National Health Service (Scotland) Act 1947 (Appendix B), which gave corresponding power to the Secretary of State, and also to hospital boards.

(Statutory powers to promote research in the medical field have been given to other ministers and authorities. Section 41 (1) (p) of the Mental Deficiency Act 1913, empowered the Secretary of State for the Home Department (later succeeded in this function by the Minister of Health) to make regulations as to "the study of improved methods of treating mental deficiency"—which might be construed as involving research. Likewise, under Section 72 of the Mental Deficiency and Lunacy (Scotland) Act 1913, district boards were empowered "to contribute annually towards any pathological laboratory having for its object or one of its objects investigation into the pathology of mental diseases", but the context suggests that little more than payment for assistance in the routine investigation of cases was envisaged; the provision was repealed in 1947. Again, and more definitely, the Minister of National Insurance (later Minister of Pensions and National Insurance, now Secretary of State for Social Services) was empowered by the National Insurance (Industrial Injuries) Act 1946 (Appendix B) to promote research into the causes, incidence and prevention of injuries and diseases against which persons are insured under the measure.)

In another field, Section 17 of the National Health Service Act 1946 empowered the Minister of Health to "provide a bacteriological service . . . for the control of the spread of infectious disease". This was in fact the Public Health Laboratory Service, which the Medical Research Council was already managing as agent in this respect for the Minister of Health in circumstances described in Volume Two.

Statutory responsibilities
Other legislative references to the Council have placed certain specific statutory responsibilities upon it. Most of them relate to the public control of therapeutic substances, a subject discussed in Volume Two. In this context, such substances are medicinal preparations "the purity or potency of which cannot be adequately tested by chemical means"; they can be assayed only by reference to biological standards, and by biological methods, and are thus outside the powers of the Food and Drugs Acts and the techniques of the public analysts.

The Council, and indeed its predecessor Committee from almost the earliest days, had been specially concerned with promoting the study of biological standardisation and the methods of biological assay, and as a result it had become responsible for applying the new techniques of testing in the public interest. Certain patent rights at first provided the only authority for imposing such tests; but, with the growing need for the latter, statutory powers became very necessary. The Council took a leading part in pressing for legislation. The result was the Therapeutic Substances Act 1925 (Appendix B). Mention of the Council was limited to the responsibility, placed upon it by Section 4(2), for appointing one member of an advisory committee to assist the joint committee of "health ministers" for the different parts of the United Kingdom. It was well understood, however, that administrative action would necessarily rest on scientific services such as only the Council could readily provide, as recognised in various references to the Council, and particularly to the National Institute for Medical Research, in the long series of highly technical regulations made under the Act and its successors.

The Penicillin Act 1947 (Appendix B) was passed to control the sale and supply of penicillin and other antibiotics—a particular class of therapeutic substances—so that excessive use of them for trivial purposes would not diminish their value for more important purposes by creating resistant strains of microorganisms. The Act applied only to penicillin in the first instance, but under Section 2(1) it empowered the health ministers to include other antibiotics by regulations made after consultation with the Council. The Therapeutic Substances (Prevention of Misuse) Act 1953 (Appendix B) amended the Penicillin Act in certain respects and extended its applicability to all substances "capable of causing danger to the health of the community if used without proper safeguards"; and again, under Sections 1(1) and (2), the Council was to be consulted before any such substances were brought within the scope of the Act or regulations were made relaxing any of the prohibitions, the Agricultural Research Council being also consulted when appropriate. (For the consolidating Act of 1956 see Appendix B.)

Two minor responsibilities have been laid on the Council by statute. Sections 6(1)a and 17(2) of the London Gas Undertakings (Regulations) Act 1939 required the Board of Trade to consult a committee consisting of representatives of various bodies before approving draft regulations made by the gas companies serving London; and the Council was named as one of the bodies to be represented (Appendix B).

Secondly, the Income Tax Act 1952 allowed tax relief to traders in respect of certain payments in aid of relevant research, provided that the receiving association or institution was approved for the purpose by "the appropriate Research Council or Committee", the Medical Research Council being named as one (Appendix B). The Science and Technology Act 1965 substituted the Secretary of State for Education and Science as the source of approval, but in practice he would presumably seek expert advice from the appropriate Council.

The Public Health Laboratory Service Act 1960 transferred the administration of that Service from the Council (acting for the Ministry of Health) to a new statutory Board, two members of which are nominated by the Council. The Radiological Protection Act 1970 transferred from the Council to a new statutory Board the responsibility for administering the Radiological Protection Service; it left the Council with the right to be consulted about the membership of the Board and the definition of its functions. Both these Services are described in Volume Two.

The Council's jubilee

The Council's jubilee, dating from the establishment of the Medical Research Committee in 1913, was celebrated on 25 November 1963, when the Council gave a dinner at the Goldsmiths' Hall in the City of London. The occasion was overshadowed by a tragedy of international impact, the assassination of President Kennedy, and the function was accordingly treated as a private one; for the same reason, HRH the Duke of Edinburgh was prevented from attending. The Chairman of the Council, Lord Shawcross, presided. In the absence of Prince Philip, the Minister for Science, the Rt Hon. Quintin Hogg, was the principal guest and proposed the toast of the Council. The reply was made by Sir Henry Dale, who had been a member of the scientific staff from the earliest days until his retirement, and later a member of Council. A company of about two hundred included members of the Government, presidents of learned bodies, and representatives of public departments and agencies, together with present and past members of Council, senior members of the scientific and administrative staff, and others closely associated with the work. The presence of Lady Fletcher and Lady Mellanby at the high table was particularly appropriate. In its issue of 23 November 1963, the *British Medical Journal* gave prominence to the jubilee with an editorial article, some pages of photographs, and contributions by Sir Henry Dale, Sir Landsborough Thomson and Sir George Pickering; the subject also received attention in other journals.

Implications of the Trend Report

From the earlier sections of this chapter it will be evident that there were no major constitutional changes during the latter forty-three years of the half-century from the inception of the original Medical Research Committee. At the time of the jubilee, however, far-reaching proposals were being made by the Committee of Enquiry into the Organisation of Civil Science, under the chairmanship of Sir Burke Trend; its report was published in October 1963. The wider implications of the Committee's recommendations are mentioned later (Chapter 8), and here it is necessary to deal only with the proposals directly affecting the constitution of the Council.

First, the Committee of the Privy Council was to be abolished, and all its powers vested solely in the Minister for Science (later Secretary of State for Education and Science). This in itself was largely a formal change, doing little more than to bring theory into line with practice. It was linked, however, with the proposal that the Minister should have a full-scale Department and not just a relatively small 'Office'; and this carried the implication that the Council would in future be dealing with the Department in financial matters, and not directly with the Treasury as heretofore. This could be helpful or otherwise, according to the spirit in which the Council's affairs were handled at the higher official level. It was in any event a change that may have become inevitable, with the increase in the complexity of the whole civil research mechanism and with the growth in the expenditure of the individual agencies. The earlier separation of the functions of the Minister for Science from those of the Lord President of the Council had pointed the way; and the eventual impossibility that these could be discharged by one individual had been foreseen by the Haldane Committee in 1918 (Chapter 4).

Second, it was proposed that the Council should have a whole-time professional Chairman, the title of Secretary reverting to an administrative second-in-command. This would have involved the disappearance of an honorary Chairman not normally possessing scientific qualifications. It also meant that the officer who, as Secretary, had been the servant of the Council would become a member of that body, and its leader. This formula recognised the reality that the whole-time and specially qualified officer must in effect always give the lead; and, further, that the position of the honorary Chairman had been somewhat equivocal, in that the Secretary dealt directly with the Minister, whose servant he was as well as that of the Council. In the event, as will be noted presently, this proposal was not accepted without some modification at the request of the Council.

It was evident that the proposals could not be implemented without legislation and changes in the Council's Charter. The substitution of the Minister for the Committee of the Privy Council was simple enough, but it nevertheless involved amendment of the Ministry of Health Act 1919. The method of appointing a Chairman and of determining his period of office involved amendment of the Charter.

Dissolution of the Committee of the Privy Council

It has already been seen that in 1959 a Minister for Science replaced the Lord President as Chairman of the Committee of Privy Council for Medical Research (and of the corresponding bodies in other fields). If this was a straw in the wind, the force of that wind became apparent when the functions of the Minister for Science, and those of the Minister for Education (England and Wales), were taken over by a Secretary of State for Education and Science on 1 April 1964; this was effected by an Order in Council of 26 March 1964 (Appendix D).

The more drastic step that followed was taken by the Science and Technology Act 1965 (Appendix B). The powers of the Committee of the Privy Council (and sister bodies) were thereby transferred to the Secretary of State. The change took effect on 23 March 1965, when the measure became law. The several Committees of the Privy Council, bereft of powers, were formally abolished by an Order in Council of 14 April 1965 (Appendix D).

The new Charter

The terms of a new Charter were closely discussed between the Department of Education and Science and the Council before being finally determined; and the resulting instrument differs in various respects from those granted to the other agencies. The Council was especially anxious to avoid being compelled to adopt the Trend formula of a whole-time scientific Chairman—the former Secretary writ large. It wished to retain an honorary Chairman; but it was agreeable to the Secretary's becoming a member of Council, with the style of 'Deputy Chairman and Secretary'. This was agreed, but in a form of words that would permit variation of practice in future.

The draft of the new Charter was approved by an Order in Council of 20 September 1966 (Appendix D); and the Charter itself was made patent on 26 October 1966 (Appendix E). The instrument, although retaining some old-fashioned legal phraseology, is a much more modern document than its predecessor. Notably, it is simpler in form and content, and more flexible in certain of its provisions.

Consequent on the Science and Technology Act 1965, references to a Committee of the Privy Council are replaced by references to the Secretary of State for Education and Science, although not always in the same respects. By reason of the repeal of the ancient 'law of mortmain' in 1960, a restriction is no longer placed on the value of land that the Council may hold. It is in respect of the membership of the Council, however, that the more material changes are made and that the new flexibility is chiefly evident.

The number of members, all appointed by the Secretary of State, may vary from twelve to sixteen. Of the total, not less than three-quarters must be appointed in respect of their qualifications in science; and, as before, these appointments are to be made after consultation with the Council and with the President of the Royal Society, and those so appointed may not hold office for more than four years or be reappointed before the expiration of one year from the end of that period. The office of Treasurer is dropped, but one of Deputy Chairman is created. The Chairman and the Deputy Chairman are to be appointed after consultation with the Council; for them and the remaining members there is no restriction on the terms for which they may be appointed, or on their eligibility for reappointment at the end of these terms.

It is thus left open whether the Chairman and Deputy Chairman, either or both, are to be appointed because of scientific qualifications or otherwise, and whether they are to be appointed on an honorary or a salaried basis. And there is nothing to prevent either office from being held together with that of Secretary. This makes possible a variety of permutations (Chapter 17).

The immediate steps taken by the Secretary of State after the grant of the Charter were the appointment of an additional scientific member of Council, and the appointment of the then Secretary (while retaining that post) as a member and Deputy Chairman from 16 November 1966. The Chairman and the other members retained their places, for the remainder of their original terms, under a provision of Clause 1 of the new Charter that validated all acts done under the provisions of the original Charter.

In 1971 certain technical amendments were made to the new Charter to give the Council wider powers of investment of its private funds and to enable a staff injury compensation scheme to be introduced.

Criticisms and new proposals

Although 'the Haldane principle' continued to be highly regarded by the Council—see an address and book by its late Deputy Chairman and Secretary, Sir Harold Himsworth (1969, 1970)—it has had its detractors. Thus Sir Solly (later Lord) Zuckerman (1970):

> Lord Haldane and his colleagues would seem to have laboured in the belief that in normal circumstances the results of scientific enquiry were not applied for useful purposes. . . . [The effect of their proposals] was to create a series of autonomous research councils which pursued their work in quasi-isolation, and whose activities in the medical, agricultural and industrial fields did little to influence the policies of those government departments which were concerned executively with related technological matters. In consequence, and contrary to what the Haldane Committee had intended, a vertical division developed between research council and university science on the one hand, and the executive activities of government departments on the other. This separation inevitably became associated in the United Kingdom with a widespread belief that the kind of work which was carried out in the universities and under the banner of the research councils was intellectually more exacting and worthy than the kind of scientific and technological work required and pursued by government departments and in industry. Science, not application, was what counted.

Sir George Pickering (1970), in a review of Himsworth's book, comments on the foregoing with special reference to the Medical Research Council:

> Personally I doubt whether Zuckerman's criticism of the government of Research Councils is just. There was certainly a good relationship with the Department of Health and the Medical Research Council when I served on it. The

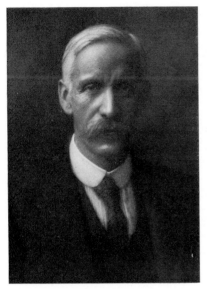

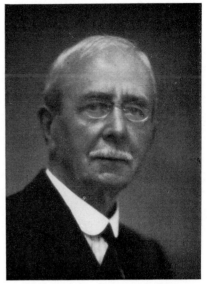

Sir Frederick Hopkins, OM, FRS

Sir Charles Sherrington, OM, GBE, FRS

Lord Adrian, OM, FRS

Lord Florey, OM, FRS

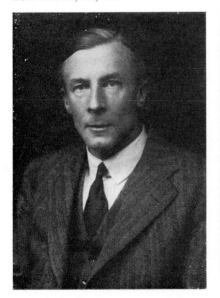

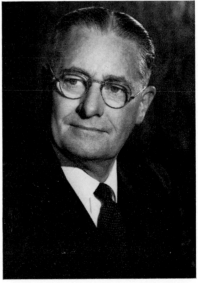

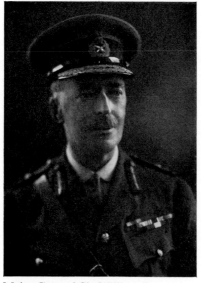

Major General Sir William B.
Leishman, KCMB, CB, FRS

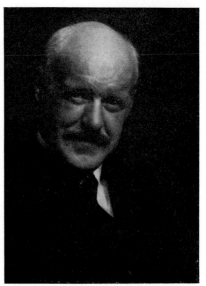

Professor T. R. Elliott, CBE, DSO, FRS

Sir Charles Martin, CMG, FRS

Professor W. W. C. Topley, FRS

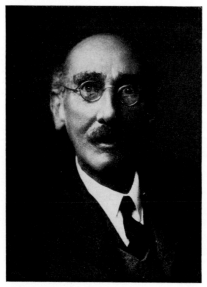

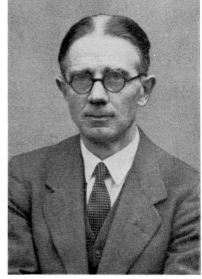

Chief Medical Officers for England and Wales and for Scotland sat with it. Requests for expert help were, so far as I know, never refused. And I believe there is nothing to prevent these relationships becoming closer given good will and understanding on both sides.

After this history had been completed for press there appeared an official document, presented to Parliament by the Lord Privy Seal (1971), putting forward new proposals greatly affecting the research councils in general, including the Medical Research Council. These were contained in reports by Lord Rothschild and by a committee under the chairmanship of Sir Frederick Dainton; they are briefly summarised in a postscript hereafter (Chapter 8). Whatever the outcome for the Council, it clearly does not fall within the purview of this history but will become manifest in an era which should in due time have its own chronicle.

Chapter 7
Official Relations

The Research Councils—Department of Scientific and Industrial Research
(and successors)—Development Commission and Agricultural Research
Council—Other bodies—Health Departments—Other administrative
departments—Defence Services—Research overseas—International
organisations—General advisory functions

The Research Councils
The constitutional history of the Council would not be complete
without some account of the relationships that have developed
between it and other governmental agencies. The subject can be
divided logically into two: relations with sister organisations
operating in contiguous scientific fields—'research councils' in time
became a collective term—and relations with administrative departments that are, so to speak, users of medical knowledge in the sphere
of government, notably the 'Health Departments' (another convenient collective term) in the different parts of the United
Kingdom.

As regards the former group, a philosophy developed that there
were three main fields of civil research with utilitarian objects
important to the state—medicine, industry, and agriculture. This
was not quite a complete picture, as it did not cover research work
in such subjects as forestry, fisheries, meteorology, astronomy, and
oceanography; for these, various independent arrangements existed
—and not improperly, on the principle advocated by the Committee
on the Machinery of Government with regard to research in subjects
falling within the scope of single administrative departments
(Chapter 4). Research on the uses of atomic energy was as yet
unborn, while nature conservation and the social sciences had not so
far been taken seriously as responsibilities of the state. Research
overseas fell into the same categories as at home, but did not greatly
concern the research councils at the outset.

Department of Scientific and Industrial Research (and successors)
The establishment and constitution of this Department, with its
Advisory Council, have already been noted (Chapter 4). It had come
into being in 1916, three years after the original Medical Research
Committee, and in 1920 it was joined by the reconstituted Medical
Research Council as a sister organisation responsible to the same
Minister. It had meanwhile developed a tendency to describe itself
as *the* 'Research Department' (without qualification), and at first

66

showed a certain reluctance to accept a partner—admittedly smaller—on equal terms; as already mentioned, there had even been veiled suggestions that the two bodies should be integrated in some way that would have placed the agency for medical research in an administratively subordinate position (Chapter 4). These early attitudes, however, were mainly personal rather than official, and they did not prevent the rapid establishment of good working arrangements.

The need for cooperation was twofold. The negative aspect, so to speak, was the avoidance of undesirable overlapping in borderline fields. Although the ultimate utilitarian aims of the two bodies were quite distinct, both were concerned to foster research in the basic sciences subserving these; and here the demarcation between physical and biological subjects did not fit. Not only were there some applications of biology to industry, but in respect of individual research and training awards the Department did not exclude work in 'pure' biology from its purview. Likewise, new knowledge in some branches of physics and chemistry was highly important for progress in medical research; the principal overlap of interest was, in fact, in biochemistry. Consultation between the two organisations, whenever one initiated or received a proposal that might impinge on the activities of the other, soon became a matter of routine. When it was thought appropriate, a proposal could be transferred from one to the other; and an application submitted to both simultaneously could be allocated to one by agreement.

The more positive aspect involved collaboration rather than coordination—in other words, joint action in matters of common interest. An early example of this was a scheme of research in chemotherapy, in which the Department promoted work by chemists on the synthesis of new compounds of possible therapeutic value; and the Council organised the biological testing of these, and clinical trials if the laboratory results justified proceeding to that further stage. One could cite other instances in which the respective resources of the two bodies were similarly pooled. An account of the Department's functions has been given by a former head, Sir Harry Melville (1962).

The Department of Scientific and Industrial Research Act 1956 put the Department under the charge of a Council for Scientific and Industrial Research. The latter was thus placed on the same footing as the other research councils, instead of being an advisory body, and was given control of its executive. By the Science and Technology Act 1965, that Council and its Department were dissolved and were replaced in large part by a Science Research Council incorporated by Royal Charter (Chapter 8). These constitutional changes did not affect the relationship with medical research.

Development Commission and Agricultural Research Council
In 1920 there was as yet no research council for agriculture. State

aid to agricultural research was mainly given in the form of block grants to a series of largely autonomous institutes engaged in research in different branches. These subsidies were administered by the Ministry of Agriculture and Fisheries (as it then was) and the corresponding departments (then separate) under the Scottish Office. In addition, there was the Development Commission, a body established under the Development and Road Improvement Funds Act 1909 (amended by various later measures). Its function was to advise the Treasury on making grants or loans for the development of rural and coastal areas; and, *inter alia*, such grants could be for agricultural research. For the time being, accordingly, the Development Commission was brought into partnership as a research council, although its responsibility for acting as such was of a restricted kind; furthermore, it was not adequately equipped to function as a scientific organisation comparable with the Department of Scientific and Industrial Research or the Medical Research Council.

This was an unsatisfactory state of affairs; and for an organisation concerned with research in human medicine the lack of a full partner dealing with veterinary medicine was a serious handicap. The two subjects have a common scientific background and many similar problems, so that each is often helpful to the other. In default, the Council found it necessary, in these early years, itself to undertake various research projects that strictly belonged to the agricultural field, particularly with regard to bovine tuberculosis.

The establishment of an Agricultural Research Council in 1931 was therefore a most welcome step. Constitutionally, this body was closely modelled on the Medical Research Council, and its instrument of foundation was likewise a Royal Charter; there was here, however, no legislative background, and this was not provided until the passage of the Agricultural Research Act 1956. At first the new Council was under the disadvantage that the existing research institutes throughout the country remained under the control, respectively, of the Ministry of Agriculture and Fisheries and of the Department of Agriculture and Fisheries for Scotland. The new Council was accordingly restricted, in respect of this major part of the research potential, to the role of advising the administrative departments. Gradually, however, this advice became increasingly effective in practice; but it was not until 1956, and then only in England and Wales, that the Council acquired jurisdiction in its own right.

Nevertheless, the new Council was able to take its place at once alongside the two existing organisations; and although it remained for a time closely associated with the Development Commission in its headquarters administration, that body dropped out of the group. Between the Medical Research Council and the Agricultural Research Council there was—as with the Department of Scientific and Industrial Research—an overlapping concern with the basic sciences. There was also an important area of common interest in the respective spheres of human and veterinary medicine. The literally 'agricultural' side of the new Council's programme was further apart; but in 1959 the promotion of research on food was added to its responsibilities (in parallel with the addition of food to the responsibilities of the administrative department, which then became the Ministry of Agriculture, Fisheries and Food), and another link with questions of human health was thus provided.

Among other matters, the Agricultural Research Council took the place of the Development Commission in an arrangement that had existed since 1922. By Cabinet instruction, meetings of the principal officers of the three research bodies were held at quarterly intervals for the discussion of questions of borderline or common interest. This was at first somewhat grandiloquently called the 'Interdepartmental Conference on the Coordination of Scientific Research'. Each body in turn provided the meeting room, and a junior officer to act as secretary; formal minutes were kept. The Biological Secretary of the Royal Society attended by invitation. The procedure served a useful purpose in bringing the organisations more closely together. On the other hand, many questions concerned two of the bodies but not all three, and others were too urgent to be left until the next fixed date; more and more, accordingly, coordination came to be a matter of day to day contact, at all levels, between headquarters staffs. A relaxation of the original instruction was accordingly approved by the Lord President in 1932; and the conference eventually dwindled to meetings of the three Secretaries on a very informal basis, held at rather irregular intervals. Latterly, however, meetings of the 'executive heads' of five research councils have been held regularly, with definite agenda and minutes.

Other bodies

In 1949 the trinity was augmented by a junior member in the shape of the Nature Conservancy, established by Royal Charter and with powers under the National Parks and Access to the Countryside Act 1949. This body operated on a relatively small scale as a research council, in the field of natural history bearing on conservation; but it had also administrative functions, including the acquisition and management of nature reserves. Its constitution was that of a research council, with a permanent secretary, although the titles used were the 'Nature Conservancy' and 'Director-General'; a 'Deputy Director-General (Scientific)' was subsequently appointed. Originally it came under the general direction of the same Committee of the Privy Council as did the Agricultural Research Council, but later a separate ministerial Committee of like status was set up—the Committee of Privy Council for Nature Conservation. In so far as the activities of the Nature Conservancy were germane to those of the three senior Councils, it was brought into the ambit of consultation already described.

In 1959 a fifth wheel was added to the coach by the establishment of an Overseas Research Council, directed by a Committee of Privy Council for Overseas Research. This Council was quite different from the others in that it was a purely advisory body, without executive functions and with only a small secretariat provided from the Office of the Minister for Science, who had meanwhile become chairman of all the Committees of Privy Council mentioned above (Chapter 6). It was charged with a general oversight of policy relating to scientific research promoted overseas, or at home for overseas purposes, by Her Majesty's Government in the United Kingdom. The execution of projects, according to their respective fields, lay with the several research councils already operating, or with the government departments concerned—latterly including the Department of Technical Cooperation (later the Ministry of Overseas Development and now the Overseas Development Administration of the Foreign and Commonwealth Office), and by this the functions of that Council were absorbed in 1964.

The Science and Technology Act 1965 brought into being a Natural Environment Research Council and a Social Science Research Council; the Nature Conservancy, already mentioned, became a subordinate body of the former.

Although the United Kingdom Atomic Energy Authority (created by an Act of 1954) is not constitutionally a research council, or concerned solely with research, it was for a time analogous to the extent of being a statutory body under the supervisory jurisdiction of the Minister for Science. From 1965 it came within the sphere of the Ministry of Technology (now absorbed in the Department of Trade and Industry). The Council's relations with it—mainly with the Research Group of its organisation—have been in respect of the supply of radioactive substances for medical purposes, and of the health hazards of radiation.

Mention may also be made here of an anomalous body that for a few years acted partly as an agency for the promotion of research, but without relation to the Privy Council. This was the Empire Marketing Board, set up in 1926 in accordance with a recommendation in the first Report of the Imperial Economic Committee. Its function was to assist the Secretary of State for Dominion Affairs in the administration of a fund voted by Parliament for furthering the marketing of Empire products in the United Kingdom, particularly raw materials and foodstuffs. The methods open to it for this purpose included the promotion of research, its only function relevant here. With such wide terms of reference, there was considerable risk that the Board might cut across the functions of existing research agencies and thus create a chaotic administrative situation. This was happily averted by agreement to work through these agencies, to which it gave grants for particular projects; these included projects for work under the Council on such subjects as the vitamin content of fruits and the hygiene of dairy produce. Its relatively large funds thus helped piecemeal to augment the resources of the then needy research councils—one scientist aptly described it as "the jug and bottle department of the Treasury". The reasons for setting up the Board had been purely political, and in 1933, when these reasons had ceased to have effect, the organisation was abolished.

Health Departments

The short life of the original Medical Research Committee was so largely dominated by the claims of the First World War that the development of relations, in the civil field, with the Local Government Board (and the equivalent Board in Scotland) was of relatively minor importance. After the war, in 1920, the reconstituted Council and the new Ministry of Health (again with Scottish counterpart) came almost simultaneously into being.

Cooperation between the Council and the Ministry was not in the early years so close as it might have been, although this perhaps mattered less in that the Ministry was at that time mainly concerned with the preventive aspect of medicine and was still heavily occupied with responsibilities—eventually shed—for such matters as housing, national insurance, and local government. The reasons why the two organisations had been kept administratively separate have already been discussed (Chapter 4); they were good reasons, but the controversy about them had left an aura of suspicion. There was the natural wariness of the small animal that had just excaped to freedom, and the corresponding frustration of the large animal that had been baulked in its spring. It was not until later that officers of the Ministry of Health came fully to realise how much more valuable to the Ministry, as well as in general, was an independent Council than some body compromised by subordination. And, in time, harmonious working was facilitated by the growth of personal goodwill, indeed often friendship, between the senior officers of the Council and of the Ministry's medical staff. The Ministry has latterly been merged in a Department of Health and Social Security.

No such difficulties hampered good relations between the Council and the Scottish Board of Health, later the Department of Health for Scotland and more recently the Scottish Home and Health Department. On the other hand, that Department naturally operated on a much smaller scale; and in matters affecting the United Kingdom as a whole it had less opportunity for taking the initiative.

As already noted, the Ministry of Health had legal power to promote research (Chapter 6); but it was allowed only a very small amount of money for this purpose, in continuation of an earlier provision to the Local Government Board (Chapter 1). It would, indeed, have been contrary to Treasury principles to make provision through more than one channel for a single purpose. The problem of delimiting the respective functions, in the field of research, was thus not a very serious one. It was resolved in 1924, at the suggestion of the Treasury, by a 'concordat' between Sir Walter Fletcher and Sir George Newman. This read as follows:

Ministry of Health	*Medical Research Council*
(1) To survey existing knowledge with a view to its applications or applicability to practical uses	(1) To survey existing knowledge with a view to right direction of new research efforts
(2) To survey by statistical or other means existing states of national (and international) health and environment, both absolutely and in relation to past history	(2) Medical research by statistical methods (primarily for the development of new methods)
(3) To provide investigation (by use of existing knowledge and recognised methods) of scientific problems arising in the current administrative work of the Ministry	(3) To give assistance to current medical research investigations, whether pathological, biochemical, or other kinds (including studies made into the better standardisation of materials or methods)
(4) To initiate research by reference to the Medical Research Council or by encouraging local authorities or other agencies to direct and carry it out, and to initiate and themselves to direct research by such investigations as can best be carried out by the Ministry, in the interests of public health administration, applied knowledge or medical services	(4) To promote new knowledge by the initiation and organisation of research in the medical sciences
(5) To propagate the results gained under all the foregoing heads by publication, by suitable information to local authorities or to the general public, and in general to promote the applications of the results in practical life, whether in the Ministry or outside it	(5) The publication of the results of research work in such a form as to aid research workers in general and to secure available application

The 'concordat', subsequently accepted also by the Department of Health for Scotland, was at first merely an official document, but in 1928 it was put on public record in the Report of the Research Coordination Subcommittee of the Committee of Civil Research (Chapter 8). It still represents the principles on which functions are divided, but as a document it largely dropped out of sight as collaboration became closer and relations were regulated by established custom and goodwill. The terms were reviewed in 1949, in the light of the changed functions of the Health Departments consequent on the National Health Service having come into operation in 1948, but no amendment was found to be necessary. In addition, however, the several responsibilities for clinical research in that Service then required formulation in some detail, as noted in Volume Two.

As already mentioned (Chapter 6), the Chief Medical Officers of the two Health Departments have served—and served actively—as assessors to the Council since 1949. They also became assessors to the Clinical Research Board, which was itself appointed in consultation with the Health Departments (Volume Two); and the Chief Medical Officer of the Ministry of Health and Local Government in Northern Ireland likewise became an assessor to the Board. Various other matters in which joint action has been taken are mentioned in Volume Two.

In the course of time, the Ministry developed a tendency to invite the Council to administer specialised scientific services on its behalf, and at the expense of its vote; and the proposals were accepted by the Council. The administration of small scientific units was of course a familiar task for the Council; the Ministry, on the other hand, was geared to deal on a large scale with local authorities, in matters of public health, and later with the hospital boards of the National Health Service. Actually, a case somewhat of this nature arose as early as 1927, when the Ministry transferred the staff of its thenceforth honorary adviser on medical statistics to the service of the Council, making an annual contribution to the cost of the unit in order to retain a claim upon its help (Chapter 9). This basis was, however, rather different from the agency type of arrangement adopted in later instances. These did not occur until during and after the Second World War; they were subject to the constitutional ambiguity that the Council became in these matters responsible to the Minister of Health instead of to the Minister concerned with its primary function.

Other administrative departments
It is perhaps not generally realised how much of the governmental responsibility for matters of health lies outside the terms of reference of the 'Health Departments' proper. The health of people in various categories—considered as members of these categories—in fact concerns a surprising number of different departments; with most of these the Council has had relations, either in an advisory capacity or in undertaking special investigations. To avoid confusion arising from concrete or titular changes in the machinery of government during the period of this history, the nomenclature of departments at the time of writing is followed in this section, except where expressly indicated to the contrary.

In England and Wales, responsibility for the health of school children lies with the Department of Education and Science; this separation of function is, however, mitigated by the fact that the Chief Medical Officer of the Department also holds the corresponding post in the Department of Health and Social Security, although below his level there are separate medical staffs. The Ministry of Social Security is now merged with that Department; while separate it was concerned with the health of pensioners and insured persons, but as these are, of course, members of the general community—

and indeed form a large part of it—the responsibility was administrative rather than medical. The same Ministry, as successor to the Ministry of Pensions, had a particular interest in special problems relating to disabled war pensioners, but the hospitals that it used to maintain for these have since 1948 formed part of the National Health Service.

The Home Office has medical responsibilities relating to certain measures of public safety (for example, regulation of the sale of poisons, control of drugs of addiction, and prevention of some types of accident), and also to civil defence, to forensic medicine, and to health in prisons. Again the Chief Medical Officer of the Department of Health and Social Security holds the corresponding post in the Home Office; there is no separate medical staff. The Scottish Home and Health Department is now a single entity.

Various other departments have, or have had, health interests in special regards: the Ministry of Public Building and Works in, for example, heating and ventilation, and the Ministry of Housing and Local Government in water supplies and sewage (both ministries now subsumed by the Department of the Environment); the Ministry of Agriculture, Fisheries and Food in the production of food; the Department of Trade and Industry in certain aspects of manufacture and importation; and the former General Register Office (now Office of Population Censuses and Surveys), and its Scottish counterpart, in vital statistics.

All these are relatively minor fields in so far as requirements for medical research are concerned, although there is none into which the Council has not been brought on some occasion. The major separate field is that of health and safety in industry. This has been largely the responsibility of the Factory Department (now HM Factory Inspectorate), originally forming part of the Home Office but in 1940 transferred to the Ministry of Labour and National Service, as it then was (now the Department of Employment). Some account of the Council's programme of research in industrial health is given in Volume Two. Other departments have responsibility in matters of health and safety in certain specialised types of industry: the Ministry of Transport (now merged with the Department of the Environment) in public vehicles, railways, and shipping; and the Department of Trade and Industry (in succession to the former Ministry of Aviation) in civil aircraft and (in succession to the Ministry of Fuel and Power) in mines and nuclear reactor plants. In the last two cases the concern is not only with employees but also with passengers, and sometimes with third parties (for example, road safety). Again, in all these matters the Council has been called upon to help with advice or investigations.

Defence Services

During the First World War the Medical Research Committee was largely occupied with emergency work for the Royal Navy and the

Army, especially the latter; and during the Second World War the Council was similarly engaged on behalf of the Royal Navy, the Army, and the Royal Air Force. These matters are dealt with in Volume Two, and it will be seen how wide were the fields of research and the applications of new knowledge.

In time of peace, research undertaken for the Ministry of Defence and its Services has naturally been of relatively very small amount and of much narrower range. It has in fact been mainly concerned with physiological questions of the health, efficiency, and safety of service personnel in special circumstances—for example, in relation to the use of equipment (including weapons, vessels, vehicles, or aircraft), to the performance of exceptionally arduous tasks, or to life in trying environments.

Research overseas

The relations between the Council and the Colonial Office with regard to research in tropical medicine are reviewed in Volume Two. From 1961 there was also the new Department of Technical Cooperation, later becoming first a Ministry and then the Overseas Development Administration concerned *inter alia* with aid to former colonial territories that are not self-sufficient in scientific resources. The role of the short-lived Overseas Research Council has been mentioned earlier. The India Office, of course, ceased to exist after independence was given to India and Pakistan; earlier the Council had had considerable contact with work in India, either through the India Office or directly with the Indian Medical Research Fund Association.

The official channel of communication between governmental agencies in the United Kingdom and self-governing territories, whether the long-established dominions or countries that have lately emerged from colonial status, is now the Foreign and Commonwealth Office. Very little business affecting the Council is in fact transacted at this level, relations between research organisations being largely on an informal and even a personal basis. Scientific liaison officers from the principal self-governing territories are housed together in the British Commonwealth Scientific Offices in London; these provide an official but informal channel of information, but one relatively little used for medical purposes. There are also periodical British Commonwealth Scientific Conferences, held in turn in different capitals; here again the Council's participation is slight, as the delegates from other Commonwealth countries are seldom appointed from the medical field—and, in fact, the need for official liaison arrangements is much less than it appears to be in respect of industrial and agricultural research.

The Council's contacts with research workers and institutions in countries outside the Commonwealth have been even less frequently on an official basis; when they were, it was through the formerly separate Foreign Office. The latter at one time had medical responsibilities overseas, when the Sudan was a condominium of Great Britain and Egypt, and the Council did have some slight dealings in that regard.

International organisations

The Council has had constant direct relations with the World Health Organisation (formerly the Health Committee of the League of Nations), and to a lesser extent with such other agencies of the United Nations as the Food and Agriculture Organisation and UNESCO. It has also been concerned with various international research undertakings (Chapters 12, 16).

General advisory functions

Especially noteworthy has been the extent to which the advisory functions of the Council have developed, considering that there was no express provision for them at the outset. By supporting research work not merely in its own establishments but in the country at large, the Council earned the goodwill of scientific men; by its methods, it gained their confidence. The Council thus became uniquely placed for obtaining the best advice on any problem of medical science that might confront departments of state; it was always in touch, through its primary activities, with those best able to advise, and it could count on receiving their help.

Furthermore, as the Council became better known and its independence appreciated, both the quality and the impartiality of advice given by it, or through it, were generally recognised. Thus its advice was of value to departments not only for its intrinsic merit, but because it could be quoted as authoritative and would be accepted as such by the public. Some examples are given later (Chapter 9).

Transcending the departmental level has been advice that the Council has been called upon to give, sometimes directly to the Prime Minister, on certain matters affecting major policy of Government. The most notable example, considered in more detail later, has been advice on radiation hazards arising from the testing of nuclear weapons or the operation of nuclear power (Volume Two).

Chapter 8
Coordination of Government Research
(1917-1971)

The Council's involvement in coordination policy—Committee on the
Machinery of Government (1917–18)—Cabinet Committee on Coordination
of Research (1919–20)—Committee of Civil Research (1925–30)—Research
Special Subcommittee of the Imperial Conference (1926)—Report of the
CCR Research Coordination Subcommittee (1926-28)—Scientific Advisory Com-
mittee to the War Cabinet (1940–47)—White Paper on Scientific Research
and Development (1944)—White Paper on the Scientific Civil Service (1945)
—Committee on Future Scientific Policy (1945–46)—Advisory Council on
Scientific Policy (1947–65)—Committee on the Management and Control of
Research and Development (1958–61)—Committee of Enquiry into the
Organisation of Civil Science (1962–63)—Council for Scientific Policy (from
1965) and Central Advisory Council on Science and Technology (from 1967)
—Postscript: Green Paper on Government Research and Development (1971)

The Council's involvement in coordination policy
The Council has naturally been affected at different times by
Government policy in respect of the organisation and coordination
of research in different scientific and territorial fields, and it has also
on occasion been actively concerned in the shaping of such policy.
Furthermore, policy in this sense has extended beyond the stage of
promoting actual investigation to that of applying the results of the
researches—and scientific knowledge generally—to the practical
affairs of Government in various branches of administration. Here
the general theme can be considered only briefly as indicating the
relations of the Council in this sphere.

(Nevertheless, it is worth noting that the subject has a substantial earlier history,
and two episodes may be particularly mentioned; they have been described by
Layton (1968) and Caldwell (1957) respectively. In the first the initiative was
taken by John, Lord Wrottesley (1798–1867), who was in turn President of the
Royal Society, of the British Association for the Advancement of Science, and of
the Astronomical Society. On his proposal the British Association decided in 1849
to form a Parliamentary Committee of its members who were also members of
the legislature; and the fourth report of this body, in 1855, recommended the
establishment of a Board of Science to advise the Government on scientific
questions and be responsible for the distribution of Government grants. This was
put forward in 1857 with the backing of the Royal Society and the British
Association; but it fell on sterile ground.

In 1868 Colonel Alexander Strange of the Royal Engineers read a paper
before the British Association "On the necessity for State Intervention to secure
the Progress of Physical Science". A committee was appointed, and its recommendations were adopted by the Council of the Association and put to the Earl
de Grey, the Lord President, on 4 February 1870. In 1872 a Royal Commission
on Scientific Instruction and the Advancement of Science was appointed, and in

77

its eighth report (1875) made proposals about scientific education and research, the latter including the provision of state laboratories, increased grants to private scientists, and the creation of a Ministry of Science and Education with a Council of Science to advise it. Again, few of the recommendations were implemented.)

Committee on the Machinery of Government (1917–18)

References have already been made to this Committee, under the chairmanship of Lord Haldane. Among other things, its report recommended the constitutional arrangements for the Council that became effective two years later (Chapter 4). More generally, it stressed the importance of scientific information for the purposes of Government. It also drew a useful distinction in principle between research work with special aims, such as might properly be the concern of a single administrative department, and research work of wider interest, such as ought to be the responsibility of special agencies serving the general needs.

Cabinet Committee on Coordination of Research (1919–20)

Towards the end of 1919 the Cabinet appointed a Committee on the Coordination of Scientific Research in Government Departments, under the chairmanship of Mr A. J. (later the Earl of) Balfour, Lord President of the Council. This body met on 16 December 1919, and again on 3 February 1920 and 21 February 1921. On the second of these occasions it appointed *inter alia* a Subcommittee on Medical Research, under the chairmanship of Sir Walter Fletcher. It does not appear that any report of the Committee or of its subcommittees was ever published; the papers were in that immediately post-war period classified as secret.

The Subcommittee on Medical Research met on 23 February 1920, and again on 6 August 1920. At this latter meeting it had before it memoranda provided by the War Office, the Home Office and the Ministry of Pensions, on their respective undertakings or needs in the field of medical research; none offered difficult problems of coordination, and to a large extent the papers represented merely an exchange of information. Of much wider significance was a memorandum, submitted by Sir Walter Fletcher, on the need for the coordination of research work at home and research work in the Colonies, India, and elsewhere, whether in the civilian medical services there or by personnel of the Defence Services posted overseas. Suggestions were made for more effective intercommunication on scientific questions and the possibility of arranging some interchange of staff. From a summary of the discussion circulated later it appears that some support was given by the representative of the War Office and others; the representative of the Colonial Office, however, was firmly of the opinion that the requirements were covered by existing arrangements and that no new coordinating machinery was necessary. Fletcher was immediately thereafter absent for some months owing to illness and there is no evidence that the subcommittee, having reached a deadlock on the major issue before it, met again; desultory correspondence continuing until 1922 indicates that no report was ever made. It was many years before satisfactory cooperation in research on tropical medicine was achieved (Volume Two).

Committee of Civil Research (1925–30)
In 1925 a new venture of an interesting and promising kind was launched. This was the Committee of Civil Research, set up at the instance of the Earl of Balfour, Lord President of the Council, who announced the Government's intention on 20 May during a debate on Kenya in the House of Lords when mention was made of the recent report of the East Africa Commission (Volume Two); further information was given by ministers in reply to questions in the House of Commons on 25 May. The formal instrument was a Treasury Minute of 13 June, and to provide an opportunity for clarification the matter was debated in the Lords on 30 June. In origin, the scheme represented a fusion of two different proposals; and unfortunately this proved to be its undoing five years later.

On 27 February 1925, Sir Frank Heath, Secretary of the Department of Scientific and Industrial Research, and Sir Walter Fletcher had put forward to the Lord President a memorandum prepared in collaboration with Sir Thomas Middleton, Vice-Chairman of the Development Commission. This was a reasoned plea for the establishment of an Imperial Development Board (later called a Council) charged particularly with coordinating the application of science to the needs of overseas territories; the object was to bring into a single focus the scientific problems of the self-governing Dominions, India, the Colonies, and the Defence Services abroad. The Lord President of the day, the Marquess Curzon, was not impressed, and in a minute of 2 March he poured cold water on the scheme. He also suggested that the Colonial Office should be consulted, missing the major point that the need was something transcending the scope of any single department.

A few days later Lord Curzon fell seriously ill, and soon afterwards his place as Lord President was taken by the Earl of Balfour. The proposal was brought to his attention and was very differently received ("George cannot understand science, indeed hates it"). At the next stage, however, it impinged on a proposal from another source. On 2 April 1925, Mr Baldwin had put to his Cabinet a proposal taken over by agreement from the preceding Government under the premiership of Mr Ramsay Macdonald, who in the year before had endorsed a Treasury memorandum on "Foresight and Coordination in Economic Enquiry". The proposal was for the establishment of a Committee of Economic Inquiry constituted as a civil counterpart of the Committee of Imperial Defence (1895–1939). There is evidence that Haldane was the instigator of Macdonald's plan, and the idea was indeed implicit in the report of his Committee on the Machinery of Government, mentioned above.

From a combination of the two ideas arose the Committee of Civil Research, as the Cabinet decided to call it on 28 May 1925. This body was "charged with the duty of giving connected forethought from a central standpoint to the development of economic, scientific and statistical research in relation to civil policy and administration and it will define new areas in which enquiry would be valuable". The Committee had the Prime Minister as its President, and in his absence a Minister nominated by him (in practice the Lord President) as its regular Chairman. Otherwise, the members were to be "such persons as are summoned by the Prime Minister or the Chairman on his behalf". The quotations are from the Treasury Minute.

The Committee of Civil Research was potentially effective, because it reported directly to the Lord President and thus to the Cabinet. Its field was as wide as could be desired, and it could deal rapidly with questions affecting more than one department or even different parts of the Empire. It was in a position either to propose new investigations or to bring existing knowledge promptly to bear on a particular problem. The procedure was admirably flexible; when the Lord President considered or agreed that any topic needed study, he summoned to a meeting the appropriate heads of departments (or their official deputies) and others; the Committee, if it approved, then proceeded to appoint a subcommittee of composition suited to the matter in hand, and this body made a report—sometimes within a very short time.

The Committee's functions did not overlap those of existing research agencies of Government, although it might initiate work in fields not so covered. It was more concerned with facilitating and expediting the later stages in bringing new knowledge into effective application in the work of administration; the results of successful research were too apt to wait long for their full and effective use in practice. In the Report for 1925–26 the Committee of Privy Council for Medical Research made comment as follows:

The past year has seen at work the first beginnings of the new machinery designed to meet present deficiencies of this kind. The Committee of Civil Research was set up to provide in the most flexible manner for the timely discussion of problems that may be common to more than one field of applied science, common to more than one administrative department, or common again to more than one part of the Kingdom or Empire. In discussions thus promoted the various scientific and administrative interests concerned can take part together. The Committee, varying in its constitution for every problem, exists only for discussion and report: it has no powers of doing or spending. Experience has already shown that the creation of this simple but new piece of Government machinery has notably facilitated the effective application of science to the administrative work of Government departments and to other activities. From our present point of view we are confident that it has aided already and will still further aid the cooperation of the Medical Research Council, among other research organisations in different fields, in the work of bringing science into its fullest application to given practical problems of administration and of human need.

The first meeting of the Committee of Civil Research took place under the chairmanship of Lord Balfour on 18 June 1925, when the questions discussed were tsetse fly and trypanosomiasis, the Imperial College of Agriculture in Trinidad, and the capacity to meet demands for credit at home and abroad. The first problem was fully discussed on the basis of a note by Fletcher, and it was agreed to set up a subcommittee under the chairmanship of the Rt Hon. W. Ormsby-Gore, MP (later Lord Harlech), Parliamentary Under-Secretary of State for the Colonies. The position in respect of the second matter was noted; and the third question was referred to a subcommittee to be set up under the chairmanship of the Governor of the Bank of England.

Several of the eventual subcommittees dealt with subjects of interest to the Council. Thus, the Tsetse Fly Subcommittee, already mentioned, considered action on the problems of human and animal trypanosomiasis in Africa; a Dietetics Subcommittee planned researches into human and animal nutrition, again with special reference to tropical and subtropical territories; and there was a Subcommittee on the Empire Supply of Quinine. These were examples of questions having imperial import.

In the field of home administration, a subcommittee considered means of meeting the growing need for radium in the treatment of disease (Volume Two); this led to the establishment of the National Radium Trust and its executive Radium Commission, bodies which functioned until the National Health Service came into being. Another subcommittee rapidly overcame opposition to the formation of an expert Pharmacopoeia Commission to supervise the preparation of successive editions of the *British Pharmacopoeia*, published under the auspices of the General Medical Council (Volume Two). Reference to the Subcommittee on the Coordination of Research is made separately below.

This useful piece of machinery was wrecked in 1930 following a change in Government in the previous year. The Ministers returning to power reverted to their original idea and a Treasury Minute of 27 January 1930 replaced the Committee of Civil Research (CCR) by an Economic Advisory Council. This latter body, as its name implies, had an orientation towards economics rather than science; the direction of activity was thus changed, and the flexibility of procedure was lost through there being a number of regular members. (One is reminded of Sir Henry Tizard's story of a committee of five economists which submitted six minority reports). It is true that the EAC had quite a strong Science Committee, and also that some CCR subcommittees remained in being until they had completed their tasks; but little interest in the potentialities of the machinery was evinced at ministerial level. The pity was that there had never been any good reason why the two concepts should have con-

D

flicted; it would have been open to the Government of the day, whether in 1925 or in 1930, to have implemented both proposals independently of each other. A further account of the CCR, based on official papers that have meanwhile become accessible, has been given by McLeod and Andrews (1969); there is also a brief summary in the editorial introduction to Thomas Jones's *Whitehall Diary* (1969).

Research Special Subcommittee of the Imperial Conference (1926)

Meanwhile, in the year following the establishment of the Committee of Civil Research, the Imperial Conference of 1926 made history, in the field of scientific administration, by for the first time having a Research Special Subcommittee. This body reported to the Conference (1926), which adopted its recommendations and referred them to Governments. The report dealt with questions of research organisation, scientific manpower, agricultural research in particular, and also with certain special matters. Medical research was involved only in general terms, but representatives of the Council took part in the work of the Subcommittee. Among other things, the report stressed the need for the designation of official representatives of each organisation throughout the Empire responsible for one of the broad fields of utilitarian research to act as 'opposite numbers' with whom correspondence might at all times be possible on scientific questions of common interest; and various other suggestions for liaison were made (Chapter 7).

The Earl of Balfour, as Lord President, made special reference to the foregoing in his covering report to the Council's Report for 1925–26. The Council itself opened its next Report (1926–27) with a section on research work in the Empire, referring to three events that it regarded as having great significance. The first was the operation of the new machinery of the Committee of Civil Research, already described. The second was the action of the Imperial Conference, just mentioned. The third was the establishment, in 1926, of the first Colonial Medical Research Committee, appointed by the Secretary of State in consultation with the Council to advise both parties (Volume Two).

Report of the CCR Research Coordination Subcommittee (1926–28)

The Research Coordination Subcommittee of the Committee of Civil Research was appointed by the Prime Minister on 29 October 1926, following a recommendation by the Select Committee of the House of Commons on Estimates (Report No. 119) that more attention should be given to the coordination of Government research with a view to economy and efficiency. The Subcommittee's report was published as a 'blue book' in 1928.

After the formal introduction, the report opens with a "Historical Outline of the Relations of Government to Research Work". This was in two sections: (A) Research in Great Britain; (B) Inter-

Imperial Research. The rest of the report consists of a full statement of the status and functions of the various Government agencies for the promotion of scientific research, and also of the arrangements for coordination between these. As a factual statement the report was useful at the time and is now a valuable historical document; but comment was incidental and generally favourable, and no drastic recommendations were made. Nevertheless, the following passage is of interest as a reasoned endorsement of the principle of having separate research councils, as contrasted with a possible unified agency for scientific research:

> We believe that a single scientific organisation would have been unwieldy and that while the optimum size and intricacy may be approached by each alone, it would be exceeded if fusion came about of two or more of the group. It may be agreed further that as each organisation has grown, or is still to grow, the development of this new kind of State machinery proceeds in large part by trial and error. Each developing along its own path is more likely so to reach the model most suited to its own work, while each, at this point or that, may gain from noting the procedure of its companion organisations and may give similar opportunities to them for sympathetic but critical attention. The most conclusive argument, however, for mutual independence among the three appears to us to lie in this, that each of the organisations in its daily work of fostering all the stages of research between primary discovery and the final applications of its results to the practical business of the professions, the trades and other interests, has to deal with a distinctive world, distinctive in its history, its psychology and its conditions of work. (This last point is then elaborated in the original documents.)

Scientific Advisory Committee to the War Cabinet (1940–47)
On 3 October 1940, it was announced that the Lord President had, after discussion with the Royal Society and with the approval of the Prime Minister, appointed a Scientific Advisory Committee under the chairmanship of Lord Hankey. The other members were the respective Secretaries of the three Research Councils and the President and the two Secretaries of the Royal Society. At the outset, Group Captain W. (later Air Chief Marshal Sir William) Elliot and Professor W. W. C. Topley were Joint Secretaries of the Committee. The terms of reference were: (*a*) to advise the Lord President on any scientific problem referred to them; (*b*) to advise Government Departments, when so requested, on the selection of individuals for particular lines of scientific inquiry or for membership of committees on which scientists are required; and (*c*) to bring to the notice of the Lord President promising new scientific or technical developments which may be of importance to the war effort. This wartime machinery remained in being until 1945.

White Paper on Scientific Research and Development (1944)
In April 1944, the Lord President presented to Parliament a White Paper on Scientific Research and Development. This was a purely factual statement of the existing Government machinery for the

promotion of scientific research and development, excluding work directed to the requirements of war production and of the Defence Services. It was intended as a background for the discussion of the part that the Government could play in the field of civil research after the war. The report dealt fully with the functions and organisation of the various agencies, and referred to the financial provision made to the universities in support of fundamental research. It also described the arrangements for coordination by the Scientific Advisory Committee of the War Cabinet (see above) and the responsibilities of the Lord President in relation to scientific research.

White Paper on the Scientific Civil Service (1945)

The full title of this publication was *The Scientific Civil Service: Reorganisation and Recruitment during the Reconstruction Period*; and to it was appended the *Report of the Barlow Committee on Scientific Staff* (1943). It did not directly affect the Council, as it was outside the organisation of the Civil Service, but further reference is made to it later (Chapter 9). What may be described as a latter-day Barlow Report was that of a Committee appointed to Review the Organisation of the Scientific Civil Service, with Sir Mark Tennant as its Chairman; this was published in 1965, but the difficulties with which it dealt had little application to the Council's service.

Committee on Future Scientific Policy (1945-46)

This body was appointed towards the end of 1945. Its first report was published in 1946 and dealt with scientific manpower. Its second report, a confidential document dated 16 October 1946, was *The Central Government Machinery for Civil Science*. This recommended that, in parallel with the creation of a Defence Research Policy Committee, an Advisory Council on Scientific Policy should be set up to deal with the civil side, replacing the Scientific Advisory Committee to the War Cabinet. It also recommended that there should be no post equivalent to that of Chief Scientific Adviser to the Government (a policy reversed by the appointment of Sir Solly (later Lord) Zuckerman in 1966).

Advisory Council on Scientific Policy (1947-65)

This body was set up in accordance with the recommendation mentioned above, and the action was the subject of a statement by the Lord Privy Seal in the House of Commons on 29 January 1947. The function of the Council was "to advise the Lord President in the exercise of his responsibilities for the formulation and execution of Government scientific policy". Its members included the respective Secretaries of the three Research Councils together with selected academic and industrial scientists and others, all under an independent scientific chairman. Later, the relevant responsibilities of the Lord President were transferred to the Minister for Science.

During this period a Scientific Manpower Committee was

appointed by the Lord President (1950); and it was later succeeded by a Committee on Manpower for Science and Technology.

Committee on the Management and Control of Research and Development (1958–61)
In 1958 the Lord President appointed a small committee "to enquire into the techniques employed by Government departments and other bodies wholly financed by the Exchequer for the management and control of research and development carried out by them or on their behalf, and to make recommendations". The original Chairman was Sir Claude Gibb; on his death in the following year he was succeeded by Sir Solly Zuckerman. The Committee reported in 1961.

The Committee was concerned with defence research as well as with civil research, and among other things with the organisation of the Scientific Civil Service. Much of its thinking was in terms of such concepts, largely alien to medical research, as the classification of 'projects' into five categories ranging from 'pure basic research' to 'applied research and development' (admittedly with intergrading). The Council thus did not find in the recommendations much that it could readily apply in its own field. It concluded, indeed, that the Committee's assessments were based on tacit assumptions widely different from the Council's own view of its needs and purpose as an official body responsible for promoting medical research on a national scale (Chapter 9). In its Report for 1960–61, the Council stated its own view in set terms. It deprecated strict classification of research, at least in its own field; it objected, for reasons given, to any prohibition of governmental agencies from engaging in so-called 'pure basic research'; and it strongly resisted proposals for methods of management that, in its belief, would be detrimental to the freedom of intellectual initiative by individual investigators without which creative work cannot fully develop.

Committee of Enquiry into the Organisation of Civil Science (1962–63)
This Committee, under the chairmanship of Sir Burke Trend, recommended some major changes in the official organisation for the promotion of research in civil science in other than the medical and agricultural fields. The Department of Scientific and Industrial Research was to be dissolved and its functions were to be distributed between new agencies—a Science Research Council, an Industrial Research and Development Authority, and a Natural Resources Research Council. The last of these (in the event called the Natural Environment Research Council) was to assume all the functions of the Nature Conservancy, and certain responsibilities for research in hydrology, fisheries, oceanography, forestry, and geology; the concept was based on the Report of the Committee on Research on Natural Resources, under the chairmanship of Sir William Slater, published as an appendix to the Sixteenth Annual Report of the

Advisory Council on Scientific Policy (1963). The Overseas Research Council, which had never exercised executive functions, was to be replaced by specialist committees advising the Department of Technical Cooperation. On the other hand, the respective functions of the Medical Research Council and the Agricultural Research Council were to remain substantially unchanged; these bodies were, however, directly affected by the proposals for constitutional changes in all members of the group of research councils. The particular impact of these on the Medical Research Council has already been mentioned (Chapter 6).

The report emphatically recommended the retention of the research council pattern that had proved so satisfactory, and its further proposals were based on the assumption that this would be accepted. The only proposal directly affecting the constitution of research councils in general was that these bodies should have whole-time chairmen with appropriate professional qualifications, and that the title of Secretary should revert to administrative seconds-in-command. At the higher level, the report recommended the abolition of the formula of Committees of the Privy Council, the powers of which would be vested by law—as already largely by custom—in the Minister for Science, who would have an actual Ministry with important functions (especially regarding finance).

The recommendations were substantially accepted by the Government, subject to modifications compatible with its intention to merge the functions of the Minister for Science with those of a Secretary of State for Education and Science and to set up a Ministry of Technology. The decisions were implemented mainly by the Science and Technology Act 1965 and by various Royal Charters. The five kindred bodies thereafter operating under the Secretary of State have already been named (Chapter 7): the Medical, Science, Agricultural, Natural Environment, and Social Science Research Councils.

Council for Scientific Policy (from 1965) and Central Advisory Council on Science and Technology (from 1967)
In 1965 the Advisory Council on Scientific Policy was succeeded by a Council for Scientific Policy advising the Secretary of State for Education and Science. This was flanked by a new Advisory Council on Technology advising the Minister of Technology.

Finally, to top the pyramid, a Central Advisory Council for Science and Technology was set up in 1967 (announced in 1966), under the chairmanship of Sir Solly Zuckerman, "to advise the Government as a whole on the most effective use of our scientific and technological resources, whether in the civil or defence fields, or in the public or private sectors". This had a membership overlapping that of the two bodies which had narrower terms of reference.

Postscript: Green Paper on Government Research and Development (1971)
It is not possible to do more than insert this postscript briefly indi-

cating the nature of changes foreshadowed in an official memorandum presented to Parliament by the Lord Privy Seal late in 1971, entitled *A Framework for Government Research and Development*. This covers a report by Lord Rothschild, Head of the Central Policy Review Staff, on "The Organisation and Management of Government R. & D.", and another by a Council for Scientific Policy working party under the chairmanship of Sir Frederick Dainton on "The Future of the Research Council System".

The Dainton report, although printed second, is the earlier of the two; it is more limited in its scope and much less sweeping in its proposals. Broadly, it favours the retention of the system of research councils, but urges the need for closer links between the several councils, and with the user departments of state, the universities and the Royal Society. The main proposal is for the establishment of an overall Board of the Research Councils on which all these parties would be represented. It would have a Chairman who would be accounting officer for the group; and it would be responsible to the Secretary of State for Education and Science. It would supplant the existing Council for Scientific Policy.

The Rothschild report deals with the whole field of Government research and development. Its most drastic proposal is the wide application of the 'customer/contractor' principle, the customer being the Government department requiring a programme of applied research and development to be carried out, and the contractor being the relevant research council or other agency undertaking the work. On this basis the cost would be borne on the vote of the customer department, which would thus call the tune. (In the case of the Medical Research Council, about one-quarter of the existing budget would be transferred to government departments in the first instance.) The research councils would be independently responsible for basic research and would derive finance for it as at present. Substantial administrative innovations for the implementation of this policy are outlined.

The Government endorsed the main thesis of the Rothschild Report and observed that this was not at variance with the Dainton recommendations. However, it allowed a period for wide discussion of the proposals—which included consideration by a Select Committee of the House of Commons (1972)—before announcing its decisions in the White Paper *Framework for Government Research and Development* in 1972. As this book went to press arrangements were being made for the detailed implementation of the proposals.

Apart from this postscript, and a paragraph referring to it at the end of Chapter 6, nothing has been inserted or changed in this book to take account of these very recent proposals. Time must elapse before they and their effects can be seen in true historical perspective.

Part II

Ways and Means:

Organisation and Administration

Chapter 9
Policy and Methods

General policy of a national body—Overall responsibility for medical research—Relations with the universities—Research in the universities: a reappraisal—Relations with other organisations—Relations with individuals—
'Pure' and 'applied' research—Discovery and development in the medical
field—Allocation of resources—Planning and coordination—Advisory boards
and committees—Methods of promoting research—Rewards as incentives?—
Publication of results—The Council's advisory role—The use of animals in
experimental research

General policy of a national body
The appointment of the Medical Research Committee in 1913
established a national body of a kind that was new in its particular
field; it had functions not previously discharged on the public behalf
to more than a slight extent; and it had potentially a scope as wide
as the farthest limits of medical science. Certain vital questions of
policy were implicit, even although they could not be fully identified
until later.

Firstly, what should be the scope of such a body's responsibility?
In terms of statutory powers, it existed to expend certain funds,
provided on an arbitrary basis for a very broadly stated purpose.
According to a legal opinion, its activities should have some relevance
to national health insurance; but this implied limitation was
unimportant even in theory, was ignored in practice, and was in any
event short-lived (Chapter 2).

This question immediately raised the further one of the proper
relationship between the national body and other organisations
operating in the same field in the United Kingdom. From this it was
a short step to consideration of the basis on which the funds available
to the national body should be allocated. This in turn raised questions about the methods to be used in promoting research, and about
the extent to which the financing agency should seek to plan or
direct, as distinct from merely assisting spontaneous projects. Later
there arose the question of the advisory role that developed as a
natural outcome of fulfilling the primary function.

Overall responsibility for medical research
It was recognised from an early stage that the Committee, and later
the Council, had a general responsibility for using all means open to
it for advancing medical research in the United Kingdom. There
was, of course, severe financial restriction in the early days, and it
was not until much later that the Council was in a position to submit
annual estimates of expenditure to the Treasury on a basis of
requirements (Chapter 15). Even so there was no reason why the

resources should not be spread thinly over a wide field, and this was in fact the policy adopted from the outset.

For the fulfilment of an overall responsibility, it was immaterial whether the necessary research work was promoted by the Committee (or Council) itself or by agencies not under its control. Nor was there any empire-building desire for power to direct, still less to absorb, the pre-existing agencies. The function of the national body was to take stock of the total effort in the country, and then to decide how best it could increase that. The resources could be used to supplement those of other institutions, or to complement them by separate enterprises where gaps appeared to exist.

In its first Report, for 1914–15, the Committee thus expressed its policy:

> It will be seen that the general plan for the future work of the Committee marks clearly a line of policy by which part, but only a part, of the new national fund for research is devoted to work in centralised laboratories under their control and carried out by a scientific staff to be directly appointed by the Committee, while the other and larger part of the fund is allocated to the support of workers and their investigations in institutes not directly under the control of the Committee.

More recently, in its Report for 1960–61, the Council restated its view of its function in these terms:

> This then is how the Medical Research Council conceive their function: to watch over the whole fields of medical and related biological research so as to foresee, to the best of their ability, the needs and opportunities; to give support to any promising research in these fields irrespective of the agent concerned; to work in partnership with the universities and professions on the one hand and the various departments of Government on the other, so that new knowledge may be made available as the need arises. It is according to this concept that we, and our predecessors, have devised our organisation and formulated our principles of working.

Relations with the universities

The other organisations to be taken into account were mainly the universities, including their medical schools and the associated teaching hospitals. With the growing costliness of many modern lines of research, university departments with small budgets were heavily handicapped in fulfilling the research part of their functions. Equally, the claims of teaching in most universities were apt to leave the staff with too little time for other work. It was therefore valuable to have a supplementary source of grants for equipment, for running expenses, and for technical or scientific assistance; and also to have the possibility of giving hospitality to additional research workers with stipends provided from extramural funds.

It was, moreover, plainly economical that such supplementary resources for research in universities should be administered by some detached body—one that could discriminate in favour of the more productive departments, and select for support approved projects undertaken by particular workers. Any method of financial provision involving allocation of funds on a basis of equal or statistically equivalent shares, among universities or among departments of a university, would have been not only wasteful but largely ineffective. Experience of applications for grants quickly demonstrated the wide extent of the local variations in research potential that exist at any particular time. The national body's activities could also be complementary to those of the universities, in that it might itself undertake projects of a kind unsuited to the academic environment.

Another factor was that the universities constituted the essential recruiting and training ground for research workers. It was therefore important that the national body should not use its resources to deflect an undue proportion of university teachers, or potential teachers, into whole-time careers in research. Moreover, many research workers find a stimulus in some contact with teaching, or with practical work in the hospitals or outside them. Likewise, there are in the universities and hospitals many leaders of scientific thought whose inspiration is of immense value to junior colleagues engaging in research. These advantages would be lost by too great a centralisation of research activity outside the academic field. At the same time, a free interchange of staff, in both directions, should be welcomed and encouraged; this has in fact become quite normal and has been accepted on both sides as desirable.

These considerations provided the basis of an enduring policy of cooperation between the Council and the universities. Sir Charles Sherrington, in his Presidential Address to the Royal Society in 1921, said of the Council:

> One of the strengths of this organisation that has arisen is, in my view, that it interlocks with the educational system of the country. It is an organisation which proceeds on the wise premise that, in the case of science, the best way to get the fruit is to cultivate the tree.

Research in the universities: a reappraisal

In 1958, the research councils reviewed with the University Grants Committee the whole question of financial responsibility for scientific research in universities and an agreed memorandum was submitted to the Advisory Council on Scientific Policy. An obvious question was why such research should not be financed by the universities themselves, with necessary additions to the grants allocated by the UGC; several cogent reasons were adduced in reply.

Firstly, if research workers in universities could obtain finance only from general university income, it was "to be feared that some scientific seedlings might fail to survive the chill blasts to which they would be exposed in competition for funds within universities". In other words, "there is inevitably an element of speculation in backing new unproved ideas, and this must be a handicap in obtaining finance if the new idea is brought, while still unproved, into competition for funds with the needs of established activities". It was therefore concluded that it was "desirable that newly-emerging lines of research should have sources of funds alternative to general university income, and thus be able to obtain outside protection against the hazards of interdepartmental competition for funds within the university".

Secondly, there were several reasons why the University Grants Committee should not be the protecting power. It had always sought to preserve university autonomy and to minimise its own intervention in the allocation of funds within universities; it was in any event not specially qualified to assess the promise of research projects. To quote the agreed document, "it is not desirable that a single governmental colossus should bestride the whole university world, but that is what would inevitably occur if the present functions of the University Grants Committee and of the Research Councils were all to be exercised by a single organisation".

On the other hand, the councils were well qualified to judge research proposals and could do so in a wider context. It was agreed, however, that when a new subject fostered in a university by a research council had proved itself it might appropriately pass to university control. Further, capital grants for new research accommodation would normally be a responsibility of the University Grants Committee; but provision for very costly items of equipment required solely for research was perhaps better left to the councils.

Relations with other organisations

Research institutes—A few more or less autonomous institutes differed from the universities in being concerned almost entirely with research; some were formally affiliated to universities and might engage in a small amount of purely postgraduate instruction. The attitude of the Council was nevertheless much the same. Specific instances are dealt with later (in Chapter 12 and in Volume Two).

Hospitals—The Medical Research Committee was from the beginning obviously dependent on the cooperation of hospitals for facilities for clinical research. Only on rare occasions has the Council been responsible for the care of patients, except in the small hospital attached to its laboratories in The Gambia (Volume Two).

Firms—Relations with the research departments of firms manufacturing medicinal products were naturally on a more restricted footing, particularly in the early days. On the one hand there were the inhibitions due to considerations of commercial security and the quest for proprietary rights; on the other hand there was the requirement that resources provided from public funds should not be used to create any monopolistic advantage. Nevertheless, in course of time satisfactory arrangements for cooperation in various projects were developed (Volume Two). Incidentally, several men who were to be leaders of the Council's research staff in the early years came from the Wellcome Physiological Laboratories, established in a commercial context (Chapter 1).

Relations with individuals

Although broad policy had to be considered in terms of institutions, as described above, in matters of detail the deliberate practice has always been to deal, as far as possible, directly with the individual research workers. There is no doubt that this was—at the outset and later—of the greatest value in gaining the confidence of the general body of those actively engaged in medical research, and in making the Committee or Council an effective instrument in fostering their work. The policy implied the development of a personal relationship between the headquarters staff and the research workers that was helpful to both.

In some spheres this type of procedure could not have been used without impropriety, but under the conditions of academic freedom enjoyed by most research workers in the United Kingdom it presented no real difficulty. There were obviously matters of major importance that had to be negotiated by the Council with the academic or hospital authority concerned. The use of official channels was more often necessary where the scientific worker was in government service or was employed in industry. In occasional instances, no institution was involved—for example, a medical man in private practice engaging in research. The Council's relations with members of its own staff are considered later (Chapter 11).

'Pure' and 'applied' research

From time to time the counsels of research organisations are vexed by considerations, usually of extraneous origin, involving a distinction between 'pure' and 'applied' research. The underlying supposition is that one kind of research is undertaken with the aim of increasing knowledge for its own sake and without any definite practical application in view, and that another kind is undertaken for the direct attainment of specified utilitarian objectives. The point has already been briefly mentioned in a more general context (Chapter 8), but its relevance to medical research in particular merits fuller consideration.

Men of science themselves are apt to find little reality in such a distinction, and less utility in attempting to draw it. Experience shows that the results of research promoted in the general pursuit of knowledge may have quite unforeseen utilitarian applications, possibly of immediate value; and on the other hand that the results of an *ad hoc* investigation may add to the general store of knowledge; the classification is thus at best a very loose one. Also, research with an immediate object must necessarily draw upon the accumulated store of general knowledge and replenishes this only to a minor extent if pursued in isolation; the process is thus a self-exhausting one, and is rewarding only for a short period such as in wartime.

Although these matters are still apt to need exposition to the uninformed, the main point was realised in Parliament two centuries ago, as witness the following extract from the British Museum Act 1753:

> ... all Arts and Sciences have a Connexion with each other, and Discoveries in Natural Philosophy and other Branches of speculative Knowledge, for the Advancement and Improvement whereof the said Museum or Collection was intended, do and may, in many Instances give Help and Success to the most useful Experiments and Inventions.

Some two centuries later the point was made by Sir Cyril Hinshelwood in his Presidential Address to the British Association for the Advancement of Science (1965):

> What would be quite useless would be any draconian edict that all scientific work must henceforth be devoted to demonstrably practical ends. There could be no surer way of rendering the future completely barren.

Or, from a generation earlier, one may cite the creed of a great physiologist, Professor E. H. Starling (1918):

> No discovery is useless, no curiosity is misplaced or too ambitious, and we may be certain that every advance achieved in the quest for knowledge will sooner or later play its part in the service of man.

It has been said that the researches of Louis Pasteur (1822–95) in France ended the separation of pure and applied science in the biological field. The balanced view was thus expressed by the Medical Research Committee in its Report for 1918–19:

> It is a truism, and now almost a familiar one, to say that the important attainments of new knowledge come from disinterested inquiry followed under the spur of free intellectual impulse, rather than from frontal attacks made in a utilitarian spirit upon problems of immediate practical interest. Disinterested or 'pure' science nevertheless yields its certain harvest of fruit, in the increase of our power over nature, but generally in the form, so to speak, of by-products often unforeseen, and commonly collected by other gleaners. Conversely, also, the application of scientific work to practical problems, in which means of power rather than gains in knowledge are the primary objects of quest, has in a multitude of instances led unexpectedly, through the hitting of some fresh paths of inquiry, to new knowledge, whether or not the immediate problem in view has been wholly solved.

Discovery and development in the medical field

Medical research has a general utilitarian aim, even although its immediate objectives lie mainly in the field of discovery. It concerns itself for the most part with elucidating natural laws bearing, nearly or remotely, on the functioning of the human organism—mind as well as body—and its reactions to the variety of inimical influences that it may encounter. This presents a wide field of study, not only of man himself but also of the processes underlying all the phenomena of life; and, further, of the physical, chemical and biological factors that impinge from the environment.

3   The four Secretaries

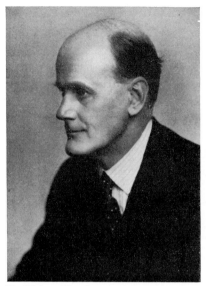

Sir Walter Fletcher, KBE, CB, FRS

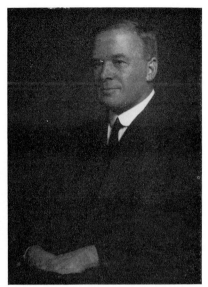

Sir Edward Mellanby, GBE, KCB, FRS

Sir Harold Himsworth, KCB, FRS

Sir John Gray, FRS

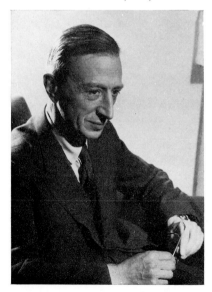

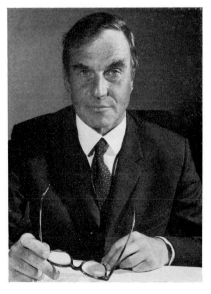

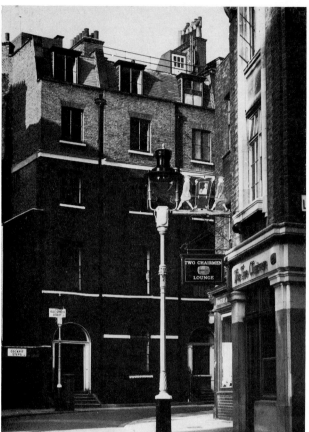

Old Queen Street, SW1

Park Crescent, W1 (*below*)

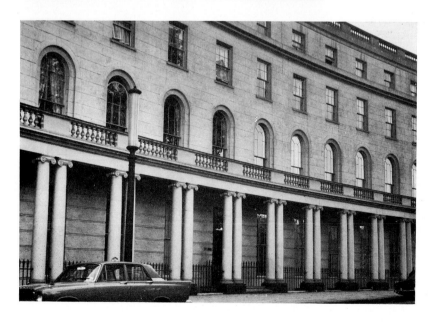

There comes a point, however, where new knowledge gained by such research is susceptible of deliberate development for a practical purpose. The point may not be sharply defined, as the purpose may have been coming more clearly into view as the research progressed and may indeed have influenced the planning of its later stages. What happens is that the main natural facts have been determined, and that the remaining problem is to find means, or the best means, of translating the knowledge into useful action. In the medical field it is usually the research that is the more difficult; the development tends to follow with relative ease.

If this be understood, it becomes clear why a medical research organisation must resist pressures to allocate resources and effort solely in terms of practical objectives. In great measure, allocation must be based on the prospects of making progress in the particular direction under current conditions of wider knowledge, the availability of investigators of the requisite calibre with appropriate experience, and the prospects of finding or creating circumstances in which the work can well be undertaken. Further, some lines of research involve the use of methods much more costly than those required in others, and a mere budgetary comparison is irrelevant where the value of the possible results cannot be expressed in financial terms.

In its Report for 1918–19, already cited, the Medical Research Committee commented on the special nature of its subject as follows:

> In no field is this interplay of disinterested or 'pure' and utilitarian or 'applied' science more conspicuous than in that of medical research. Here every branch of science is called upon to aid the study of the organism and of its environment, and of their interaction. Nowhere are offered more suggestions for disinterested intellectual effort, and in no other field at the same time are there given problems of more immediate, of literally vital, practical significance. The spur to gain knowledge is offered as in all natural inquiry, but there is an unparalleled call for increased power through applied knowledge, for it is given by the presence everywhere of removable pain and waste of life.

Allocation of resources

The deployment of money, material, and manpower to the best advantage, avoiding both serious gaps and undesirable overlapping, can be successfully undertaken only by those who comprehend the nature of the problem. Up to a point, the statesman or administrative official can indicate priorities, although perhaps least of all in the medical field; by priorities he means those subjects on which further knowledge would, in his estimation, be of the greatest practical benefit and for which the strings of the public purse may, therefore, be most readily loosened. On the other hand, he is unlikely to be in a position to judge for himself whether a particular problem is at the moment susceptible to frontal assault or must await the success of outflanking movements; whether the prerequisite conditions for staging the attack already exist or must be developed; whether highly specialised manpower can, in fact, be switched at will from one effort to another; and whether financial provision should be related more to the cost of particular types of investigations than to the supposed value of the results that might be obtained. There is thus a certain ideological conflict between those who deem it obvious that greater resources and effort should be devoted to this or that problem because it is important and those who more clearly appreciate the requirement for effective research.

Planning and coordination
It may be asked how far the promoting agency can itself plan investigations and direct their performance, as distinct from deciding whether to support proposals made to it; but the question overlooks the distinction between tactics and strategy. Research tactics are a matter for the leaders in immediate touch with the problems, in the laboratory or the ward; but behind them there is a prime necessity, in any enterprise on a national scale, for a grand strategy of research promotion. Neither chance nor individual predilections will ensure that the attack as a whole is sufficiently comprehensive, that the various efforts are properly balanced, and that the total resources are deployed to the best advantage. Planning is essential for filling gaps in the subject cover, and for creating opportunities where these do not already exist.

Accordingly, although the whole of medical science has always been the Council's field, from time to time more than ordinary attention has been deliberately given to particular subjects that have appeared to be ripe for intensive research. Thus, it was natural that tuberculosis should bulk largely in the original schemes of research, even had this been merely for historical reasons (Chapter 2). Then also, the pioneer work of Gowland Hopkins on the fat-soluble vitamins was a main reason for an early concentration on nutritional problems and deficiency diseases. Situations arising indirectly from the First World War stimulated programmes on biological standardisation and on radiotherapy in malignant disease. All these fields of research, and those mentioned below, are discussed in Volume Two.

In the 1920s there was a deliberate selection of virus diseases for special attention. In the 1930s there was an important project for work on chemotherapy, although by the 1940s antibiotics had become the focus of interest in the treatment of infections. In the 1950s some of the main developments were in such basic subjects as genetics, biophysics, and molecular biology.

The evolution of research projects in some of the broad fields of medical work has been either instigated or facilitated by administrative changes. Thus, problems of the health of munition workers during the First World War heightened interest in social and industrial medicine. After the Second World War, the existence of the Public Health Laboratory Service, under the Council's wing until it became independent in 1961, opened up new opportunities for research in preventive medicine; the creation of the National Health Service helped the further development of clinical research; and attention to work in tropical medicine was greatly extended under the joint auspices of the Colonial Office (as it was) and the Council.

Although planning has in the main been strategic, it is understandable that the original Committee—with an open field before it—should have planned more closely in drawing up its first schemes of research (Volume Two). For this purpose the members of the Committee, severally or together, visited all the chief centres of medical research in the country and received reports on the needs and opportunities of various departments. It came to be recognised, however, that the glib word 'coordination' has little meaning in the field of medical science when used of research performance rather than of strategic planning; the idea that it requires great mental agility on the part of administrators and committees to keep scientific workers aware of what their fellows are doing is an illusion where research is conducted in an atmosphere of academic freedom with no barriers to discussion or publication.

Advisory boards and committees
The Council has always greatly depended on a system of committees in special fields. The more specialised branches of medical science cannot all be directly represented in the membership of the Council itself; and even the more general fields cannot, for the most part, have more than a single representative. It is therefore important to broaden the basis of expert advice. Although individual opinions are obtainable from almost any appropriate quarter, it is often desirable to have a forum in which specialised subjects can be discussed. An advisory committee need not consist wholly of specialists in the particular subject; indeed it is commonly preferable to have a few such specialists together with others who can bring their knowledge of different disciplines to bear on the problems, and perhaps others again chosen for their general wisdom or breadth of outlook.

Of these bodies, some are standing committees giving advice from time to time, on their own initiative or on questions specifically referred to them by the Council. Such a committee usually covers a particular field indicated by its title, and as a rule it has no formal terms of reference other than "to advise and assist the Council" in dealing with problems in that field. The Council periodically considers whether particular committees should be continued in being, should be reconstituted with changes in membership, or should be discharged; and to facilitate reconstitution without embarrassment, the members are commonly appointed for a stated period such as three years. Other committees, of a more temporary nature, are appointed to assist the Council in particular projects.

The members of committees are appointed by the Council, which also selects the chairman and secretary in each case. When a new committee is being set up, it is customary to appoint a chairman first and then consult him about the further membership. In appropriate circumstances, other organisations may be invited to nominate representatives. On the whole, however, members of committees serve as individual counsellors, and they commonly include members of the Council's own staff as well as experts in other employment. The members mostly serve without special remuneration.

Certain of the standing advisory bodies, because of the special importance or nature of their functions, have the status of Boards. These cover broad fields of research rather than specific subjects; and there has been a greater tendency for the Council to delegate authority to Boards than to Committees, subject only to formal approval of action recommended. These Boards, which are considered at more length in Volume Two, are (in chronological order) the Industrial Fatigue (later Health) Research Board, the Public Health Laboratory Service Board, the Clinical Research Board, the Tropical Medicine Research Board, and the Biological Research Board.

A few committees are appointed jointly by the Council and other organisations to advise on questions of common interest. Notable examples (all discussed in Volume Two) have been the Accessory Food Factors Committee appointed jointly with the Lister Institute, the Chemotherapy Committee at one time appointed jointly with the Department of Scientific and Industrial Research, and the former Colonial Medical Research Committee appointed jointly with the Colonial Office. Such a joint committee naturally advises both, or all, of its appointing bodies. The Clinical Research Board is purely advisory to the Council but nevertheless half its members are appointed in agreement with the Health Departments, and there are departmental assessors in addition. Similarly, the Tropical Medicine Research Board is appointed in agreement with the Overseas Development Administration (and formerly the Colonial Office) and has assessors from it.

Advisory boards and committees, except joint committees, form part of the domestic machinery of the Council; they have no external relations of any formal kind and do not tender advice directly to any other quarter. Nevertheless, the Council is often glad to make it clear that its actions or recommendations are based on the advice of a certain committee; and reports made to the Council by committees are frequently published as such, as the special qualifications of the members give scientific weight to the conclusions.

Methods of promoting research

Partly on lines recommended by the Departmental Committee on Tuberculosis (Chapter 2), the Medical Research Committee initially defined the main methods by which it proposed to promote research

(Chapter 3). They may here be restated in terms, not essentially different, of the practice of the present day:

1. By maintaining a central research establishment, the National Institute for Medical Research, with a whole-time permanent staff and facilities for visiting workers (Chapter 10); and, more recently, a Clinical Research Centre attached to a hospital (Volume Two).

2. By employing a research staff, mainly whole-time, for work in institutions not under the Council's own control, such staff being either placed as individuals or grouped in 'research units' and the like, sometimes with their own separate accommodation (Chapter 11).

3. By providing temporary research grants and other awards (fellowships, scholarships, studentships) for the support or assistance of individual workers not in the Council's employ; and also by providing longer-term grants to individuals as well as block grants to autonomous institutions (Chapters 12, 13).

The development of each of these methods is considered in the succeeding chapters.

Rewards as incentives?
The offer of money prizes as an incentive to discovery was never contemplated by the Committee or Council as a method of promoting research. This negative fact calls for brief notice, however, as there was at one stage some external pressure in favour of adopting the procedure; and there were historical precedents.

In 1807, Napoleon Bonaparte offered a prize of 12 000 francs, in open competition, for the best work on 'croup', a condition which had just caused the sudden death of his nephew and godson, Napoleon Louis Charles, at the age of four. Seventy-nine essays were submitted and the prize was equally divided between two authors, from Geneva and Bremen respectively; three others received honourable mention. These five essays were all published subsequently, and many of the others were presumably among the numerous treatises on the subject appearing about that time. Of this whole output the authors of the Council's monograph on *Diphtheria*, giving a fuller account of the episode, remarked that "one searches in vain for new views or even for new facts of clinical observation, well recorded".

What appears to be the only similar action ever taken by the British Government was not in implementation of any offer made beforehand. In 1802 Parliament voted £10 000 to Edward Jenner for his discovery of a successful method of vaccination against smallpox. This precedent was not followed by further awards, and of it the Medical Research Committee, in its Fifth Annual Report, said: "Its fitness is not here discussed; it is only noted that the general economic discouragement given to research in medicine is not counterbalanced by any lottery in which high stakes may occasionally be won".

There are, of course, some honorific prizes in the award of various institutions and bodies, usually endowed as memorials. Such an honour may be given substance by a money gift, or by a handsome fee for a special lecture or lectures, but the amount is seldom large. The chief exceptions are the Nobel Prizes awarded annually in physics or chemistry by the Swedish Academy of Science and in physiology or medicine by the Royal Caroline Institute in Stockholm; the very substantial value of the prizes and the truly international field of selection have made these awards famous. Such rewards are certainly not to be grudged to the outstanding research workers fortunate enough to receive them, and the Council has been gratified that many of its staff have been among the number (Volume Two). It would be naïve, however, to suppose that any research worker has ever changed his course or increased his effort in the hope of such an eventuality.

The Council, like the Committee before it, has steadfastly regarded its function as that of creating opportunities for research and of supporting work in progress by the methods already discussed. That it should, in addition, offer substantial money prizes for notable discoveries was proposed by Sir Ronald Ross to the Departmental Committee on Tuberculosis when plans were being formulated (Chapter 2); he continued to press this view on the new Committee, and on its successor Council in its early days, but it found no acceptance.

The question of research workers sharing in the profits of patentable inventions is covered in Volume Two.

Publication of results

Whatever methods may be used to promote research, the function is not fulfilled until the results of the work are made known. Ensuring publication is, therefore, an essential part of the responsibilities of the research organisation, and the Council's policy in this respect is given separate consideration (Chapter 14).

The Council's advisory role

The proposition may seem self-evident in retrospect, but there is nothing in the very early record to suggest that anyone foresaw how the public promotion of research on a national scale would almost inevitably engender the reciprocal function of bringing scientific advice readily to the government (Chapter 7). But so it proved; and the agency established for the one purpose was also well suited to the other. The original intention had clearly been to entrust the promotion of research to a body that was both expert and independent; and these attributes were likewise precisely those required in a body playing an advisory role.

In performing its primary function, the Council had necessarily to acquire detailed, up-to-date information on the interests and qualities of the research workers currently active at 'the growing points of knowledge'; and it had to gain the confidence, and possibly gratitude, of those in the front rank of relevant scientific inquiry. Thus, it was able to call upon the best advice in the country whenever it required this either for its own purposes or on the government's behalf. When more than specialised knowledge was needed, the Council itself was well constituted to give a final assessment on general scientific grounds.

Realisation of the possibilities came quite soon, and perhaps more quickly than would have happened in time of peace. In its Fifth Annual Report, covering 1918–19, the Medical Research Committee wrote:

> Experience during the war has taught the Committee, and must equally teach their successors in the new constitution, the ease with which fertile cooperation can be arranged with the scientific services of the different Government Departments in activities of the kind that will now progressively fall to the Ministry and Boards of Health. This cooperation during its development has displayed one of the most striking boons given by the original institution of the Medical Research Fund, and one hardly foreseen. A centralised department, in touch with all the scientific work at the Universities and other centres contributing to medical progress, has offered a new link with this national work and the administrative services of the country. It has allowed an effective and rapid mobilisation of any given scientific effort needed upon occasion by Government Departments. Through this mechanism an administrative department can, so to speak, lay its hand upon effective instruments or available knowledge in a manner possible no doubt before, but only possible after longer delay for inquiry and special adjustment, and open to attendant risks of disturbing or reduplicating work needed in other directions at the same time.

In the event, government departments, especially those most concerned with health, increasingly requested advice from the Council as the years passed. Sometimes the request was for a statement on the basis of existing knowledge, taking the latest findings into account. Sometimes it was for special investigation of a problem; or the Council might itself find such an investigation to be necessary before the question could be adequately answered. To arrange for such investigations has always been a recognised function of the Council (for financial implications see Chapter 15); and during both World Wars a large part of the resources of personnel and material were devoted to short-term research with immediate practical objectives (described in Volume Two).

The Council in time became well known as a body that was mainly composed of, and largely staffed by, scientific men; that was free from external administrative commitments; and that could be counted on to resist political pressure. Its pronouncements were thus accepted as impartial where those of departmental officers or committees would always be suspect in some quarters, however intrinsically sound and unbiased they might in fact be. The Council's independent position was indeed advantageous, not only to the general public interest but also to the special interests of the departments coming to the Council for advice.

Relations of this kind between the Council and the Ministry of Health, in particular, were always important (Chapter 7); they became notably close and frequent after the Second World War. Among the more important questions, for a time very much in the public eye, were recurring technical difficulties relating to the manufacture, importation, testing, and use of vaccines for prophylaxis against poliomyelitis, especially from 1954 onwards. (This and the subjects referred to in the next paragraph are discussed in Volume Two.)

Another important field was that of industrial medicine, including industrial physiology and psychology. Here a whole programme of research was undertaken largely for the assistance of the administrative department concerned—originally the Home Office, but later the Ministry of Labour—although the results were also made directly available to industry by publication. In extension of this, much help was given to the Defence Services in what was termed 'personnel research', particularly during the Second World War and immediately before and after.

The outstanding example of advice given to the Government as such, formally through the Lord President of the Council but sometimes personally to the Prime Minister himself, concerned hazards to safety and health from nuclear and other radiations. Early in 1955 there was public alarm about the possible effects of world-wide fallout from the nuclear explosions then being practised by the great powers; and this drew attention also to the risks of exposure to radiation from more ordinary sources. The Council, acting on a direct request from the Government, thereupon appointed a Committee on the Hazards to Man of Nuclear and Allied Radiations. This was a large body, composed of specialists in the appropriate branches of physical, biological, and medical science; it reported to the Council, which, in turn, reported to the Government. In addition to statements quoted publicly by Ministers, the full report of this Committee was published as a Command Paper in 1956. This was followed in 1958 by another Command Paper, in which the Committee gave its comments on a scientific report made to the General Assembly of the United Nations, and in 1960 by the Committee's own Second Report. Also issued by the Council, from 1960 onwards, was a series of short 'monitoring reports' giving the latest figures for the assay of strontium-90 in human bone in the United Kingdom. The Council was peculiarly well placed to deal with this whole subject of radiation hazards, because of the substantial organisation that it had built up for research into the value and methods of radiotherapy, and more fundamentally into the biological effects of radiations (discussed in Volume Two).

The use of animals in experimental research

The use of living animals for experiments plays a necessary part in many aspects of biomedical research, as also in the control and testing of many preparations used in the diagnosis, treatment and prophylaxis of human and animal disease. Inevitably the Council is exposed to a share of the adverse propaganda launched against so-called vivisection by those who are opposed to the use of animals in this way. (The Council has not considered itself generally responsible for countering this flow of propaganda but has left the matter mainly to the Research Defence Society, which performs the valuable task of keeping the public informed of the true facts about animal experimentation is rigorously controlled by law under the Cruelty to Animals Act 1876. Under this, the permissible purposes of Council acts with the conviction that the use of living animals for experiment is essential for the advance of biomedical research and that the practice, if under proper control as in Britain, is justifiable. This stand is taken by the Council on two main points.

Firstly, the advancement of medical knowledge is an agreed aim of public policy and the research necessary to this end inevitably entails animal experimentation. Secondly, in the United Kingdom animal experimentation is rigorously controlled by law, under the Cruelty to Animals Act 1876. Under this, the permissible purposes of experimentation are defined; places where experiments are performed must be registered and open to official inspection; the person performing an experiment must hold a licence from the Secretary of State, and additional certificates in respect of any procedures not covered by its general conditions. Among the latter is that no experiment involving pain may be performed unless the animal is kept under an anaesthetic; and that if the pain is likely to persist the animal must be killed before emerging from anaesthesia. The Act was based on the report of a Royal Commission appointed in 1875. The position was reviewed by a Royal Commission appointed in 1906 and reporting in 1913; and again by a Departmental Committee appointed by the Home Secretary in 1963 (reporting in 1965).

Although the Reports of the Council naturally contain numerous references to research work involving experiments on animals, these have rarely been the subject of any general discussion. The Report for 1922–23 includes a notable exception, in a passage relating to the part played by animal experimentation in the discovery and use of insulin:

This potent agent for the diminution of suffering is the outcome of a long series of experiments upon animals. The functions of the pancreas in the control of diabetes were first elucidated by the study of diabetes artificially inflicted upon dogs. At every subsequent stage in progress, animal experiment has been necessary, if only for the simple reason that insulin itself, the chemical composition of which is at present unknown, cannot be identified, its presence detected, or its qualities measured, without the use of an animal for test. Now that it is made available, every batch that is manufactured for the relief of sufferers must be tested upon animals for the assessment of its potency, so that the physician may know what he is giving and how much he is giving under particular conditions.

This statement may be regarded as a postscript to a memorandum presented to the Government by the Medical Research Committee in 1919, and printed as a Command Paper, in opposition to a Dogs Protection Bill introduced into the House of Commons by a private member and aimed at excluding dogs altogether from experimentation. Apart from the principle that was at stake, dogs are in fact necessary for certain types of experiment, although the numbers used are relatively small. The point was stated as follows in the memorandum mentioned above (as verbally amended in a revised edition in 1927):

> Many reasons have made it necessary, and will always make it necessary, to use dogs instead of other animals for some of this experimental work. Considerations of size are important, and in this respect the only animals giving a practicable alternative are the sheep, the pig, the goat, or the ape. The dog, unlike these animals, can be kept completely healthy and comfortable in the laboratory and in near association with man. He is not afraid of close and friendly observation. His long domestication has assimilated his natural diet to that of man. Many of his bodily structures provide the nearest approximation among available animals to those of man. The study of diet, and the collection and chemical study of the excreta, can be carried out readily in the dog, and the results of these are in the main directly applicable to the case of the man or of the child. The actions of drugs and of anaesthetics are in the main identical for the dog and the man.

The Bill failed to make progress, but similar measures were thereafter introduced with tedious frequency in one or other of the Houses of Parliament. They seldom came to a vote, but on 31 March 1925 the motion for such a Bill's second reading in the Lords was taken to a division and lost by 77 votes to 8.

In general, it is axiomatic that no scientific worker would use so complex a test system as an animal if any simpler one would meet his need. For example, greater knowledge of the constitution of vitamins has made it possible to use chemical instead of biological tests for the assay of these substances; and from the earliest days of the technique the Council has encouraged the development of tissue culture methods in place of animal tests. The large number of animals still used (especially of mice, rats and guinea-pigs for testing purposes) is accordingly a true measure of their indispensability. The provision of so many animals for laboratory purposes raises a variety of administrative and technical questions, and these have tended to become increasingly important. Moreover, the nature of many of the current purposes has created special requirements for animals conforming with definite specifications and often of particular genetic constitution. In neither numbers nor quality can such a demand be met by purchase in an uncertain market or by haphazard breeding.

The solution of this problem of supply has lain in two directions. First, there is control over the trade, a control which the Council is in a position to exercise over dealers and commercial breeders because it, together with institutions likely to follow its lead, effectively represents the laboratory market for animals. Thus, Dr W. Lane-Petter of the Council's staff was able to effect much needed improvements by identifying animal breeders who were in a position to supply well-cared-for animals in a good state of health. Secondly, there is breeding by the research laboratories themselves, to meet their own needs and possibly those of other institutions; this method has been increasingly used, at the National Institute for Medical Research and elsewhere, and is almost mandatory where special strains are required.

The Council has also taken a lead in effecting an improvement in the quality of the care given to animals awaiting experiment or undergoing prolonged observation. Both on scientific and on humanitarian grounds, test animals must be healthy and well nourished; appropriate housing and diet are important. Tending the animals must therefore be regarded as a skilled occupation, and it has for long been the Council's policy to encourage this view, and to act upon it by raising the status of such employment in its own service. Much is due to the efforts of Mr D. J. Short of the Council's staff, with other leading animal technicians inspired by him, which resulted in the formation of the Animal Technicians Association, followed by the introduction of training courses and recognised qualifications as well as by the publication of a comprehensive manual (Short & Woodnott, 1963). These steps, during the past quarter of a century, have completely altered the standard of the work.

Apart from the political aspect, the Council's chief instrument in dealing with all these matters of animal supply, breeding and management, and in undertaking relevant research work, is its Laboratory Animals Centre (originally Bureau). This was established in 1947, at first in the Council's Laboratories at Hampstead and later in those at Carshalton (Chapter 11; also Volume Two).

Chapter 10
The National Institute for Medical Research

The need for a central institute—Acquisition of a building—First staff appointments—Proposals from the Lister Institute for amalgamation—Temporary accommodation in wartime—Assembly of the original departments—Statistical Department—Direction of the Institute—Deputy Directors—Farm laboratories—Evolution of the internal organisation—Removal to Mill Hill—Major trends in the research programme—Biological standardisation and assay—World Influenza Centre—Library—Academic status

The need for a central institute

As already said, the need for a central institute had been envisaged even before the Medical Research Committee came into being (Chapter 2); and one of the Committee's first decisions was to declare such an institute (in London) to be a prime essential, and one of its first actions was to acquire premises for the purpose (Chapter 3). Yet the reasons underlying this view were never deliberately formulated at any early stage. The question can thus be approached only with some degree of hindsight, and with the present knowledge that the venture continues to justify itself by immense success.

In 1958 Sir Charles Harington, the second Director, reviewed the question in a Linacre Lecture at Cambridge; he dealt generally with the place of research institutes in medicine but largely with reference to the particular instance. In this lecture, published in full, Harington made the point that a research institute implies two things for the scientific worker within it. Firstly, he is enabled to devote his whole time to research, free from the demands of teaching duties. Secondly, he becomes part of an organisation for research, and thus subject to certain restraints in respect of his part in it. Whereas the former circumstance may be welcomed by the worker, the latter may be accepted only with some reluctance. As Harington said, "it may well be felt that original investigation must remain a purely individual intellectual activity that can only be properly pursued in conditions of complete freedom, inconsistent with any form of organisation". He believed, however, that this feeling "is based on a nostalgia for the time when the body of scientific knowledge was such that one branch at least could be fully comprehended by an individual, when techniques were simple and when the practical applications of scientific research were less urgently sought after". That era is past, and scientists as well as others must accept the conditions imposed by the more highly organised society of today; and "as time goes on the importance of the work of any one person in the total of scientific effort becomes inevitably less".

Pioneer ventures of the kind were the Institut Pasteur in Paris (1888), the Institut Robert Koch in Berlin (1891), and the Lister Institute of Preventive Medicine in London (1891; see Chapter 1). These had specialised terms of reference, chiefly related to inoculation against infective disease, although in time they broadened the basis of their work. The first general institute for medical research, from the outset without restriction of field, was the Rockefeller Institute in New York (1901). Even this had some initial bias towards the study of infectious diseases. In his history (1964), Dr George Corner refers to the original staff as "a corps of investigators chosen primarily to solve problems of infection and epidemic diseases"; and the Director for the first thirty-four years, Dr Simon Flexner, was a bacteriologist.

There can be little doubt that these notable examples influenced the Medical Research Committee. There was, further, an implied intention that a central institute should be more than a well equipped place of work with whole-time posts for a number of selected investigators. It was to be a centre, as was said in a Council memorandum of much later date, for "a collection of related disciplines, under single control, directed to a coordinated and planned purpose". The idea was to have an institute divided into departments for administrative purposes but with no barriers to working contact. The nature of many biological problems calls for attack by variable groupings of workers with different qualifications; and a research institute should be so organised as to make it easy for such groupings to be arranged, or indeed to form spontaneously. As Harington put it:

> The prerequisites are: (1) that the institute should be large enough, in the sense that the scientific staff will include men covering a sufficiently wide range of disciplines; (2) that the internal organisation should be flexible; and (3) that personal relations are such that members of the staff are willing, for a time at least, to set aside their individual preoccupations in order to collaborate with their colleagues.

There was thus justification for thinking that a new central institute could make a contribution different in kind from that attainable by reinforcing the universities in their own vital role of advancing knowledge. At the same time it was fully realised that, in promoting medical research on a national basis, a proper balance must be maintained between the two types of action (Chapter 9).

Acquisition of a building

In 1913, as already mentioned, the Committee acquired an option to purchase accommodation that seemed likely to be suitable for the purpose (Chapter 3). This was a building at Hampstead, in the northern part of London, that was being vacated by the Mount Vernon Hospital on its removal to another location. The contract for the purchase of the freehold site of $2\frac{3}{4}$ acres, comprising the hospital, a nurses' home (the original manor house of the estate), and grounds, was completed on 25 March 1914. The price was

£35 000, spread over five years (but in the event paid up in 1915).

According to the First Annual Report, "the structure of this building made it suitable for conversion into an institute for research, and its position appeared to the Committee to give it exceptional advantages in amenity and convenience". Utilisation of the building was delayed, however, by two events in 1914. First of these was the intrusion of an alternative proposal, presently to be mentioned, and next came the outbreak of the First World War.

First staff appointments

Meanwhile, the Committee had decided that the 'central institute' should comprise three departments of experimental research and one of statistics; this implied that the Statistical Department was to be part of the central institute and not a separate entity as earlier suggested. During the summer of 1914, the Committee was able to give effect to the following appointments of directors and other senior staff:

Bacteriology: Sir Almroth Wright, cb, md, frs, with Captain S. R. Douglas, mrcs (late ims)

Biochemistry and Pharmacology: H. H. Dale, md, frs, with G. Barger, dsc, and A. J. Ewins, dsc.

Applied Physiology: Leonard Hill, mb, frs, with B. Moore, dsc, frs, and M. Flack, mb

Statistics: J. Brownlee, md, d sc

For the time being, the bacteriologists continued to work in the Inoculation Department of St Mary's Hospital, London, from which they had been appointed. Dr Hill similarly remained for a time at the London Hospital Medical College, where he was joined a few months later by Dr Moore from Liverpool. Dr Dale and Dr Barger were, after the outbreak of war, given temporary quarters at the Lister Institute; so also was Dr Brownlee for a few months.

Proposals from the Lister Institute for amalgamation

In March 1914, the Committee received from the Governing Body of the Lister Institute (see Chapter 1) a suggestion that its property might, on conditions, be offered to the nation to become the central institute under the control of the Committee; incidentally, it seems to have been in this context that the title 'National Institute for Medical Research' was first suggested. The proposal was an attractive one, as the Lister Institute already had well equipped and conveniently situated premises of a suitable kind, with a distinguished scientific staff; and it had an established reputation in the world of medical research. A further attraction was added by the generous offer of Lord Iveagh to provide, at his own expense, a research hospital of fifty beds, to be built on a site next to the Lister Institute and transferred as part of the property. The Committee was therefore most willing to enter into negotiations, in spite of its commitment to the Hampstead site; it was believed that the latter could, if necessary, be disposed of without loss—but one idea was that it might be used as a research hospital, with clinical laboratories attached.

A detailed plan of amalgamation was worked out between the Governing Body of the Lister Institute and the Committee; and later this received ministerial approval, after consultation with the Advisory Council. Among other points, the large majority of the Lister Institute staff was to be given continued employment, mostly in an additional Department of Experimental Pathology to be directed by Dr C. J. (later Sir Charles) Martin; and two members of the existing Governing Body were to be added to the Committee, their successors being appointed by the Minister on the nomination of the Council of the Royal Society.

Ultimately, when all seemed to have been agreed between the responsible parties, the recommendation of the Governing Body of the Lister Institute failed to obtain the constitutionally necessary support of the ordinary members at a meeting on 18 November 1914. Whether the matter would have been further pursued, but for the war that had by then broken out, it is now impossible to say. In fact, the negotiations were never reopened, and soon after the war the increasing commitment to the Hampstead site made any such course permanently impracticable. Nonetheless, many forms of friendly cooperation have continued throughout the years between the Lister Institute on the one hand and the Committee and its successor Council on the other. Five successive Directors of the Lister Institute have had periods of service as members of the Council.

As a fuller account of these negotiations can be found in the First Annual Report of the Committee, it is unnecessary to go into greater detail here. Nevertheless, those who know the National Institute and its record may be allowed to smile at Sir Rickman Godlee's complacent comment in 1917: "The view of those who hold that official red-tape strangles original research prevails; and the [Lister] Institute has escaped the fate of being merged in a Government Department"—evidently, one of those fates worse than death!

Temporary accommodation in wartime

Meanwhile, war had broken out on 4 August 1914 and the Committee offered the Hampstead building to the War Office for use as a hospital. As the Hampstead Military Hospital it was the site of work on disordered action of the heart ('soldier's heart') by Dr Thomas Lewis, with which the Committee was closely concerned (Chapter 11). In 1917 these investigations were transferred to Colchester, where Captain Lewis continued the work, and the building at Hampstead became the Central Hospital for Flying Officers, at which other work of special interest to the Committee was done until 1919.

The indefinite postponement of occupation of the building made it necessary to extend the arrangements for temporary accommodation. The Department of Bacteriology remained at St Mary's Hospital, but its staff was in fact doing much of its work in an Army laboratory at No. 13 General Hospital, Boulogne. Among other things, there was an agreement that the Committee should pay St Mary's at the rate of £2500 per annum for twenty-five research beds at the disposal of Sir Almroth Wright; this remained in force until 1917.

The Department of Biochemistry and Pharmacology was accommodated at the Lister Institute. The Department of Applied Physiology also came to the Lister Institute, from the London Hospital, in 1917. After a few months at the Lister Institute, the Statistical Department occupied a rented house at 34 Guilford Street, Bloomsbury, near the location of its main wartime work in the basement of the British Museum (Volume Two).

The fact that the several departments developed in isolation during their first six years had an effect, as will be noted, that lasted for some time after they were eventually brought physically together at Hampstead in 1920.

Assembly of the original departments
The reconditioning of the Hampstead building was a responsibility of HM Office of Works, which also undertook the task of equipping it for its intended purpose. The building had been released in June 1919 and was ready for full occupation in April 1920. The four Departments could then for the first time be assembled under one roof; the question of an associated research hospital had meanwhile been solved in another way (Chapter 11). In its Report for 1920–21 the Council first definitely used the title 'National Institute for Medical Research', incidentally mentioned six years earlier; the provisional term 'central institute' had clearly no validity in a wider context.

The Department of Bacteriology came without its original Director, Sir Almroth Wright, in circumstances mentioned below; Dr (later Sir) Alexander Fleming, who had joined the staff temporarily during the war, also remained at St Mary's Hospital, where he was later to make his fame. The second-in-command, Captain S. R. Douglas (late Indian Medical Service), was made Acting Director of the Department in the first instance and was later confirmed as its Director. There was also Dr Leonard Colebrook, another of Wright's men who had joined the staff temporarily during the war, but most of his subsequent career with the Council lay outside the Institute (Chapter 11). The Department was brought up to strength by several new senior appointments, made either immediately or within the next few years—Dr W. E. Gye, Clifford Dobell (protistologist), Dr P. P. (later Sir Patrick) Laidlaw, and Dr (later Sir) Percival Hartley; of these, more is said in Volume Two.

The Department of Biochemistry and Pharmacology also arrived without some of its original staff; but Dr Dale (who had been Director of the Wellcome Physiological Laboratories for ten years before joining the staff in 1914) was fortunately still at its head. Dr Barger went to a university chair, and Dr Ewins had already taken a research post in the pharmaceutical industry. The new senior recruits were Dr H. W. Dudley (biochemist) and Dr Harold King (organic chemist), both of whom did very distinguished work although the former's career was cut short by an untimely death.

The head of the Department of Applied Physiology, Dr (later Sir) Leonard Hill, had made a reputation by distinguished research in pure physiology. During his time at the Institute he was mainly occupied with practical problems of ventilation and heating, and this programme failed to attract recruits of adequate scientific calibre to provide for a succession. (He was given to inventing gadgets that integrated recordings of different environmental and physiological factors, and one of these he regrettably christened the 'comfimeter'; it was said, however, that he introduced this term into his reports to the Council solely to annoy the Secretary—which it never failed to do.) The second-in-command, Dr Benjamin Moore, soon left to take a university chair of biochemistry; and so the early death of the third original member, Dr Martin Flack, meant that there was nobody left to succeed Hill on his retirement, as the interests of Dr R. B. Bourdillon, who had meanwhile been appointed to the Department by the Council, lay in another direction. Work on heating and ventilation, however, was continued in a research unit accommodated elsewhere (Chapter 11); and later on a Division of Human Physiology was recreated at the Institute, in the first instance to deal with problems referred to the Council from the Army after the Second World War. The tradition set by Hill was thus continued.

The Statistical Department, being independent of laboratory services, was the first to move in, at the end of 1919, together with the Council's Publications Section (Dr Edgar H. J. Schuster) and the beginnings of the Library. Of the Statistical Department's short period of inclusion within the Institute something is said below.

The four original departments were in 1919 augmented by a small additional one of Applied Optics, which much later developed into a Division of Biophysics. This was created to utilise the abilities of a remarkable man, James Edwin Barnard, who not only gave his services on an honorary basis but brought with him costly apparatus that was his private property. His development of optical methods, particularly the ultraviolet microscope (forerunner of the electron microscope), was of great value to his colleagues engaged in virus research. Although not a scientist by training, he became a Fellow of the Royal Society. He was, in fact, the proprietor of a men's hat shop in Jermyn Street, where he spent his mornings before going to Hampstead for the afternoon, a transition facilitated by his habit of lunching only on alternate days.

E

Statistical Department

The original fourth method of promoting research was the maintenance of a statistical department. The concept, as expressed in the first "Scheme of Research" in 1913 (Chapter 3), was that of a permanent staff engaged in "all statistical investigations useful either as preliminary to research or confirmatory of its results". These were to include "enquiries relating to diet, occupation, habits of life and other matters bearing upon the incidence of disease". Another function was to "collect and deal with all types of vital statistics", including particularly those with an epidemiological bearing. This concept was linked with another, never so clearly formulated, of an Information Bureau, to which further reference is made later (Chapter 14).

It seemed to be implied that a statistical department of this kind would play a major role in showing where the problems lay, and perhaps later in providing a basis for measuring the progress of research in terms of practical application. This would explain the special status then accorded to it. In the event, the department did make important investigations of the kind envisaged; but it was never called upon to advise or assist in the planning of research over a wide field, and any idea that it should do so was probably impracticable.

Whatever may have been the original thought, the Committee came to see the functions of a statistical department as being: (*a*) to undertake statistical research into problems of epidemiology and the like, and (*b*) to advise and assist other research workers in applying statistical treatment to a wide variety of data. Such a department could well be provided either as a division of the Institute or as a unit of external staff; both these forms were adopted in turn.

Brownlee had latterly been Physician Superintendent of Ruchill Hospital, Glasgow, where there is now a laboratory named in his honour. He was a disciple of Karl Pearson and one of the pioneers in applying statistical methods to medical problems. He was a widower, a kindly man and a genius; he had various foibles that endeared him all the more to his friends. He set store by his "administrative principles", one of which appeared to be never to answer letters—well, hardly ever. He had an endless flow of talk displaying a wide variety of knowledge.

A Statistical Department in charge of this wayward genius met the practical requirement only in part. Brownlee considered it to be his function to devote himself to original research almost to the exclusion of giving advisory help to other workers. Fortunately, the opportunity arose of placing another statistical team alongside. This was headed by Dr Major Greenwood, who was statistical Medical Officer on the staff of the Ministry of Health but worked at the Lister Institute; by arrangement with the Ministry, he was moved in 1920 to the National Institute and was there provided by the Council with additional assistance. In this way a useful collaboration began, the Council having the services of two distinguished experts and their respective staffs; and for consultative purposes Greenwood was "the key that unlocked Brownlee's mind". The arrangement was rationalised by the establishment of a Statistical Committee under Greenwood's chairmanship, with Brownlee among the members. The Statistical Department was discontinued as a separate entity after Brownlee's death in 1927, and the two staffs were merged in what later became the Council's Statistical Research Unit, with Greenwood as Honorary Director.

Direction of the Institute
It was at an early stage intended that the Institute should have an overall Director; and this would seem to have been an essential condition both of administrative efficiency and of successful functioning as an integrated organisation for research. On 22 October 1913, as already noted, the Medical Research Committee minuted that "at the head of all these [departments] should be a Chief Director who should be the best man obtainable at any price"; and at an adjourned meeting next day, that Sir Almroth Wright was considered to be "the only man satisfying the requirements of such a post". On 30 April 1914, moreover, it was significantly minuted that Sir Almroth Wright should have first refusal of the tenancy of Mount Vernon House. This was the original manor house but needed reconversion from its latter use as a nurses' home. It in fact became the official residence of successive Directors; and so it remains at the present time, even with the main Institute some miles away at Mill Hill.

Soon afterwards, however, the Committee apparently changed its view. On 27 May 1914, Sir Almroth Wright was formally offered "engagement on their permanent staff for research in bacteriology"; and on 24 June he was given explicit assurance that the appointment carried the directorship of the Bacteriological Department at the Institute. Meanwhile he had written referring to an alleged promise that if it were decided to appoint a Chief Director he would have a lien on the post. On 16 July he was informed that it had been decided that no such post would be created; that the Institute would comprise the scientific departments, with a research hospital as soon as possible, and also the office of the Secretary. The Directors would have equal status, each responsible to the Committee. Domestic affairs would be in the hands of a staff committee, consisting of the Directors and the Secretary; and of this Wright was invited to become chairman.

In principle this was a retrograde decision. The record is discreet about the underlying reasons, but one may readily surmise that personal considerations were largely involved. Perusal of the correspondence and minutes conveys the impression that the Committee was finding it very difficult to deal with this eminent scientist as a man of affairs. In the negotiations over appointment to the staff he was exacting in his personal demands about conditions of service; and the Committee's refusals on various points led to further argument. He also never ceased to maintain that he and the other departmental heads should have seats on the Committee. He also claimed the power of direction over all external workers in bacteriology supported by the Committee, unless these were in fact under local directors who were themselves of high standing. His expressed opinions indeed extended to the Committee's general conduct of its affairs; thus, on 21 January 1914, just before Dr Fletcher was appointed: "I think that there should be no Secretary in the sense of a superior officer who administers in the name of or under instruction of the Governing Committee"—and he reiterated this view five years later. It would thus scarcely be surprising if the Committee had come to feel that Wright was not the man to represent it as single chief of its central establishment.

Wright has been described as a large bear-like man, a dominating personality and aggressive in disputation; withal, he had an undoubted capacity for inspiring intense loyalty in his assistants, of whom some themselves became eminent. He was a friend of George Bernard Shaw, and is generally accepted as having been the prototype of the character Sir Colenso Didgeon in the latter's play *The Doctor's Dilemma*. He was already a man of great scientific reputation when he joined the staff. "Almroth" was the maiden name of his mother, a Swede who was one of Florence Nightingale's volunteer nurses at Scutari in 1854; her father, Nils Almroth, enjoyed the honour of being a Knight of the North Star. Further references to Wright's views are made later (Chapters 13, 17).

One can sense that after the war it was not without relief that the Committee received, in March 1919, Sir Almroth Wright's request to be allowed, on terms, to remain at St Mary's Hospital. This was certainly accepted with alacrity, as Wright's letter was written and sent by hand on the morning of the Committee's meeting on 14 March 1919, and the reply was posted in the evening of the same day. He was given what might nowadays be called a 'golden handshake', in the form of a personal research grant of whole-time dimensions supplementing his relatively small salary as Director of the Inoculation Department of the Hospital; this arrangement continued until he was 66 years of age. Thus, for a dozen years Wright was either employed or largely paid by the Committee or Council; the fact needs to be stated, because Wright himself avoided public acknowledgement of this support and his biographers have tended to follow in minimising the connection (Colebrook, 1954; Cope, 1966).

Wright's departure left open no easy choice of an overall Director. The most suitable of the departmental heads was clearly Dr Dale; but he was also the most junior in years. The Council accordingly continued to rely on the expedient of treating the departments as separate entities, each head being directly responsible to the Council. For the administration of the building as a whole, and of its common services, the Secretary of the Council was at first represented on the spot by an Assistant Secretary appointed for the purpose. This arrangement had worked while the building was still in process of conversion and equipment, but proved to be unsatisfactory under conditions of full occupation. In 1923 the compromise was adopted of having a Committee of Directors jointly responsible to the Council in all general matters, with an administrative officer under them. Dr Dale was chairman of this body and exercised in practice many of the functions of a Director. In time, the retirement of senior colleagues made it possible to dispense with this formula.

In 1928 Dr Dale, while retaining charge of his own department, was accordingly appointed by the Council to be Director of the Institute (the title 'Director-in-Chief' never had wide currency). From this date the full integration of the Institute began, and in the fourteen years of Dale's tenure of office it developed greatly in strength and reputation. His own laboratory, in particular, attracted highly qualified investigators from all over the world to spend periods of voluntary work alongside the regular staff. His many personal honours, then or afterwards, included a Nobel Prize (1936), the Order of Merit (1944), and election as President of the Royal Society (which had already awarded him the Copley Medal). His term as Director included the planning of a new and larger Institute at Mill Hill; but the advent of another war baulked the Council of their hope that he would still be in office when the move took place. He retired in 1942, and afterwards served for a term as a member of Council and for much longer helped it in many ways. His ninetieth birthday, in 1965, was widely celebrated; his speech at the principal banquet, at which he was to have been guest of honour, was all the more remarkable for being delivered by the sound-track of a cinematograph film showing him sitting up in bed with a bandaged head, the result of his having fallen down a flight of stairs a few days beforehand. Dale continued to be active as Director of the Royal Institution for a time, and as Chairman of the Wellcome Trustees, before retiring completely. He died at Cambridge on 23 July 1968, aged 93, and was commemorated by a service in Westminster Abbey. There is an admirable and extensive biographical memoir by Professor W. S. Feldberg.

In choosing Dale's successor the Council decided, after much heartsearching, that a medical qualification was not essential in a post concerned solely with the laboratory branches of science subserving medicine; and that it was indeed undesirable to limit the field of selection by imposing any restriction in this respect. The appointment was given to a distinguished biochemist, Professor C. R. (later Sir Charles) Harington, FRS, who had already served as a member of Council but not previously on its staff. Although not himself a medical man, his personal research work had been in the basic field of medicine—notably on the hormone of the thyroid gland (thyroxine). He had held appointments in the Universities of Edinburgh and London, in the latter becoming not only professor of chemical pathology at University College Hospital Medical

School but eventually head of its whole department of pathology, which included also the professors of morbid anatomy and of bacteriology. He became a Royal Medallist of the Royal Society in 1944.

In Harington's twenty years as Director, the National Institute continued to develop, and more than ever as an integrated entity. Early in his time came the removal to Mill Hill. When he retired from the post of Director in 1962, he became attached to the head-quarters of the Council as a scientific adviser, and for a time acted as Second Secretary (Chapter 17).

Harington was succeeded as Director by another non-medical biologist, Professor P. B. (later Sir Peter) Medawar, who had held the Chair of Zoology and Comparative Anatomy at University College London. Medawar had for long been doing biological research work, at Oxford and in London, with direct bearing on medical problems. He had received a Royal Medal of the Royal Society and a Nobel Prize in Medicine (1960). For reasons of health he retired from the post in 1971, for less exacting work with the Council, and was succeeded by Professor A. S. V. Burgen, who had held the Chair of Pharmacology in the University of Cambridge and had been Honorary Director of the Council's Molecular Pharmacology Unit.

Deputy Directors
A post of Deputy Director of the Institute was not created until 1930, and it was in abeyance from 1940 to 1948. It was successively held by a number of departmental heads: Captain S. R. Douglas (1930–36), Sir Patrick Laidlaw (1936–40), Dr A. A. (later Sir Ashley) Miles (1948–52), Dr C. H. (later Sir Christopher) Andrewes (1952–61), and Dr J. H. Humphrey (from 1961).

Of the two early Deputy Directors, Captain (late Indian Medical Service) Stewart Ranken Douglas died in 1936, shortly before he was due to retire. He had joined the Council's staff in 1914 with Sir Almroth Wright, whom he eventually succeeded as head of the largest department of the Institute. Of him the Council said, in its report for 1935–36:

> He was able to follow his own natural instinct for friendly and unobtrusive co-operation, to maintain a wide contact with general progress in the fields in which his colleagues were occupied, and to give full play to his real genius for encouragement and for quietly lubricating the wheels of collaboration. There was no item in the programme of work on the pathological side of the Institute's activities, and no success achieved there as a result of these researches, which did not owe much to his long and varied practical experience and to his wise judgement.

Socially one remembers him as a genial companion, fond of the good things of life.

Sir Patrick Playfair Laidlaw died suddenly in 1940 at the age of 59, after eighteen years at the Institute. The Council said in its Report for 1939–45:

He was one of the greatest investigators in medical research of our time, and to mention the chief discoveries with which he was associated gives but a partial idea of the wide influence he exerted in his subject; . . . [he had] great ability and knowledge, with an exceptional command of laboratory technique in many branches of medical research.

He was a quiet, unassuming man, notable for his readiness to help other research workers who might be in difficulties over their problems—and self-effacing to a fault with regard to his share in the outcome. He is best known for his distinguished work on viruses, notably those of distemper in dogs and influenza.

In its Report for 1939–45 the Council referred to the deaths of Sir Patrick Laidlaw and Sir Thomas Lewis, and to the retirement of Sir Henry Dale, in these words:

As the question of attracting the best brains to scientific work in the Government service is so important that various official committees have been sitting and reporting on it continuously in recent times, it is worthy of note that three such men as Laidlaw, Lewis and Dale, of the highest international fame in medical research, gave their best years, with an average period of a quarter of a century, to the service of the Medical Research Council and the predecessor Committee.

Farm laboratories

A minute of 30 October 1913 reaffirmed the Committee's view that the central institute should be in London itself, but with a rider considering the possible later purchase of a country house with grounds in which further buildings could be erected. It was thus envisaged from an early stage that the resources of an institute in an urban area would need to be augmented by farm laboratories. These would provide opportunities for work with large animals, when required, and also for breeding stocks of small animals under spacious conditions and for growing some of the food. Implementation of this policy was delayed by the First World War; but it will be seen later that in 1918 the Committee was able to set aside £7000 for the capital cost (Chapter 15).

Early in 1919 the Committee minuted that there was an urgent need for a breeding and standardisation establishment, as an annexe to the Institute; some possibilities were investigated, but no purchase resulted. It was not until the summer of 1922 that the Council was able to buy, for £6000, a property at Mill Hill known as 'Rhodes Farm'. This site, six miles further out than Hampstead to the north-west of London, then comprised 39 acres of agricultural land, much of it steeply sloping, without any substantial buildings; it had a frontage of about 900 feet to a road called The Ridgeway. The surroundings were at that time relatively rural, but have since undergone much development as a residential area. A plot of about 6 acres on the east side of the property was almost immediately leased to the Imperial Cancer Research Fund as a site for new laboratories. This lease was surrendered to the Council in 1934 in return for a longer one of an adjoining estate of 8 acres and a large house then

known as 'Burton Bank', which the Council had just bought for
£8300, thus extending the whole property eastwards to another road
frontage.

The farm laboratories (sometimes called field laboratories) were
from the beginning treated as part of the organisation of the National
Institute, and the Veterinary Superintendent was responsible to the
Director (or, at first, the Committee of Directors). A small ancillary
staff was also resident, but the research workers came out from
Hampstead as necessary.

The cost of developing the site had to be met by the Council out
of current income, and only cheap wooden buildings could at first be
afforded. Further wooden buildings were later erected for the
research programme on canine distemper. The first more permanent
structures were a house for the Superintendent and a small laboratory
that was for a time used by Dr W. E. Gye and J. E. Barnard for their
work on chicken sarcoma. A more substantial one was the Clark
Building, put up in 1932 at the charge of a benefaction (Chapter 16),
as a breeding house for small animals. Generally speaking, there was
a gradual replacement of the original wooden buildings by others of
a more durable and more pleasing type.

An important addition was the Nutrition Building, completed in
1940. This was a long, low series of laboratory and animal rooms,
incorporating also a minute residential flat, which was put up in the
first place to fulfil the Council's promise to Dr (later Sir) Edward
Mellanby, when he accepted appointment as Secretary in 1933, that
he would be given facilities for continuing his personal research work.

Evolution of the internal organisation
In its report for 1919–20 the Council said:

> The several departments which during the war have been geographically
> isolated in temporary quarters provided elsewhere are now brought together in
> accordance with the original design of the Committee. The expected advantages
> of this close association of workers in the different technical branches of research
> have already been realised; daily intercourse between bacteriologists and bio-
> chemists, between physiologists and statisticians, or of other kinds, has given
> abundant opportunity for the exchange of intellectual stimulus or of technical
> help, and the Council look forward with confidence to the fruit of this free
> association between men of different minds engaged in different methods of
> work.

It was, however, not until the appointment of Dale as overall
Director in 1928 that the process of full integration gathered
momentum. Looking back in 1963, he wrote of the early days from
the Institute's point of view:

> One steady source of encouragement, of which we were all fully aware, was the
> broadminded policy of successive Councils, with their distinguished Secretaries
> and administrative staff, in assuring for us so continuous a freedom of oppor-
> tunity, and in their generous appreciation of our efforts. And I believe that all
> of us would have given a special place, among the many reasons for our grati-

tude, to the readiness shown by the Council and its staff so to modify the administrative pattern of the Institute, in the light of experience, as to enable us eventually to pass it to our successors, as still, indeed, a young and immature, but already a vigorously viable and intimately cooperative organism.

His successor, while still Director in 1949, stressed the advantages of a flexible internal organisation for securing cooperation in research. The programme of work on viruses served as an example; and Harington explained how the cooperation was brought about:

It is perfectly clear that the field of scientific effort covered by the research as a whole has been so wide that no man unaided could have made much progress. On the other hand, at the outset of the investigation it was quite impossible to predict the devious paths which would have to be followed and the different branches of science into which excursions would have to be made. In these circumstances the course which was actually followed seems to have been the best, the essential feature being readiness at all times to extend the investigation in any desired direction by the addition of the help of an appropriate worker. In this way there is in fact ultimately formed a team of investigators whose efforts are all generally directed to the same end; but the team is never rigidly defined; it grows only in response to the demands of the work, and the individual members retain a considerable degree of scientific independence and scope for initiative.

The evolution of the scientific organisation of the Institute towards greater flexibility involved a replacement of the original main departments by more numerous small 'divisions', each with a senior worker as its head. These divisions represented groupings of staff that had no essential permanence but met the needs of the current programme, placing the available personnel to the best advantage. Regrouping was relatively simple; and divisions changed their designations to match shifts of emphasis in their scientific interests. Like organic evolution, this process is still going on.

As has been seen, the original Departments were Bacteriology, Biochemistry and Pharmacology, Applied Physiology, and Statistics, to which was added the Department of Applied Optics in 1919. Statistics ceased to be a department of the Institute in 1927; and the Department of Applied Physiology was dissolved in 1928. The Department of Bacteriology changed its title more than once, to acknowledge the inclusion of workers in Experimental Pathology and Protistology. A Department of Biological Standards was interdigitated in an informal way from 1920 onwards; it had at first no senior members other than its Director (see below).

The Report for 1930–31 gives a consolidated list of the scientific staff at the Institute, under departmental headings. These then were: Physiology, Pharmacology and Biochemistry; Experimental Pathology and Bacteriology; Microscopy and Physical Methods; and Biological Standards. In the following year a new Department, Physiology of Sex Hormones, was added when Dr A. S. (later Sir) Alan Parkes joined the staff; but afterwards this was treated as a

E*

subdepartment of Endocrinology (later to become the Division of Experimental Biology). The accession of Parkes and his associates to the Institute's staff in 1932 followed a meeting held at the Institute under the auspices of the Health Committee of the League of Nations. This was attended by leaders from different countries in the developing science of the oestrogenic hormones and their chemistry; Dale was chairman, with Parkes as secretary. The latter has given an amusing description of the meeting in his book *Sex, Science and Society*.

During the period 1930–36 there was a progressive regrouping into two main departments, headed respectively by the Director (Dale) and the Deputy Director (Douglas) of the Institute. Within the Department of Physiology, Pharmacology and Biochemistry there was a Subdepartment of Endocrinology; and within the Department of Experimental Pathology and Bacteriology there were Subdepartments of Protistology and of Microscopy and Physical Methods (formerly Applied Optics). The Department of Biological Standards continued to have its special relationship with the others. All this represented a step towards greater integration, the main dichotomy implying no barrier.

After the end of the war, in 1945, Harington introduced a more decentralised pattern of ten divisions: Biochemistry; Chemotherapy (Chemical); Chemotherapy (Biological); Physiology and Pharmacology; Applied Physiology; Endocrinology; Bacteriology and Virus Research; Protistology; Biophysics and Physical Chemistry; and Biological Standards. The names of successive heads of divisions are given in an appendix to Volume Two.

Subsequent changes reflect reorientations in parts of the research programme. By 1948, Endocrinology had become Experimental Biology; Biophysics and Physical Chemistry had become Biophysics and Optics; and Applied Physiology had dropped out. By 1950, Protistology had also gone, but new Divisions of Human Physiology, of Physical Chemistry, and of Bacterial Chemistry had been formed, in the last case through absorption of the formerly external Bacterial Chemistry Research Unit (Chapter 11); this brought the number to eleven.

By 1953, an Instrument Division had been recognised. By 1954, Chemotherapy (Chemical) had become Organic Chemistry (later simply Chemistry), and Chemotherapy (Biological) therefore simply Chemotherapy. By 1955, Bacterial Chemistry had become Bacterial Physiology, and the Instrument Division the Engineering Division. By 1958, a Division of Immunology had been added; by 1959, a Laboratory Animals (later simply Animals) Division had been recognised; by 1960, Biophysics and Optics had become simply Biophysics. By 1961, Chemotherapy had become Chemotherapy and Parasitology; a Laboratory (later Division) of Cytopathology and a Laboratory of Human Biomechanics had been added; and Biological Standards had been supplemented by a Division of Immunological Products Control (see below).

By 1965 the Common Cold Research Unit near Salisbury had been recognised as a separate division instead of as an annexe of Bacteriology and Virus Research; it had always been part of the Institute's organisation, and never an external research unit in the usual sense (Chapter 11), but in 1967 responsibility for it was transferred to the new Clinical Research Centre (Volume Two). In 1965, also, Bacterial Physiology became Microbiology; Bacteriology and Virus Research became Virology and Bacteriology; Chemotherapy and Parasitology became simply Parasitology; and a Division of Biomedical Engineering was set up.

In 1967 a Laboratory for Field Physiology was added, and in the following year one for Physical Biochemistry. In 1969 a Genetics Division and a Developmental Biology Division were established, these being regarded as central to a programme framed by Sir Peter Medawar after he became Director of the Institute. Also in 1969 a Laboratory for Leprosy and Mycobacterial Research was established.

Removal to Mill Hill

Inevitably, as one can now see, the building at Hampstead became in time too small for the expanding needs of the Institute; but two things helped to stave off a crisis. Firstly, some rooms had been released for other purposes by the departure of the statisticians, mentioned above. Secondly, further space became available in the main block when all animals were removed to the new Ronan Building alongside, in 1929. This last had been designed specially as an animal house and was connected with the main building by bridges at different levels. Maxwell Ayrton was the architect; and the cost, about £18 000, was provided from the Ronan benefaction (Chapter 16). To many contemporary eyes this annexe was more pleasing than the original Victorian building (although the architect of that had, in his day, received a medal for it). The addition, however, did not escape objection by neighbours. One of these was Mr Ramsay Macdonald, about to become Prime Minister for the second time, who wrote to the press in January 1929 protesting that the building was an 'atrocity'; the effect of this was somewhat diminished by photographs showing that the scarcely completed structure was as yet shrouded in scaffolding.

Of the Ronan Building, the Council optimistically said in its Report for 1928–29:

Its completion now brings the National Institute as a whole, including the associated Farm Laboratories at Mill Hill, to a stage of development at which the Council have been aiming from the beginning, and it can now be expected to provide all the main requirements for the research work centralised here that can be foreseen for a long period of years.

In fact the problem of providing additional space became acute as soon as 1936, with the Council's decision to embark on a new major programme of research on chemotherapy. There were cogent reasons for placing this work at the Institute, beside its existing chemical and bacteriological laboratories and with access to its general facilities. Funds were available, and could be used in the first instance for the cost of building (Chapter 15). Only a site was lacking.

The possibilities of placing additional buildings on the Hampstead estate were thoroughly explored, but the conclusion was inescapable that the property was unsuited to further major development. Moreover, the main building, constructed as a hospital in 1890 and never perfectly meeting the requirements of a research institute, was already of some age—and is in fact now near the end of its useful life.

A drastic decision thus became necessary: no addition was to be made to the capital stake in the Hampstead property, but an entirely new and larger Institute was to be erected on a different site. This building would be designed especially for its purpose and would be large enough to house all the existing activities at Hampstead, plus a chemotherapy department, with some margin for further expansion. The proposal received ministerial approval, and in due course the Treasury provided funds for the capital expenditure (Chapter 15).

Inquiries were made about possible sites, almost inevitably further from the centre of London but desirably in the same northwesterly direction; one rural site was in fact inspected. In the end, however, it was decided to build on the Council's own land at Mill Hill, where the Institute would have its Field Laboratories immediately around it and would still not be too far from the centre of London. This solution may in retrospect seem to have been obvious, but the lie of the land was at first thought to be an obstacle. The property was of ample extent, but the favourable building site was a relatively narrow strip fronting the road appropriately named The Ridgeway. Behind this the land fell steeply to lower ground in the bottom of the valley; and this ground was somewhat inaccessible by road and below the level of main drainage. The Council was, however, advised by HM Office of Works that the apparent difficulty could be overcome.

Indeed, when Maxwell Ayrton was appointed as architect he said that he regarded the configuration of the ground not as an obstacle but as a challenge. In his first design, a series of blocks was arranged continuously in the form of a hexagon—which the scientists predictably dubbed "the benzene ring". On this plan, what was the ground floor at the front had an increasing number of storeys below it towards the back. This design was eventually discarded, but something of it still remains in the one actually adopted.

In the eventual structure, there is an oblong main block parallel to the frontage, and at each end of this two wings diverge obliquely in Y-formation. The central block rises seven storeys above ground-level; the wings rise only three storeys above the level at the frontage, but those running downhill have additional (and well illuminated) floors below as in the earlier design. Backwards from the middle of the centre block extends the Fletcher Memorial Hall, at ground floor level, with the main store in its basement. The furnishings and equipment of the Hall, which can be used both for scientific meetings and for social occasions, were provided in part from the fund subscribed in memory of the first Secretary of the Council, Sir Walter Fletcher, whose posthumous bust by Miss Dora Clarke stands in the foyer.

A nowadays unusual characteristic is that, to reduce vibration from large high-speed centrifuges or the like, the building has no steel frame; the brick walls actually bear the weight and are therefore immensely thick at the bottom. There are many other special devices that resulted from close consultation between the architect and the prospective users; no trouble was spared to make the building fit its purpose. A noticeable architectural feature, incorporated for sound practical reasons, is the copper sheeting on the sloping roof of the central block.

Construction began in 1937, and it was hoped that occupation might be possible within three or four years. Again, as in 1914, fulfilment was deferred by the outbreak of war; when this occurred on 3 September 1939 the building was as yet only a shell. Again, also, the building was to be made available for emergency purposes, although it was not until 1942 that a use was found for it; the Council then lent it to the Admiralty, which completed it for temporary occupation as a training establishment for the Women's Royal Naval Service. So until 1945 the future National Institute for Medical Research flew the White Ensign as one of His Majesty's ships, with a 'quarterdeck', a 'fo'c'sle', and 'cabins', while the Wrens housed there went on 'shore leave' and 'came on board'. An unconnected circumstance of war was the probably groundless apprehension of local residents that so conspicuous a building might attract enemy bombers to the neighbourhood, but a proposal to ruin the appearance of the building by pointlessly applying an indelible 'dazzle' camouflage was happily averted.

The building was handed back to the Council in 1945, but the work of completing it for its intended purpose was beset by many frustrations, arising from the aftermath of war; not only were there delays over materials and difficulties over labour, but financial control was constantly being stultified by rapid rises in costs—to an extent that caught the attention of the Committee on Public Accounts (Chapter 15). There was the further complication that important changes had to be made in the internal layout to meet previously unforeseen requirements, including new research techniques that had been developed in the interval.

Eventually, the work was sufficiently near completion for the Institute to begin moving from Hampstead to Mill Hill on 20 November 1949. The removal, spread over nearly two months, was in itself a considerable operation in logistics, which needed elaborate planning and in the event worked smoothly. An opening ceremony was performed on 5 May 1950 by HM King George VI, accompanied by HM the Queen, in the Fletcher Memorial Hall.

The total working space in the building was approximately 90 000 square feet, excluding the Hall and the stores beneath it. The laboratories for various subjects were mainly on the first and second floors (and later on the third floor of the central block, which was for a time left undeveloped). The accommodation for experimental animals was on the first and second floors of the north-west and south-west wings. In addition to some laboratories, the ground floor housed the administrative offices, conference room, and instrument shop; and the lower ground floor held engineering services and stores. The fourth floor and its mezzanine, in the central block, were devoted to the library, the fifth floor to the canteen, and the sixth floor attics to club-rooms for staff.

The building was heated by hot-water floor panels supplied from oil-fired boilers. The illumination was mostly by fluorescent lights. The services to the laboratories included pressure-water, steam, compressed air, and direct current electrical supply of various voltages. There were numerous hot and cold rooms. Various ancillary buildings, old and new, stood on adjacent parts of the site. Other works have since been added, including two monkey-houses capable between them of holding some 800 animals, and also an insectarium. A very recent major expansion has provided room for two new divisions, much increased animal accommodation of modern design, and improved general amenities; this involved conversion of the fifth floor of the main building and construction of a new 'north building' as an extension.

The old Hampstead building was not given up by the Council as had originally been intended, but was instead retained to provide accommodation, then very difficult to obtain, for some of the growing number of research units (Chapter 11); for this purpose it was renamed 'Medical Research Council Laboratories, Hampstead', but one division of the Institute still occupied part of the building. In the course of time the various units were disbanded or moved, and the vacated space was taken up by the expanding needs of the Institute itself.

At Mill Hill the Council acquired, with funds of private origin, a few houses close to the Institute, for letting to members of the staff. A block comprising fourteen flats has been acquired at Hampstead for letting to visiting workers who come from a distance to work at the Institute and have great difficulty in obtaining temporary accommodation.

The Nutrition Building at Mill Hill, of which the origin has already been mentioned, has until recently continued to be regarded as 'extraterritorial' in relation to the Institute. When Sir Edward Mellanby retired from the Secretaryship of the Council in 1949, he and Lady Mellanby retained their occupation of the laboratory and he was free to give his whole time to research. It was actually in the garden of the laboratory that he died, very suddenly, in 1955. Afterwards, the Council's Human Nutrition Research Unit under Professor B. S. Platt moved in (Chapter 11). Still later, in 1967, the building provided temporary accommodation for 'shadow departments' of the Clinical Research Centre, then under construction a few miles away. It is now being converted for purposes of the Institute.

Major trends in the research programme
Although about certain of the projects more is said in a wider context in Volume Two, it is not possible here to do more than indicate broadly the nature of the investigations that have been undertaken at the National Institute. Dale, referring in 1963 to the early 1920s, wrote:

> It seemed natural to expect that the Council would from time to time find it proper to bring special directions to our notice, in which the research qualifications of one or another of our departments might find new opportunities. This was in fact to happen, and in more than one direction, when we were still in our early years at Hampstead; but all such requests and proposals were made with a sympathetic understanding of the needs and the possibilities of true research, so that the result was in every case to strengthen the Institute's contribution to the general advance of medical science.

Dale clearly had particularly in mind the Council's proposal to the Institute of a major programme of research on viruses, with the initial opportunity of working on canine distemper in a big way. Such occasional initiatives by the Council were not incompatible with the freedom that it allowed its staff in developing their own ideas. Looking back in 1965, Harington wrote:

> The Medical Research Council have consistently taken the broadest view of their responsibilities and in particular they have been at pains to avoid the prescription of projects of research to their staff; moreover they have regarded it as necessary that their scientific staff should have the greatest degree of freedom in the choice of their field of work that can be provided within their very broad terms of reference; in the general selection of problems an eye is kept particularly on subjects that are at an early stage of development but show promise of increasing importance in the future. These principles are well illustrated by the way in which the present activities of the National Institute have developed.

The Medical Research Committee did in fact create a framework for the initial programme when, in 1914, it decided on the main subjects for which provision was to be made in the Institute and selected the first leaders. As has been seen, it put bacteriology in the first place; but it could not have foreseen how significantly the study of the infective agents of disease would develop along the lines of virus research. Also in the forefront were the linked subjects of biochemistry and pharmacology, about which Harington remarked in 1965 that the "Committee showed unusual prescience in the importance which they attached to chemistry and biochemistry"; the dividends have certainly been great.

Some of the subjects of research represent programmes on broad lines that have continued over many years and have involved a number of investigators either simultaneously or in succession. Thus, distinguished work in neurophysiology was for long done in the Institute, largely in elucidating the intervention of certain chemical substances in the natural control of bodily functions by nerve-impulses, as in the transmission of excitation across nerve-junctions in ganglia or from nerve-fibre endings to muscle fibres, by the liberation of tiny doses of acetylcholine. Such findings provided a stimulus for King's brilliant chemical elucidation, in the same Department, of the structure of the natural alkaloid muscarine; and also for his work on curare alkaloids. A further outcome of the latter work was the research of Paton and Zaimis on the methonium bases; this joint effort of the Divisions of Organic Chemistry and of Physiology and Pharmacology led to the first effective drugs for the treatment of hypertension. There was also Dudley's isolation of the useful alkaloid ergometrine, following the clinical demonstration by Chassar Moir of a hitherto unknown principle in ergot. These various pharmacological advances are mentioned more fully in Volume Two.

There was also work on the structure of cholesterol that reorientated the chemistry of the steroids, substances of great biological importance. One member of this group was shown, in another investigation at the Institute, to be activated by ultraviolet light into a form of vitamin D (antirachitic factor). Recent interests on the biochemical side have centred on the problem of the synthesis of protein in the body.

The Institute has throughout been the main centre of the programme of work on filter-passing viruses that the Council launched in 1922. This began with canine distemper, proceeded to the discovery of the virus of influenza, and has later concerned itself with many other viruses, including those of the common cold (the first of which were isolated at the Institute's outstation established for the purpose of this research near Salisbury). There was also work on the virus factor in transmissible tumours. Hand in hand with all this has gone the development of physical methods of investigation, such as differential microfiltration and forms of ultramicroscopy.

Although virology continues to hold a major place in the Institute's work on infective agents, more recent developments are studies of bacterial physiology and of immunology, in both cases essentially biochemical in their approach. Protistology had a distinguished but decidedly one-man part from the earliest days at Hampstead until the death of Clifford Dobell at the end of 1949.

The discovery of insulin at Toronto in 1921 was quickly followed up in the Institute, where work was done on methods for the purification and biological assay of this hormone. Its availability also stimulated a series of investigations of intermediate carbohydrate metabolism. Among the later results of these was the successful

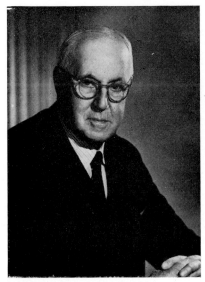

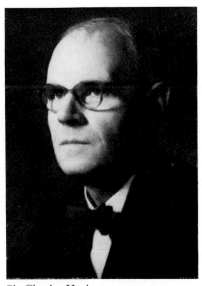

Sir Henry Dale, OM, GBE, FRS

Sir Charles Harington, KBE, FRS

Sir Peter Medawar, CBE, FRS

Sir Landsborough Thomson, CB, OBE

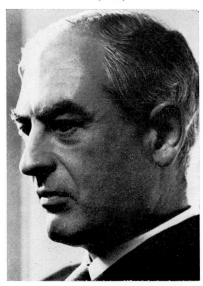

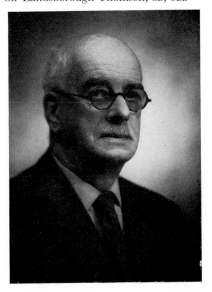

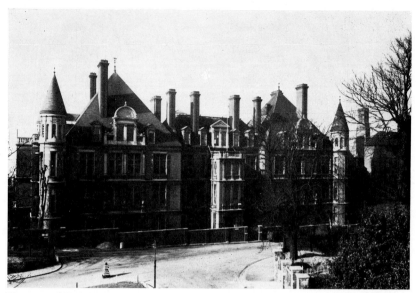

Hampstead Building

Mill Hill Building

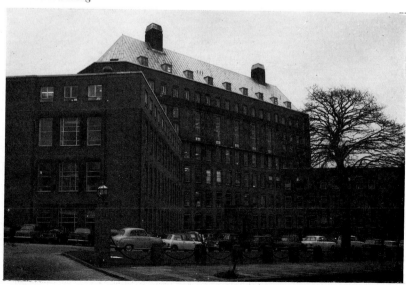

production, for the first time, of hormonally induced diabetes in the experimental animal by injection of extracts of the anterior part of the pituitary gland.

Another programme, from 1932, was concerned with the sex hormones. These studies in reproductive physiology eventually broadened out into a wider field of experimental biology. Among the subjects investigated was the effect of extreme cold on the body, with applications of hypothermia to surgical procedures and the preservation of living tissues.

Reference has already been made to the Council's inauguration, in 1937, of a more intensive programme of work in chemotherapy. The Council's decision was partly an acceptance of proposals from the Institute itself, and the latter was chosen as the main scene of operations. The work involved the cooperation of chemists, pharmacologists and microbiologists, but later became increasingly centred on the biological problems rather than on the search for new synthetic drugs.

As has been mentioned before, an early interest in environmental physiology lapsed in 1929, but was succeeded in 1941 by a new programme on questions of special interest to the Defence Services.

Increasingly, biochemistry has become a necessary associate of the other disciplines; and new biophysical methods have extended the technical possibilities of investigation in different fields. In addition to phase-contrast and electron miscroscopy, the methods include high-speed centrifugation, ultrasonics, the use of radioisotopes, electrophoresis, and methods of separation such as gas chromatography (for which Dr A. J. P. Martin had received a share of a Nobel Prize). The facilities of the Institute in these directions are made available to external workers as well as to the staff.

Summing up in 1949, when the Institute was on the point of moving to its new and larger quarters at Mill Hill, Harington wrote as follows:

> Looking in more detail at the process of expansion of the work at the Institute from the early days of the three laboratory departments to the present very much larger and more complex establishment, we see an increasing emphasis on biochemistry and biophysics on the one hand together with a broadening of the biological research through endocrinology to more general aspects of experimental biology on the other. In these respects the development is a true reflexion of the general trend during the past thirty years of medical research in the laboratory, which must make ever wider demands on the whole field of scientific effort if it is to progress. The very increase in the range of work which has to be covered, with its accompaniment of multiplication of departments with differing immediate interests, adds weight to the principle laid down by the Council in the early days of the Institute that there must be the freest contact between the different laboratories.

Biological standardisation and assay

In addition to its general programme, the Institute has a special and largely unique function which involves both research and the performance of a service. The function is that of determining and maintaining standards for the biological assay of certain medicinal preparations of which the properties cannot be measured by ordinary chemical tests. The uniqueness lies partly in the pioneer role that the Institute has played in developing the subject, and partly in the international responsibility that the Council exercises in many instances. This special activity of the Council receives fuller description in Volume Two.

Regarded as a function of the Institute, the standards work is peculiar in a further respect; although it is now segregated in a particular department, the work during its development was spread over a wide spectrum of staff. Since 1930 there has been a Department of Biological Standards, later renamed as a division, but its senior staff at first consisted solely of its Director. He was able, however, to call on specialist colleagues for cooperation in dealing with substances of different types. Latterly, the necessity for safety testing of live poliomyelitis vaccine made it necessary to add a Division of Immunological Products Control, the cost of this more routine function being borne by the Ministry of Health (as it then was). At the close of the period of this history, however, the whole policy has been reviewed in the light of expected further increase in the demand for work of this kind, following the Medicines Act 1968 and the development of a European Pharmacopoeia. It has been agreed that the work of the Divisions of Biological Standards and Immunological Products Control should be brought together in an autonomous National Institute for Biological Standards and Control responsible to the Health Departments (with the Council represented on the Board), and that it should then be carried out in a building separate from the National Institute.

World Influenza Centre
Another form of control work undertaken at the Institute, within the Division of Virology, is the maintenance of type strains of various respiratory and arthropod-borne viruses for the rapid identification of specimens from outbreaks of disease. In particular, there has been in the Institute since 1947 a laboratory known as the World Influenza Centre, maintained on behalf of the World Health Organisation. Strains from outbreaks are sent here by central laboratories in other countries, and this makes possible a continuing study of the epidemiology of the disease. Early identification of a strain causing a spreading epidemic facilitates the production of appropriate vaccines; and a perpetual watch is kept for the appearance of any strain showing unusual virulence.

Library
The Council's principal library is at the Institute, of which it is of course an indispensable part. Its purpose is to make available to the Council's staff, both in the Institute and elsewhere, the scientific literature of the world, either from its own resources or through the

various inter-library lending schemes. The formation of the library was put in hand in 1920, when the departments of the Institute came together in the building at Hampstead, but the move to Mill Hill provided an opportunity for replanning on the most modern lines. The present library is notable for its excellent design and almost perfect lighting. It contains about 30 000 volumes, including 800 sets of periodicals (700 of them current), and 6000 books; there are also some 30 000 reprints and several hundred administrative and statistical reports.

During the last few years there have been developments in the use of the computer to store and retrieve references to the medical literature. The library staff now devote much time to searching the literature in this way for the research workers.

Academic status

As stated at the outset of the chapter, the Rockefeller Institute for Medical Research in New York was a principal model for the incipient National Institute for Medical Research in London. The younger institute never vied in size with the other; neither was it autonomous, being part of a wider organisation. Since 1914 the patterns have diverged in two respects. One is that whereas the Rockefeller Institute had its own hospital, immediately adjacent, the idea of a similar arrangement for the National Institute was—as already mentioned—dropped at an early stage; and the Council has progressively made different provision for clinical research.

In another respect the Rockefeller Institute has developed in a direction that the National Institute does not seem likely to follow. After half a century as an establishment purely for research, with a whole-time staff free from academic duties, the Rockefeller Institute became a university in its own right in 1954, although of a limited kind. Dr Detlev Bronk, President of the Rockefeller Institute, wrote as follows in his foreword to Corner's history, already mentioned: "The Rockefeller Institute for Medical Research had so successfully fostered research in the academic world that a career of teaching and research in a university had become more desirable than life in an intellectually limited research institute that lacked the vital stimulus of eager graduate students".

The nearest equivalent status possible for the National Institute would be that of a school of the University of London—as already held by the Lister Institute and by the Institute of Cancer Research, to mention two examples in the particular field. The Council has in fact been content with a less close form of association which does not in any way abrogate its own authority as parent body. The purpose is that junior members of the Institute's own staff, and also visiting workers, should be eligible to qualify for higher degrees (usually PhD). Accordingly, almost from the beginning at Hampstead, and subsequently at Mill Hill, the Institute has been specially recognised by the University as a place where those aiming at higher degrees may register as 'internal students'; and certain senior members of the staff have been recognised as teachers under whose supervision such students may work.

More recently this particular arrangement has been rendered obsolescent by regulations made by the University in 1966; under these, there is greater freedom in some respects but closer University control in others. An alternative has latterly become available, however, and has become the method of choice at the National Institute. The Council for National Academic Awards, constituted by Royal Charter in 1964, has power *inter alia* "to grant and confer degrees to and on persons who shall have carried out research under the supervision of an educational or research establishment other than a university under conditions approved by the Council."

One may note a suggestion behind the recent change at the Rockefeller Institute that, in spite of its immense productivity and reputation, it had not acquired advantages of a special kind to offset the lack of an academic atmosphere for its staff. Corner says that "the system of distinct laboratories, each devoted to the work of an eminent investigator and his personal associates, had sometimes led to cloistral exclusiveness of these groups". On the other hand, the National Institute has fortunately been able to break down inter-departmental barriers and develop an integration of disciplines that would be impossible, at least in Britain, within a university organisation; and this characteristic will surely be cherished by the Council in the foreseeable future.

Chapter 11
External Staff and Research Units

External staff—Research units—The Department of Clinical Research—
Additional clinical research units—Other early external establishments—The
unit concept—Wartime and immediate post-war units—Nomenclature of
units—Further development of the unit system—Eventual policy on research
units—Transfer of units to universities—Individual members of external staff—
Total staff numbers—The employment of research staff

External staff

The peripheral employment of staff has always been the Council's
second main method of promoting research (Chapters 2, 9). The
term 'external staff' eventually came into use, meaning staff outside
the National Institute for Medical Research; but it later had a
narrower use, for those who were placed individually in other
institutions as distinct from those who were members of organised
'units'.

It is not clear from the record how closely the idea of an external
staff was originally linked with the special needs of clinical research,
for which facilities might not be—and, in the event, were not—made
available at the central institute (Chapter 10). Certainly this soon
became an important consideration, and was for a time the main
one. There were, however, other reasons for having an external staff,
although these reasons may not have been fully appreciated until
later. There was the advantage of being able to exploit some local
opportunity, such as the inspiration of a university department
active in a particular line of research, or the guidance of an outstanding leader of research holding an academic post. There might also
be more material factors in the opportunity—some unusual equipment it might be, or access to some special material. Conversely, the
'seeding' of a whole-time research worker of quality might be helpful,
perhaps stimulating, to the university department in which he was
placed, and possibly encouraging to the recruitment of young graduates to the research field.

Research units

The formation of organised teams of external staff under the general
title of 'research units' was a later development; and the particular
form of unit was peculiarly a Medical Research Council concept. In
its Report for 1936–37 the Council referred to "a gradual development of an intermediate type of arrangement"—intermediate
between the central institute and individual workers elsewhere—in
the establishment of "a number of special units or departments", and

not only for clinical research. Rationalising retrospectively, it might be tempting to suggest that the separately housed departments of the future National Institute (Chapter 10) were the first research units; but there is no evidence of contemporary thought on these lines.

The Department of Clinical Research

It is nearer the mark to say that the Department of Clinical Research, attached to University College Hospital Medical School in London, was the first of the Council's research units, although it did not have that term in its title. The unit concept was as yet not fully developed; and the original plan for this Department had been to treat it as an integral part of the central institute, although the problem of providing it with hospital beds had never found any definite solution. Even after the attachment to an existing hospital had been decided, the Department continued for a short time to be regarded as an outlying part of the National Institute. In the event, the title 'Department' came to relate to the Hospital (although not formally until 1930) and not to the National Institute; and from the Council's standpoint it came to rank as an establishment of the external staff. Of its role more is said in Volume Two.

Additional clinical research units

In 1933 and 1934, respectively, the Council established two further clinical research units attached to medical schools of teaching hospitals in London; and both were 'units' by title. The first was in the specialised clinical field of neurology—a field especially notable for the quality of the research work that had been done in it. The initiative came from the National Hospital for Nervous Diseases, in Queen Square, London, with an offer of accommodation for a research department, including adequate beds and laboratory facilities, on the condition that the Council would provide a whole-time director and an assistant staff. Agreement was quickly reached, and Dr E. A. Carmichael, already an honorary Assistant Physician to the Hospital, entered the Council's service as Director. The Halley Stewart Trustees agreed to provide two or more studentships tenable in the Unit; and further staff was added later by the Council.

Even before this, a change had taken place in the Department of Clinical Research at University College Hospital, through the generous action of the Rockefeller Foundation in permanently endowing the post of Director. Thus Sir Thomas Lewis passed technically from the service of the Council, although the latter remained under obligation to meet any part of his remuneration not covered by the income of the endowment; this was at first a small matter, although it eventually grew to be the greater fraction. At the time, this liberated a large part of the annual cost of the Department, hitherto borne wholly by the Council, which accordingly regarded it "as an honourable obligation to use the funds thus set free within the same sphere of work, clinical research, as being that which the

Foundation have thus come forward to aid" (Report for 1931–32).

Accordingly, the Council decided to approach Guy's Hospital with a proposal to establish a Clinical Research Unit there, under the direction of Dr R. T. Grant, from Sir Thomas Lewis' Department. The basis of the understanding thereafter reached with Guy's Hospital was that:

(i) The salaries of the Director and of his assistants, and the cost of all apparatus and material used by the Unit, were to be provided by the Council (of whose staff the personnel would be members).

(ii) Suitable laboratory accommodation was to be provided free of charge by the Hospital. At least six beds (three male and three female) were to be placed at the disposal of the Unit and maintained by the Hospital; the Director was also to have out-patient facilities.

(iii) The Director was to give whole-time service and not to engage in private practice. He was to be free from all ordinary duties, but might be allowed to take some small part in teaching. He was to be *ex officio* a member of the visiting staff of the Hospital, and to have a seat on the medical and school committees.

(iv) The whole scheme might be terminated by either party at twelve months' notice.

The agreement became a prototype for similar arrangements in future, although each had to be adapted in detail to suit local circumstances. In this case the negotiations took some months to conclude, as a proposition of a then novel kind was being made entirely from the outside to an institution rather noted for its independence; moreover, the nominated Director was a graduate of another university (Glasgow) working in another hospital (University College Hospital). In the two earlier cases the unit had developed within the hospital concerned and the nominated director was already a member of its honorary staff. It is thus understandable that Guy's Hospital insisted that the appointment of the Director should be considered by a special advisory committee consisting of members nominated by the Council, by the Hospital, and by the President of the Royal College of Physicians of London. This body was duly formed, and it unanimously recommended the appointment of Dr Grant.

The respective units at the National Hospital and at Guy's Hospital were both maintained for more than twenty years. Each was eventually dissolved on the retirement of its original director, and other arrangements were made for the remaining members of the Council's staff working therein.

One further clinical unit was set up before the Second World War—namely, the Unit for Clinical Research in Surgery, which was established in 1938 in the Royal Infirmary and Royal Hospital for Sick Children, Edinburgh, with Mr W. C. Wilson as Director. This step was mainly due to the initiative of Sir David Wilkie, Regius

Professor of Surgery in the University, but the project came to an early end when Mr Wilson was appointed to the chair in Aberdeen.

Other early external establishments

Outside the clinical field, four further establishments of the unit type were set up by the Council between the wars, although the term was not applied at the time. (Certain minor groupings of external staff that were later recognised as establishments also date effectively from this period.) In 1926 the Council founded the Dunn Nutritional Laboratory on a leased site at the University Field Laboratories, Cambridge. The capital cost of a modest building was provided to the Council by the trustees of the late Sir William Dunn, who also made substantial capital grants for special purposes to the Universities of Oxford (pathology) and Cambridge (biochemistry), and to certain teaching hospitals in London (clinical laboratories). The motive here was to provide for additional work under the inspiration and guidance of Professor (later Sir) Frederick Gowland Hopkins.

As already noted, an organisation for statistical work had a special place in the original schemes of the Medical Research Committee (Chapter 9), and first took shape as Dr John Brownlee's department of the National Institute for Medical Research, where it was later augmented by a small staff under Dr Major Greenwood as chairman of the Statistical Committee (Chapter 10). In 1927, after Brownlee's death and Greenwood's appointment as Professor of Epidemiology and Vital Statistics at the London School of Hygiene and Tropical Medicine, the combined staff acquired the status of a separate establishment, eventually known as the Statistical Research Unit. The working integration of this staff with that of the School's department continued after Dr A. (later Sir Austin) Bradford Hill succeeded Greenwood in 1945. On Hill's retirement in 1961, the Statistical Research Unit, under the direction of Dr (later Professor Sir) Richard Doll, became an entirely separate entity and other accommodation for it was found by the Council. In 1970 most of the staff were transferred to the new Clinical Research Centre for its Division of Epidemiology. An entirely new Statistical Research and Services Unit had subsequently to be created. The application of computer science to medical research was a separate development, late in the period under review; the Council now maintains in London both a Computer Unit (mainly for research) and a Computer Services Centre.

In 1932 the Council were able to place a malaria research unit (a description that later became a title) in the London School of Hygiene and Tropical Medicine. The purpose was to utilise the experience of Sir Rickard Christophers after his retirement from the Indian Medical Service. Provision for his post took the form of a Leverhulme Fellowship, specially placed at the Council's disposal; apart from that, the cost of the project was shared by the Leverhulme Trustees, the School, and the Council. Christophers relinquished the appointment in 1938, and the project terminated with the outbreak of war in the following year.

In 1934 the Council offered a whole-time appointment to Dr (later Sir) Paul Fildes, bacteriologist at the London Hospital, and invited him to form what later became the Bacterial Chemistry Research Unit. This was set up in the Bland-Sutton Institute of Pathology at the Middlesex Hospital, by arrangement with the authorities of the latter. Additional staff was provided by fellowships placed at the Council's disposal by the Leverhulme Trustees (two) and the Halley Stewart Trust (one). After the war of 1939–45, the Unit was reorganised at the Lister Institute; and on the Director's retirement it was absorbed by the National Institute for Medical Research.

Two other establishments, both set up at an early stage and each directed by a member of the external scientific staff, had special functions widely different from those of a unit engaged wholly in research—the Standards Laboratory for diagnostic suspensions and sera set up at Oxford in 1915, and the National Collection of Type Cultures of microorganisms set up at the Lister Institute in 1920. They were both eventually moved to the Central Public Health Laboratory at Colindale; and they passed entirely from the Council's jurisdiction in 1961.

Some pre-war elements of external staff would certainly have been given establishment status had they continued into the period when that became the normal practice. For instance, Dr A. Stanley Griffith, who had formerly been an investigator for the Royal Commission on Tuberculosis (Chapter 1), worked until 1940 as a member of the external staff at the University Field Laboratories, Cambridge, on the bacteriology of tuberculosis. And there was Dr Leonard Colebrook, who was appointed in 1919 to the staff of the National Institute, became in 1922 an external staff worker at St Mary's Hospital, Paddington, and in 1930 was given the status of Honorary Director of the new Research Laboratories of Queen Charlotte's Hospital, Hammersmith, at the head of a team studying puerperal infections and the application to them of chemotherapy. Also as a member of the external staff, from 1937 to 1939, and grant-aided before that, Dr L. S. Penrose had his own laboratory for the study of mental defect, attached to the Royal Eastern Counties' Institution at Colchester, Essex; this was a joint project of the Council, the Darwin Trust and the Institution; and it was continued for some time after Dr Penrose's own departure. In 1933 the Council joined with University College London in setting up a subdepartment on the physiology and pathology of vision, headed by Dr R. J. Lythgoe.

The unit concept

By the beginning of the war of 1939–45, the Council had thus created several establishments of the research unit type, although in some cases the status and title were conferred retrospectively and not at the date of foundation. A formulated policy and standard nomenclature grew only gradually; a good deal of subsequent rationalisation was indeed applied to what had been a series of pragmatic decisions. Four of the earliest research establishments were set up to provide facilities for clinical research. One other represented only an administrative redeployment of statistical staff that already existed; three created new opportunities for research in special subjects outside the clinical field—nutrition, bacterial chemistry, and experimental chemotherapy of malaria. Most of the numerous later units were founded for like reason, but another motive eventually played a part—namely, the need to provide special opportunities overseas for research work in tropical medicine.

It was later enunciated as a principle that a unit was built round a chosen leader. He might already be a member of the Council's staff, or might be appointed thereto as director; or, again, he might hold and retain a professorship or other academic post and serve the Council as an honorary director. In the main the thesis was true in these early cases, although a general policy had not yet been formulated; either the selection of the director was the initial step, or a particular man was in view from an early stage in the deliberations. Sometimes it was necessary to meet the sensibilities of the host institution by leaving open the formal appointment of a director until this could be made in accordance with academic protocol; but the other party can scarcely have been under the illusion that the Council would whole-heartedly support any choice different from its own. On rare occasions a director was not chosen in the first instance, even informally, but was sought only after the main decision had been taken.

That a unit is built round a man implies that it should cease to exist as such when the man retires or dies, or even if he moves to another post unless he can take the team with him; but this does not hold in every instance. The reason for continuing to maintain a unit may be the presence of an obvious successor to the departing director, or the persistence of a strong need for the particular line of work, or some element of permanence in the available facilities. Certainly there was at the outset no express policy concerning the long-term future of these early units.

It was for long considered as axiomatic that accommodation for a research unit was provided by the host institution, and that the Council had no commitment in 'bricks and mortar'. The Dunn Nutritional Laboratory, just mentioned, was an early exception, owing to the availability of a capital benefaction. Other exceptions were made later because the necessary size of the unit made the provision of additional accommodation inevitable. Sometimes the need was not apparent at the outset, but the unit had outgrown its allotment of space or the latter had been withdrawn or restricted by, say, the arrival in the institution of a new departmental head with interests different from those of his predecessor. Latterly, pressure on university space has made it almost normal for the Council to provide special accommodation.

In some instances there has been no host institution, the unit being maintained by the Council as a separate establishment. Several unattached units in the London area have been grouped in two buildings controlled by the Council—the MRC Laboratories, Hampstead, and the MRC Laboratories, Carshalton; these are the titles merely of buildings, not of establishments, although some common services are shared by the tenant units. The building at Hampstead was that originally acquired to house the National Institute for Medical Research, later moved to Mill Hill (Chapter 10). That at Carshalton was built by the London County Council as a serum laboratory to supply its hospitals, but became government property—and redundant for its original purpose—by reason of the National Health Service Act 1946.

As regards the organisation of a research unit, the interrelations with the host institution tend to be especially intricate where a clinical subject is involved. Professor Sir Aubrey Lewis (1965), for long the Honorary Director of the Council's Social Psychiatry Research Unit, has described its organisation. He points out that such a unit needs contacts both with a hospital and with a university. The first are necessary "because illness provides the stimulus and the testing ground for study of its crucial problems"; the second in order to attract recruits to the subject from among promising undergraduates and also to give "access to workshops, libraries, computing, and other services rarely available on a large scale to isolated research centres". Moreover, a research unit "needs the spur of extraneous criticism, intellectual forays, and uncovenanted reinforcements to its stock of ideas and methods".

Wartime and immediate post-war units

Reverting to the chronological account, it has been seen that only one establishment of the research unit type existed before 1926, and that between then and 1939 only a few more were set up. During and immediately after the Second World War, on the other hand, there was a great proliferation of establishments of this kind.

Only two establishments can be strictly termed 'wartime', in that they were set up not only during the war but in fact to meet certain of its special demands and were no longer required after the emergency had ended. These were the Physiological Research Laboratory (1941) attached to the Armoured Fighting Vehicle Training School, and the Wound Infection Unit (1942). Other establishments that were brought into being during the war period represented the continuing development of the Council's normal programme, in so far as conditions permitted; some of these indeed had immediate wartime tasks in view, but of a kind that would continue to have relevance to national needs, including those of industry.

The number of establishments began to grow so rapidly, from this stage, that the treatment here must necessarily be selective. A complete chronological list, with locations and directors' names, is given in an Appendix to Volume Two, and the mention of initial dates in this chapter will facilitate consultation. Many of the establishments are referred to again in Volume Two, in respect of their role in the general programme of research promoted by the Council.

During this period, which may be taken as 1940–46, new research units were still mostly in the clinical field, although often with a substantial laboratory element. They were, however, more specialised than their prototypes, and several of their subjects had industrial applications. Thus, there were the Radiotherapeutic Research Unit (1941), the Burns Research Unit (1942), the Department for Research in Industrial Medicine (1943), the Otological Research Unit (1944), the Pneumoconiosis Research Unit (1945), the Department for Experimental Medicine (1945) in the University of Cambridge with human nutrition as its main interest, the Clinical Endocrinology Research Unit (1946), the Clinical Chemotherapeutic Research Unit (1946), the Industrial Medicine Research Unit (1946) studying industrial injuries and later combined with the Burns Research Unit already mentioned, the Electro-Medical Research Unit (1946), the Blood Transfusion Research Unit (1946); and the Council's first Dental Research Unit (1946). The locations of these units ranged from London and the provinces to Wales and Scotland. Two of the units named were large establishments with premises specially built for them—the Radiotherapeutic Research Unit in London and the Pneumoconiosis Research Unit at Cardiff.

In one instance the arrangements were of an unusual kind, in that the University of Cambridge was provided by the Council with an additional department, but one having minimal responsibilities apart from research. The Department of Experimental Medicine was both a department of the University and a research unit of the Council; and the professor at its head was likewise its director on the Council's behalf. Rather different was the arrangement whereby the Council placed a Department of Industrial Medicine in the London Hospital, by arrangement with the authorities there; in this case the head was already a part-time consultant physician on the staff of the Hospital, became a part-time member of the Council's staff, and retained another fraction of his time for private consulting work.

Outside the clinical field was the Applied Psychology Research Unit (1944), in terms of scientific manpower one of the largest of the Council's external establishments. This was placed within the Department of Psychology, University of Cambridge, at the instance of Professor (later Sir) Frederic Bartlett, at that time a member of the Council. Its creation was to a large extent an act of consolidation, as many workers in the Cambridge laboratory were already employed or grant-aided by the Council.

The Human Nutrition Research Unit (1944) was set up mainly to investigate nutritional problems in or affecting tropical countries, and was to be associated with the training of personnel for work overseas on the practical applications of nutritional science. Responsibility for the educational aspect was accepted by the London School of Hygiene and Tropical Medicine, but as the School had not accommodation for the research work the Unit had to be housed, in three successive locations, under arrangements made by the Council. Much of the research work was done overseas, and for six years the Unit had its own field research station in The Gambia; in 1953 this last became an establishment directly under the Council, as is recounted in Volume Two.

Other units set up in the same period were the Chemical Microbiology Research Unit (1944), the Cell Metabolism Research Unit (1945), the Blood Products Research Unit (1945), the Blood Group Research Unit (1946), and what was later called the Group for Research on the Building Industry (1946).

Nomenclature of units

At this point it may be noted that up to the time of the Second World War the Council used the title 'unit' almost exclusively in the clinical field, where the term was being applied to new teaching departments in London medical schools headed by whole-time professors. (There was one transient exception, the Malaria Research Unit, late in the period.) Thus in the Council's Report for 1938–39 the headings of two main parts were "Clinical Research Units" and "External Scientific Staff", the latter covering non-clinical establishments. From 1943 it was applied, sometimes retrospectively, to non-clinical establishments founded before the war, and it was thenceforth used freely for new establishments.

From 1947 it became customary to designate minor aggregations of external staff as 'research groups'; more recently the term disappeared in this sense, when it came to be applied in quite a different context (Chapter 12). Groups were in general smaller, less formally constituted, and more obviously temporary than units, but the distinction was ill-defined. The selection of individual members of the external scientific staff as directors of nominal groups, possibly including no senior staff but themselves, was likewise somewhat arbitrary. One titular director petitioned, unsuccessfully, for the promotion of his research group to the rank of research unit, on the ground that he was its only member and would therefore be more correctly described as a unit than as a group!

Exceptionally, a few establishments that were in effect units were given different titles for special reasons. Thus, a few have had the title 'Department'—as in three instances already mentioned. A few have had the title 'Laboratory' or 'Laboratories', indicating the existence of separate premises (but in the plural usually attached to a building in which two or more units were housed). The terms 'Bureau', 'Centre' 'Collection', 'Station' and 'Service' have been used for establishments that were not typical research units, although administratively equivalent.

In 1969 a general change was made in the system of naming units. 'Medical Research Council' or 'MRC' was prefixed to the title of each establishment, and the word 'Research' was omitted before 'Unit'; thus, 'Toxicology Research Unit' became 'MRC Toxicology Unit', and so on. This ensured that the status of a unit as an establishment of the Council would not be overlooked; as before, the name of the host institution, if any, formed part of the address.

Further development of the unit system

By 1947 the Council was fully embarked on a policy of building up a staff organisation largely made up, in addition to the National Institute for Medical Research, of research units and the like. In that year the number of new ones set up was considerable, and at the same time several already existing elements of staff were given similar status. The process of creating units has continued since then, until at the time of writing just over one hundred establishments of this type have been instituted, counting from the very beginning. The number of these existing at any one moment has naturally never been so large, many units having meanwhile run their course. At a point in 1970 there were 77 units in being (including four overseas); of these, 59 had direct links with universities, 7 others had informal links, and 11 had none. The chronological list indicates the rate of development and turnover, as well as giving some particulars of each establishment (Volume Two).

Eventual policy on research units

Early in 1961 the Council devoted some time to reviewing its methods of supporting research. This resulted in the adoption of a prepared statement "as a general standard of reference on future policy for the support of research", including certain points relating particularly to research units.

It was laid down that, in considering a proposal for a new unit, the Council would give deliberate consideration to the following questions:

(a) whether the field of work is appropriate and whether, in view of the total national effort, this field is in need of extra support;
(b) whether the research proposed requires such strong continuing support as a unit or group in the sense defined [Chapter 12] and cannot adequately be supported under the research grants scheme;
(c) whether the man proposed is of the requisite ability to direct research; and
(d) whether the programme of work is of the requisite quality.

Acceptable reasons for providing support in the form of a research unit, rather than of a group (in the newer sense), were stated to be:

(a) the existence of an outstanding man for whom no other post as suitable is available;

(*b*) the apparent emergence of a new subject, for example one which has not yet proved its suitability for inclusion in the university curriculum;

(*c*) the need to set up a research team independently of a university or teaching hospital;

(*d*) the existence of a public need requiring research which is either unsuitable for a department of a university or hospital or which requires development on a scale that would distort their organisation;

(*e*) the need to develop a subject that is being neglected by other organisations.

It was further agreed that a unit would normally be set up for a trial period of seven years, unless the director had already proved his ability to lead an independent team and the Council was certain that the particular line of work proposed was of continuing importance. Before the end of any such trial period it would be decided whether to disband, to renew for a further limited period, or to continue until the director's retirement. In the case of a unit set up for a limited period, appointments of staff would, as far as possible, coincide with this period, but the director and possibly other senior members might be granted appointments of unlimited tenure provided that they met the normal criteria for such appointments (see below).

Transfer of units to universities
The formulation of future policy on the creation of new research units was only one aspect of the question. The Council already had on its hands the problem of older units that had in the course of time become virtually an integral part of the academic structure in their respective universities. In 1958 the Council, after some discussion of wider principles (Chapter 7), agreed with the Advisory Committee on Scientific Policy and the University Grants Committee that units which had reached this stage in their development should preferably be transferred to the universities concerned. There were, however, various practical difficulties in implementing this principle; but these are likely to arise less frequently in future, as the Council will to an increasing extent have the eventual disposal of the units definitely in view.

Individual members of external staff
As already mentioned, 'external scientific staff' eventually came to mean those employed as individuals outside even the Council's minor establishments such as research units. Each of these individuals deals directly with the Council's headquarters in the same way as the director of an establishment. From the earliest days of the Medical Research Committee a few research workers were employed on this basis, although the category was not given its name until several years later.

This type of arrangement originally catered for the experienced worker who was essentially a lone hand, and who usually already had an academic or hospital environment suited to his needs. Even if he held a whole-time appointment from the Council, the latter encouraged him to take a limited part in the general activities of the department in which he worked. Latterly, also, such arrangements have often been found suitable for members of a research unit that has been disbanded on the retirement of its director. There has likewise been a demand for part-time research appointments for the holders of part-time clinical posts in the National Health Service.

In June 1971 there were 106 members of the external scientific staff placed in other institutions as individuals or small teams; of these, 12 were part-time in the service of the Council. These 106 were divided between 47 departments of 28 different universities or other institutions in the United Kingdom and 5 overseas. These figures are not quite so high as they were a few years previously, since new forms of grant-aid have latterly been introduced to meet much of the need (Chapter 12); indeed it is now the policy of the Council to seek other means of support in preference to the multiplication of scattered posts, tending towards an unwieldy staff structure.

It is obviously impracticable to list even the senior members of the external staff of recent years; but it seems proper that the pioneers in this category should be named, for in the days before the prolifera-tion of research units they played a relatively large part in the Council's programme. Dr A. Stanley Griffith and Dr Leonard Colebrook have already been mentioned. Dr (later Sir) Alan N. Drury, from 1920 with the Department of Clinical Research (see above), became in 1928 an individual worker in the Department of Pathology, University of Cambridge; he left the Council's service in 1943 on appointment as Director of the Lister Institute. Dr Matthew Young was a member of the Council's staff from 1922 until his death in 1940, at first with the Statistical Department of the National Institute for Medical Research (Chapter 10), and from 1927 in the Institute of Anatomy, University College London. Dr H. M. Vernon and Dr May Smith came into the direct employ of the Council in 1920 as investigators for the Industrial Fatigue (later Health) Research Board.

Dr Mervyn H. Gordon worked for the Council on virus infections at St Bartholomew's Hospital, London (1923–36); Dr Helen M. M. Mackay on paediatrics (part-time) at the Queen's (later Queen Elizabeth) Hospital for Children, Hackney Road, London (1933–51); Dr Julia Bell on human genetics at the Galton Laboratory, University College London (1933–44); Dr (later Professor) Dorothy S. Russell on the pathology of the nervous system at the London Hospital (1933–46); and Dr S. S. Zilva (1919–49) and Miss E. M. Hume (1926–52) on vitamins at the Lister Institute.

Total staff numbers

In this section and the next the Council's staff is considered as a whole, including those at the National Institute for Medical Research (Chapter 10). The records surviving from the earliest years are inadequate for exact comparisons, but the total scientific staff numbered barely 40, of whom almost half were at the National Institute. By 1954 the figure had risen to 484, and by 1970 to 1054; and at the latter date the proportion at the National Institute had fallen below a sixth.

On 1 April 1970 the total staff of all categories stood at 3948, of whom 357 were employed part-time; in addition 161 were employed locally overseas. Of the 1054 scientific staff, rather less than a third were medically qualified. At the same date the total technician staff was 1630, the maintenance staff 451, and the administrative and clerical staff 813 (including medically and scientifically qualified officers at Headquarters).

The employment of research staff

HM Treasury exercises, now indirectly, not only financial control over the Council's actions but also control in establishment matters, concerning itself with rates of pay and conditions of service for members of the staff. In an *Administrative Handbook*, printed for the Council in 1963, the nature of this control was described in the following terms informally agreed with the Treasury at the time:

> The relationships between the Council and the Treasury in this field are governed by certain understandings reached from time to time, designed primarily to ensure that the pay and conditions of service of the Council's staff are consistent with those of comparable staff in certain other employments that have been designated for the purpose in respect of different categories—the universities for scientific staff (medical and otherwise, except that clinicians have the equivalent of NHS hospital appointments), the Civil Service for administrative staff, and so on; this obviates embarrassment to the Treasury in respect of other employments financed from public funds. In certain respects where convenience calls for common treatment of all categories, the Civil Service model is followed. Responsibility in the first instance for ensuring that the understandings are properly applied rests with the Council, but the Treasury are kept informed of the Council's practice through the provision of the Establishment Code, amendments to it as they are issued, and other relevant notices. The Council consults the Treasury in advance about changes in the pay of the various categories of staff, but is not required to obtain prior Treasury approval for its detailed interpretation of conditions of service in the particular circumstances of its own work, except where there is doubt whether a particular action proposed is consistent with the relevant general understanding, or where it may in other respects be of concern to the Treasury—for example, where there is a risk of embarrassment in relation to other employments financed from public funds. Such prior consultation might be necessary when the action in question affects the whole category of the Council's staff, or where it would make an exception from the Council's standard practice in favour of a particular individual or individuals.

One freedom of vital importance to the Council is the absence of an 'establishment' of scientific staff that would fix the numbers in each salary grade. On the Council's research staff, between the levels of assistant and director, there are no 'posts' to which definite

F

degrees of responsibility can be permanently attached; each member of the research staff in effect creates his own job and impresses his personal value on the position that he holds.

All this is foreign to the concept, appropriate enough in different circumstances, of a 'rate for the job'—implying a series of graded posts of increasing responsibility and a system of promotion from one such post to another as vacancies permit. On the contrary, the requirement is for flexible arrangements for promotion on assessments of merit. A scheme of salary grades is convenient, but there should be the possibility of accelerated promotion within a grade and from grade to grade, even to the extent of by-passing a grade altogether. Except at directors' level, there should be no arbitrary limitation on the number of staff in a given grade at any one time—no 'waiting for dead men's shoes'. It is highly undesirable that a progressive research staff should have imposed upon it the rigid structure of a grade-by-grade 'establishment'.

This has been the Council's policy from the earliest years, even before principles of the kind were explicitly formulated. It is noteworthy that much of it has since been adopted for the Scientific Civil Service on the recommendation of successive special committees—the Barlow Committee reporting in 1945, the Tennant Committee in 1965, and the Fulton Committee in 1968 (Chapter 8).

The retiring age for staff in all categories is 60, but service may be continued by mutual consent up to age 65 and exceptionally beyond that; in no case has whole-time employment been continued beyond age 67. New appointments are commonly made for a limited period, such as three years, but they may be renewed on the same or other conditions. Unlimited tenure, subject only to retiring age, is not usually given before the staff member is over 30 years of age, has been with the Council for five years (except for workers appointed directly to senior posts after approved service elsewhere), and has (apart from certain highly specialised assistants) attained a status equivalent to that of a senior lecturer, reader or professor.

The printed *Conditions of Service on the Council's Staff* (revised 1961) are more notable for what they permit than for anything that they prohibit.

Chapter 12
Grant-aided Research

Status of research grants—Characteristics of research grants—Types of research grant—The award of grants—Research fellowships—Long-term support—Research groups—Programme grants—Block grants—Contributions to international projects

Status of research grants

The third method of promoting research has from the beginning been the award of grants, payments of one kind or another to workers not employed by the Council. This has come to be known as the 'indirect' support of research; definitions of current methods are given in the Report for 1969–70. During the earliest years, however, a sharp distinction was not always drawn between the members of the external staff and the holders of personal grants; both were on occasion loosely described as "working in the service of the Committee" (or Council). There was still no general superannuation scheme to raise administrative questions of status in acute form, and possible legal difficulties over employer's liability had not yet been clearly envisaged. It was also not always explicit whether a grant was being made for the performance of duties assigned to the investigator or to support him in independent work of his choice. These early uncertainties arose mainly during time of war, when makeshift arrangements to meet special conditions were a common necessity. Serious misunderstandings did arise later from a few early awards where a substantial personal grant had been given without sufficiently precise definition of its terms, and in 1938 one ex-grantee ill-advisedly resorted to litigation.

Gradually a clear concept developed, at first in practice and later in stated principle. A member of the staff was an employee of the Council, working as it might direct (although in scientific terms such direction would be only of the most general kind); he must have a definite contract of service and as a rule be eligible for superannuation benefits. On the other hand, the holder of a grant, even one for whole-time personal remuneration, was to be regarded as an otherwise employed, or 'self-employed', person, receiving financial help from the Council to do what he himself had proposed to do.

Late in the period covered by this history, the practice was changed. Grants were still sought by and awarded to individuals, but the great majority of grants came to be paid through the institutions in which the work was being done. In this way, any responsibilities as employer devolved on the institution, which explicitly accepted them and could impose its own conditions on the holder of a personal grant, even including him (at the Council's charge) in its own superannuation scheme.

Characteristics of research grants

In the 'research schemes' presented in 1914 it was stated that "The Committee have not thought it wise to frame for the present any rigid policy to govern the general or particular conditions under which grants should be recommended. In some directions the right lines of policy will be settled best in the course of time by experience". It was in fact not until 1929 that the first edition of a pamphlet on *Conditions Applicable to Research Grants* was printed, and about the same time a standard form to be completed by applicants was introduced.

Nevertheless, three primary characteristics of a research grant had already come to be recognised as normal: it was made to an individual and not to (although occasionally through) a department or institution; it was awarded for a specific purpose and not for the support of a general programme; and it was on a temporary basis and without long-term commitment.

The ordinary research grants have always been made to, or at least in respect of, individual research workers; this is one facet of a more general policy already discussed (Chapter 9). Any person exercising independent responsibility in his research work, as distinct from a research assistant working under continuous direction, is eligible to hold a grant in his own name. The applicant must already have a place of work, in fact or assurance, as the Council cannot undertake to find this for him.

A grant is made for a specific purpose—a strictly limited project or programme of investigation; in the last few years the term 'project grant' has been used to distinguish these grants from the longer-term ones discussed below. The award is decided on the basis of a proposal submitted; and if this be approved it becomes the main condition under which the grant is held. This principle was sometimes breached in the earlier days, when a grant might in fact be a thinly veiled subsidy for the general research programme of some specially deserving but impoverished academic department; but such relaxations of principle were apt to create new difficulties.

Grants are expressly temporary, or short-term, and the tendency has been towards greater strictness in this respect; the fact that a grant is made for a clearly defined purpose, as just noted, makes this easier to enforce. Grants may be terminated at short notice if necessary; even subject to that, they were until quite recently not normally made for longer than one year at a time, although an intention to renew for one or more further years might be indicated where appropriate. They are now normally awarded for a period of three years, and extension beyond that can be made only after special review. The general aim is to prevent the establishment of 'freeholds' that would tend to lock up the available funds in a series of long-term commitments of possibly diminishing fruitfulness.

It was always a principle that grants should not be made retrospectively as payment for work already done or as reimbursement for committed expenditure; slight exception might sometimes be made where the decision had been rather long delayed through no fault of the applicant. The purpose of research grants was, in fact, to enable new work to be done; the question of rewards for discoveries has already been discussed (Chapter 9).

Types of research grant
At the outset, in the 'research schemes' submitted to the Minister in 1914 (Chapter 3), the Medical Research Committee strongly recommended that grants for personal remuneration and grants for expenses should be kept entirely distinct; the principle may seem to be an obvious one, but apparently it was by no means universally observed in the practice of other bodies at that time. Eventually, three categories of grants were defined—personal grants, grants for assistance (originally 'scientific assistance'), and grants for expenses. A research worker might receive grants under any or all of these headings.

A personal grant provides remuneration for the research worker himself, in respect of either whole-time or part-time work. At one time a grant for scientific assistance often had a dual motive—to provide the professor, it might be, with an extra pair of hands in his own investigations, and simultaneously to give some training to a potential recruit to the research field; this ambiguity ended with the later establishment of a definite scheme for training awards (Chapter 13).

Grants for expenses could originally cover, among other things, the cost of any laboratory or clerical assistance specially required, scientific assistants being placed in a separate category because they were potential future research workers of independent standing, but latterly this distinction has not been maintained. These grants might also, and still do, cover such items as the cost of special apparatus or materials that could not be provided from departmental resources. The nature of the expenses that may be charged to the grant is determined at the time of award, on the basis of an itemised budget included in the application; and the grant is not a lump payment, but a maximum amount up to which proper claims will be met.

Two points about expenses were decided at the outset, in the 'research schemes' already mentioned. One was that the ordinary equipment of the laboratory, and normal quantities of the usual consumable supplies, must be at the free disposal of the research worker; and where no special expenditure was involved in the research work, no grant for expenses would be made. The Council has also always taken the view that when the number of research workers in a university department grows as the result of personal grants, any increase in the overhead costs is not a matter for the grant-giving body, which does not purport to do more than contribute.

The other principle was that when apparatus or equipment of permanent and separate value was purchased from an expenses grant, it should remain the property of the Council; but application of the rule was always flexible. It might often be in the general interests of medical research that the apparatus should remain where it was. There was also the point that a piece of equipment might have been repaired or partially renewed by the laboratory at its own cost. Nevertheless, items on loan remained on record, and subject to annual check, until such time as they were written off as being no longer of significant value.

This policy about the ownership of permanent apparatus was reversed in 1965, when it was decided that this should normally become the property of the institution, the latter being "responsible for accommodating the apparatus, for operating costs and insurance and for maintaining it in efficient working order so long as it is economical to do this". It was a condition that the investigator for whom the grant had been made should "have free and unfettered use of it until the conclusion of the approved research project"; and exceptionally the Council might require it to be transferred to another institution to which the investigator moved before completing the work.

The new ruling about ownership applied also to items bought under a class of 'special departmental apparatus awards' which had been instituted in 1959 for the provision of expensive apparatus for general research purposes in university departments; although this was considered to be only a secondary responsibility of the Council, it was recognised as a service of great value in the furtherance of research. This complete change in policy reflected the great increase in the complexity and cost of research apparatus since the time when the original views on the subject had been formulated.

The award of grants

The administration of research grants at one time bulked largely in the work of the Committee or Council and of its office. In 1920 the Council had a grants programme to which about two-thirds of its total recurrent expenditure (excluding administrative costs) were deliberately allocated; and an even greater proportion of its attention was devoted to this, as the external staff was still quite small and the business of a largely self-contained central institute was more speedily dealt with than a large number of separate items.

So it was that for a good many years the Council kept the award of grants very much in its own hands, delegating only emergency powers to the Secretary and using specialist committees purely in an advisory role. It was not until 1946 that the detailed discussion of applications for grants and for renewal of grants was delegated to an Appointments and Grants Committee meeting earlier on the same day as the Council; but even this body was a 'committee of the whole house', although in practice the non-scientific members of Council did not normally attend. From 1954, appropriate applications were dealt with, except purely formally, by the Clinical Research Board; and from 1962 the remainder similarly stood referred to the Biological Research Awards Committee (later the Biological Research Board). Both these latter bodies consisted in part of Council members and in part of others, so that the load was spread without serious loss of control. Since 1969 these Boards have had their own Grants Committees, two in each case. The Tropical Medicine Research Board advises on applications within its field. In 1970 a further committee was set up to consider grant applications—the Medical Research Council/Cancer Research Campaign Committee for Jointly Supported Institutes, whose function is to advise the Council and the Cancer Research Campaign on the scientific merits of the applications for support that either body receives from the jointly supported institutes. Like the Council's Research Boards, to which it is similar in status, it also examines and advises on progress reports.

During the greater part of the Council's existence, applications for grants have been considered at any time of year; each has been brought to the next meeting following the completion of any preliminary inquiries by the office and any reference to an advisory committee. From time to time, however, there have been attempts to confine this function to two occasions in the year; but in practice it has been found that too many exceptions have to be made, on grounds of urgency, for any such rigid arrangements to be workable. The chief objection to sporadic consideration has been that, in periods when financial limitations are particularly stringent, it is desirable that applications should be judged competitively and not by a standard that may vary to some extent from meeting to meeting according to the size of the current list. In 1915 the Medical Research Committee had another reason, having to submit its 'schemes' to the Minister, after reference to the Advisory Council, which could not be done piecemeal.

The Council has in fact usually found it possible to maintain an even standard, from meeting to meeting, such as enables it to accept all applications of normal magnitude and high quality. The Council recorded in its Report for 1962–63 that in the period 1953–63 the percentage of grant applications that were successful varied annually from 80 to 93; the high average acceptance rate was thought to reflect a widespread realisation that only applications of good scientific standard have any prospect of success. More recently the acceptance rate has usually been around 50–75 per cent.

The growth in the number of research grants is shown in the following table giving figures at ten-yearly intervals. The figure in each case represents the number of grants in being during the academic year from 1 October; grants of different kinds (personal, assistance, expenses) to the same worker for a single project are reckoned as one grant:

1923–24	176	1953–54	271
1933–34	205	1963–64	715
1943–44	(*wartime*)	1970–71	1216

Increase both in the number of grants and in their nominal values is reflected in the expenditure figures. In the financial year 1923–24 expenditure on grants amounted to £65 944, and in 1970–71 to £2 884 000. The earlier figure represented 48 per cent of total recurrent expenditure, and the latter only 13 per cent; but against this apparent fall must be set the enormous growth, over a like period, of expenditure on research units and external staff, with the addition of a programme of training awards and different forms of long-term support—all of these being different ways of aiding research work in universities and other institutions.

Research fellowships

A fellowship awarded to enable the recipient to devote himself for a period to his own chosen line of research—or sometimes to one specified in the terms of foundation—is something between a whole-time personal grant and a staff appointment. The conditions are not tailored to the man, but are predetermined; but the award does not imply employment in the strict sense and does not usually carry any inherent prospects of permanence or advancement. Further characteristics are the special titular status that is given and the potentially competitive aspect owing to the limited number of places available on each occasion.

Other fellowships are intended for training selected candidates for careers in research, and to promote the recruitment of investigators to particular fields; all the fellowships spontaneously instituted by the Council have been primarily of this second type and are accordingly discussed under the heading of training awards (Chapter 13).

There have been three research fellowships of the first type, placed in the Council's gift by private benefaction:

(1) The Kathleen Schlesinger Research Fellowship was instituted in 1935 under an endowment by Mr and Mrs Eugen M. Schlesinger, in memory of their daughter, to enable the recipient to devote himself to research on cysts of the brain and allied conditions. The endowment took the form of an annuity for 25 years, and the fund is now exhausted.

(2) The Mapother Bequest Research Fellowship in psychiatry was provided, from 1950, by benefactions under the wills of Dr and Mrs Edward Mapother. This came to be treated as a training award.

(3) In 1960 the Trustees of the Nathan Bequest for Cancer Research agreed to make funds available for the Council for the award of a fellowship for at least two years to a British medical

graduate who would undertake an investigation of bone sarcoma. The arrangement has expired.

Long-term support

Some other forms of grant-aid were adopted by the Council relatively late in the period under review. The system of project grants left unsatisfied a need for longer-term support for research in universities and other institutions; and although the difficulty could sometimes be overcome by exceptional treatment of one kind or another, too frequent resort to such expedients is undesirable. To meet this situation, a category of 'special grants' was introduced in 1959, following a lead by the Department of Scientific and Industrial Research. Grants under this head were made in respect of men whom their host institutions wished to retain as research workers but could not immediately appoint to their own staffs. From 1965–66, however, this category of grants lost its separate identity and was merged in the ordinary programme, special conditions being attached when desirable.

Research groups

When the Council wishes to promote a certain line or programme of research in a particular institution, on a scale transcending the work of an individual worker, it may make a long-term or 'programme' grant, as defined later, or it may arrange either to place there a research unit of its own staff organisation (Chapter 11) or to support a research group by means of a grant to the institution. This is a recent use of the title 'research group' conforming with a terminology adopted by the Department of Scientific and Industrial Research—earlier, as has been seen, the Council applied it to the lesser sort of research unit; such changes in nomenclature tend to confuse history.

The grounds for choosing the unit formula have already been stated, both historically and in terms of present policy (Chapter 11); when these do not apply, either the group formula or a programme grant now provides an alternative. In 1961, the Council minuted a resolution that "in all cases in which the primary need is to accelerate the development of a line of research in accord with the purpose for which the recipient university or hospital department was created, support will be by means of a group". It was at the same time laid down that "a prerequisite to the establishment of a group is that the university or other institution concerned should undertake to absorb the group into its normal structure at the end of the agreed period, if it wishes the work to continue". The pamphlet *Long-Term Support for Research*, printed in 1964, set forth the Council's policy. It stated that the purpose of the research group scheme is to assist the development of research programmes in university departments on a longer-term basis than is possible under the scheme of temporary research grants; it is operated when the Council sees need to accelerate the

F*

development of a particular field of research. The Council's acceptance of any request for help under the scheme depends on the merits of the research programme proposed and the presence of an outstanding worker to direct it.

If the leader of a research group moves to another university, the Council will normally transfer the arrangement with him, provided the second university in turn undertakes to assume financial responsibility in due course. Support is thus normally granted for an initial period related to the end of the current quinquennium of the University Grants Committee, or some point in the one next succeeding; and the award is based on an undertaking by the university that it will, in its application for UGC support, include provision in the category having priority equal to or next after that for the continuance of its own existing projects, and before that for entirely new projects. Exceptionally, the Council may give support for longer periods.

The Council approves the number and salary gradings of members of a new research group, but the appointments are made by the university and on its own usual conditions of service. The director under whom it has been agreed to form the group nominates the other members of its staff; in the case of graduate staff, the names of those appointed by the university are subsequently reported to the Council. The budget within which the Council will meet claims for reimbursement also includes provision for equipment and for running expenses; any permanent apparatus purchased remains the property of the Council, on loan to the university for the period of the arrangement and subject to discussion of its subsequent disposal. All administrative negotiations are conducted between the authorised officer of the institution and the Council's headquarters office. The host university is expected to find the accommodation and services required for a research group. At the discretion of the director, members of the graduate staff of the group may take a limited part in university teaching. A full report on the work of a research group is expected by the Council at the end of every period of three years of its support.

The whole scheme is primarily applicable to the assistance of particular medical research programmes in the universities, or in colleges or schools thereof. At the end of 1970 there were 25 research groups in being, as compared with 47 in 1966, and since then numbers have been declining further. The place of research groups is to some extent being taken by the newer programme grants.

Programme grants

The Council's scheme of programme grants is intended to provide long-term support for programmes of work that the Council feels it is in the national interest to pursue. Grants are usually made for five years in the first instance and may be renewed. Programmes should be designed to achieve some broad objective, and preference in providing support under this scheme is given to fields that the Council particularly wishes to develop, although support can be given to other work as well. In either case programmes must be of outstanding scientific merit to qualify for award. At the end of the period covered by this history this form of support was becoming increasingly important.

Block grants

In the spectrum of forms of grant-aid, the block grant to an institution lies at the opposite end from the ordinary research grant. Apart from their common object of promoting research work, the two are strongly contrasted; the block grant is impersonal, more general in its purpose, and semi-permanent in effect even although in form subject to annual renewal. On all these grounds the concept was anathema to the Council in earlier days; and latterly it has been applied only in a very few exceptional instances. The first of these involved no great sum of money and developed without any deliberate change in policy; for long it was not formally acknowledged as a new departure. The second instance involved finance on a major scale, and the arrangement was approved only with some reluctance and after very careful consideration. Three others, of lesser dimensions, were later added on the precedent of the second. Incidentally, anyone consulting the contemporary record in the Council's reports may find that the terms 'special grants' (later restricted in meaning as shown above), and for a time 'special (block) grants', were applied to this category.

The objection in principle to a block grant is that it involves, for the Council, a derogation of responsibility if the administration of a substantial fraction of its resources be entrusted to another authority. As a Treasury official put it, in respect of the second instance mentioned below, the procedure in effect creates "a grant in aid within a grant in aid"—meaning that it placed the expenditure at two removes from close control by the Treasury and might thus be doubly suspect in the eyes of the Public Accounts Committee of the House of Commons. The formula is accordingly one to be invoked only for very good reasons, and even then subject to a close financial control on the part of the Council. Another objection is that a block grant inevitably tends to become a permanently earmarked commitment in all but name, and even to attract progressive augmentation. Nevertheless, it was found that exceptional cases do arise in which a block grant is the only practicable form of support that can be given to a valuable research programme. In three out of five of the instances that have occurred, the special circumstances arose from the history of important institutes for research in cancer, these having developed in association with voluntary hospitals later incorporated in the National Health Service.

The Strangeways Research Laboratory, Cambridge. This was the earliest case in which the Council made a long-term recurrent grant to an institution as such. The payment was at first treated as a grant for research expenses of the ordinary kind, but was not tied to any particular worker or specific project; later it gradually became recognised as a block grant towards the total cost of the Laboratory. The Council has given further help by appointing some of the workers to its own external staff. These arrangements began, in a small way, in 1927 (although some grant-aid had been given from 1917); the annual amount of the block grant had risen by 1969–70 to £36 673, not including £55 462 paid directly to workers there as personal remuneration.

The Laboratory developed from what was originally the Cambridge Research Hospital, founded in 1905 by Dr T. S. P. Strangeways (Huddersfield Lecturer in Pathology in the University) and rehoused in a new building, the nucleus of the present one, in 1912; the purpose was an intensive clinical and pathological study of rheumatoid arthritis and allied conditions. The whole history of the venture is one of personal endeavour, voluntary service, and struggle to obtain financial support from a multiplicity of sources. Mr (later Sir) Otto Beit was a principal benefactor in the early stages. In 1923 it was decided, for scientific reasons mentioned in Volume Two, that the clinical investigations should cease, so far as Cambridge was concerned, leaving the laboratory research work to be continued there. Dr Strangeways died at the end of 1926.

In 1927 the Hospital Trustees, assured of continued and increased support from the Council, decided that the work should be carried on; and in 1928 the Laboratory was given its present name in memory of its founder. In that year, also, Dr (now Dame) Honor Fell was appointed as Director while holding a Senior Beit Fellowship, and later her salary was provided by the Royal Society (still later augmented by the Council); Dr F. G. Spear was Deputy Director from 1931 as a member of the Council's external staff. The research programme was broadened to cover a wide range of work on cell biology, some of it particularly relevant to fundamental problems of malignant disease. As the Laboratory's scientific reputation grew, financial support was secured from a variety of foundations and trusts, from the British Empire Cancer Campaign (as it was then called) and public bodies, and from private benefactors. This aid included some large capital grants for expensive apparatus or additional buildings, notably from the Rockefeller Foundation and the Wellcome Trust. The facilities now include well equipped laboratories for the several disciplines that are relevant to the problem; and up to thirty resident or visiting research workers, with commensurate ancillary personnel, may be taking part in the programme at any one time.

Institute of Cancer Research, London. This is the outstanding example of an institution to which the Council gives major support by means of a block grant; and it was in respect of it that the procedure was first explicitly recognised. The Council's contribution represents the greater part of the current resources of the Institute; the other regular income includes a large annual grant allotted by the Cancer Research Campaign. The parent institution was renamed "Royal Marsden Hospital" at about the same time as the Institute became a separate entity; but the old name, to which a long tradition is attached, was deliberately retained in the title of the Institute, and appears in the formal instrument of incorporation as "Institute of Cancer Research: Royal Cancer Hospital". The original title, when the Institute was evolved from the Pathology Department of the Hospital in 1909, had been "The Cancer Hospital Research Institute" (see Brunning & Dukes, 1965; Haddow, 1961). Another point of nomenclature is that the Institute of Cancer Research includes, as its largest element, the "Chester Beatty Research Institute"; but this is the title of a building, adjacent to the Hospital, and not of an institutional entity. The other elements are, in respect of their research activities, the Hospital's Departments of Physics, Biophysics, Clinical Research and Radiotherapy (and to a minor extent those of Pathology and Medical Records). The Institute has an outlying research station at Pollards Wood, in Buckinghamshire, and a section of the Physics Department is now housed in the Surrey branch of the Royal Marsden Hospital at Sutton, on the southern fringe of London.

Originally, the research activities were regarded as a function of the Hospital and were financed by it out of private grants and subscriptions. When the National Health Service Act 1946 came into operation, in 1948, the Hospital became the responsibility of the Ministry of Health. It was soon concluded, however, that it was inappropriate to make an administrative department of the government responsible for financing research on this scale, representing a proportion of the total expenditure much greater than is usual in hospitals. It was accordingly proposed that the research activities should be hived off, much as the medical schools had been administratively separated from the teaching hospitals, and that the new institution thus created should become the responsibility of the Council.

At first it was intended that the Institute should be administered by the Council as one of its own establishments, and that the staff should be brought into the Council's employ. The senior members of the staff, however, were anxious to preserve the independence of the Institute and also their own academic status; the Institute was recognised as a postgraduate school of the University of London, although not receiving any financial support from that source, so that some members of the staff held university titles and workers there could qualify for higher degrees. A suggestion that the University Grants Committee should become the future arbiter of finance was not pursued, as it became apparent that the objections to this alternative were even stronger. It was eventually agreed, with the approval of HM Treasury, that from 1951 the Council would make an annual block grant towards the support of the Institute; that the latter should retain its place within the British Postgraduate Medical Federation of the University of London; and that it should be incorporated under Articles of Association (completed in 1954) similar to those granted by the (then) Board of Trade to the undergraduate medical schools attached to London teaching hospitals.

The Council was thus presented with an administrative situation of some delicacy. Since the grant in aid represented more than 50 per cent of the Institute's total income, the Treasury looked to the Council to exercise financial control over the whole of the expenditure, maintaining the standards of economy and propriety applicable to expenditure of public funds and aligning rates of pay and conditions of service with those approved for the Council's own staff. This control was, in practice, not easily accepted by a body that had until recently formed part of an entirely autonomous institution, free from the usual inhibitions placed on those entrusted with the expenditure of Exchequer funds. The connection with the University was slender, involving no material control except over the manner of appointment to a small number of higher posts, but its existence involved a method of internal administration by a Committee of Management, a Finance Committee, and an Academic Board; there were also relations with the Board of Governors of the Hospital. A screen of committees and honorary officers was thus interposed between the Council and the Institute's staff, in a way quite alien to the Council's normal practice of dealing immediately, through its headquarters office, with the directing staff of its establishments. There was also a divergence in budgetary methods, characterised by a tendency to incur lasting expenditure commitments on the strength of short-term augmentations of income from special sources. The Council had the right to appoint one-third of the members of the Committee—in practice it never appointed so many—but even this could be a cause of embarrassment, as the presence of persons apt to be regarded as 'representatives' (especially if they were administrative officers) was sometimes taken as implying the Council's concurrence in decisions taken.

The Council was never in doubt that the research work of the Institute was of high quality, some of it very high indeed; and there was no suggestion of overall extravagance, despite deviations from orthodox financial practice as understood in the public service. Had it been otherwise, the Council could scarcely have retained its responsibility without insisting on some radical constitutional change. These difficulties are recorded here solely to make the general point that the block grant formula, where its proportion demands oversight of total expenditure, is not an appropriate method of financing an autonomous institution with an academic form of internal government.

The Council's grant provided £150 000 towards the Institute's estimated total expenditure of £230 000 in the first year of the arrangement; and this had increased to £494 000 (towards an estimated total expenditure of £1 157 675) in 1969–70. In 1957 the Council, after consulting HM Treasury, had agreed to a large capital expenditure by the Institute, from endowment funds, for the provision of additional accommodation for the Chester Beatty Research Institute.

In 1968 the general question came again to a head when the Institute transmitted to the Council a report by an internal committee under the chairmanship of Sir Edward Hale. This led the Council to seek once more to transfer responsibility for administering the block grant to the University of London; but this proved to be impossible. In the following year a special subcommittee of the Council examined the work of the Institute in some detail and made recommendations for the future. (By this time Sir Alexander Haddow had been compelled by ill-health to retire as Director of the Chester Beatty Research Institute.) It was agreed that the laboratory and clinical studies should continue to be kept together within a unified Institute for Cancer Research; and that there should in future be an overall scientific Director. Some parts of the work currently being done in the laboratories were considered by the subcommittee to be of a lower standard than the rest, and the question of discontinuing these was therefore for consideration. In general, the Council agreed to remain responsible for arrangements for support of the Institute, but decided that its block grant should be reduced by about half and the other portion converted into support for specific research programmes; this would give the Council more control. Detailed arrangements implementing this policy were agreed in 1970. Professor Thomas Symington was appointed to the new post of Director of the whole Institute.

Cancer Research Department (now Beatson Institute for Cancer Research), Royal Beatson Memorial Hospital, Glasgow. A similar problem presented itself here in 1955, although on a much smaller scale. The Cancer Research Department had been supported by funds from the Glasgow Western Hospital Board of Management (National Health Service), from the Department of Health for Scotland (as it then was), and from private sources. After consultation with the Western Regional Hospital Board (Scotland), and the British Empire Cancer Campaign, the Council assumed major financial responsibility for the programme of cancer research directed by Dr P. R. Peacock. A block grant was first made in the financial year 1957–58 in the amount of £12 000; by 1969–70 this had increased to £34 560. After Dr Peacock's retirement in 1966, the arrangement was continued, with Dr John Paul as Director.

Paterson Laboratories, Christie Hospital and Holt Radium Institute, Manchester. The title of these laboratories dates only from the retirement, in 1962, of Professor Ralston Paterson from his post as Director of the Holt Radium Institute: before that they constituted the six research departments of the Christie Hospital. From 1953 to 1962 the Council maintained here a Betatron Research Unit (at first called a Group) under the honorary direction of Professor Paterson; at the end of that time this was transferred to the Manchester Regional Hospital Board (Volume Two). In 1956 the Council assumed responsibility for financial support formerly given to the research departments from National Health Service funds through the South Manchester Hospital Management Committee. Three of the senior research workers were appointed to the Council's external staff, and a block grant of £10 000 per annum was made towards the cost of the activities; further support was given by a large grant from the British Empire Cancer Campaign and by a contribution from hospital endowment funds. In 1969–70 the Council's block grant had risen to £90 320, but this included all salaries, among them that attached to a new post of Director of the research departments; to this Dr L. G. Lajtha, a member of the Council's external staff elsewhere, was appointed.

Davy Faraday Research Laboratory, The Royal Institution, London. Under the direction of Sir Lawrence Bragg, the research work here was principally concerned with the structure of protein molecules and involved close collaboration with the Council's own Laboratory of Molecular Biology at Cambridge. The Council had made grants in support of the programme from 1955, and two years later appointed three of the workers to its external staff. In 1960 the Council added a block grant to enable the work to be expanded and developed. A sum of £55 750 was in this way provided to meet expenditure, at varying annual rates over a period of five years; the items included further scientific and technical staff, equipment and running expenses, and the purchase of computer time. The arrangement was subsequently continued until the retirement of Sir Lawrence Bragg in 1966.

Other block payments. Certain other payments to institutions have been temporarily administered under the block grants formula; two of the more substantial instances may be mentioned. From 1961 a payment of £21 000 per annum (increasing to over £36 000 in 1969–70) was made to the War Office for work undertaken on the Council's behalf at the Microbiological Research Establishment, Porton, Wiltshire, on the production of various substances by or from microorganisms; this was in continuation of work that had been done at the Council's own Antibiotics Research Station at Clevedon, Somerset, until that unit was closed down. The new arrangement was, however, more by way of reimbursement for services rendered

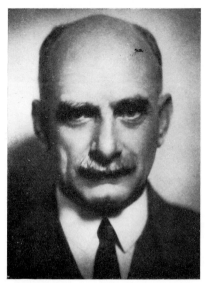

Sir Thomas Lewis, CBE, FRS

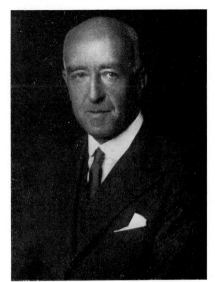

Sir Paul Fildes, OBE, FRS

Sir Patrick Laidlaw, FRS

Sir Percival Hartley, CBE, MC, FRS

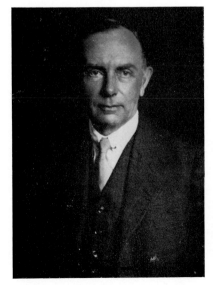

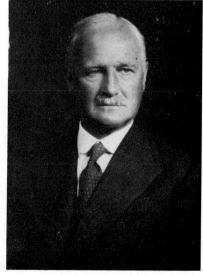

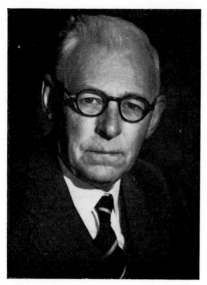

Sir Alan Drury, CBE, FRS

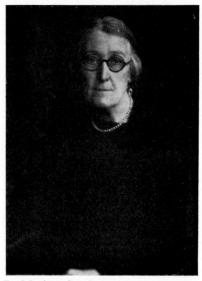

Dr Marjory Stephenson, FRS

Dr Leonard Colebrook, FRS

Professor John R. Squire

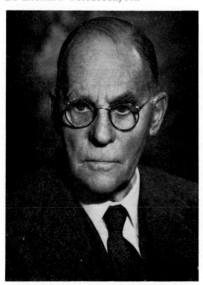

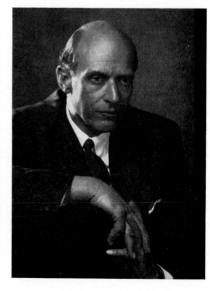

than a grant in aid in the usual sense. In 1962 a grant of £6000 per annum (increasing to over £20 000 in 1969–70) was made to the East Grinstead Memorial Trust for a programme of work at the McIndoe Memorial Research Unit in the Queen Victoria Hospital, East Grinstead, Sussex.

Since 1969 the Council has made some small contracts for the promotion of research and development work which could not be undertaken in its own establishments or under existing methods of research promotion. Under a contract an external institution (e.g. a university department, independent research organisation or commercial firm) carries out, on a reimbursement basis, a project specified by the Council.

Contributions to international projects
An entirely new type of grant was instituted in 1965 in a then unique case. The Council is responsible for providing, from its grant in aid, the United Kingdom's contribution to the cost of the new International Agency for Research on Cancer. The payment, standing at £79 568 per annum in 1970–71, has not to be accounted for in detail to the Exchequer and Audit Department, and no unexpended balances are returnable to the Council. Sir Harold Himsworth was appointed by the Secretary of State for Education and Science to represent the United Kingdom on the Governing Council of the Agency; and his successor, Sir John Gray, has been appointed Chairman of that body. The other countries supporting the Agency are the USA, the USSR, France, West Germany, Italy and Australia; Professor John Higginson was appointed Director of the Agency, which has its headquarters in Lyon.

This enterprise arose from proposals made by the French Government in 1963 for an international cancer research organisation to be financed by governmental grants. The original scheme envisaged a research institute for experimental research, but great doubt was felt about the advantage of placing a large international group of laboratory workers under one roof, to the impoverishment of the existing institutions all over the world. It was accordingly decided that the appropriate role was mainly on the epidemiological side, and the Agency's plans include such studies in several parts of the world, with centres in East Africa, Asia and South America.

Chapter 13
Training and Travel Awards

The principle of training awards—Awards in special fields—Studentships or scholarships for training—Senior awards—Travelling fellowships—Travel awards of limited scope

The principle of training awards

Sir Almroth Wright, doyen of the scientific staff of the original Medical Research Committee, held decided views on (among many other subjects) the training of research workers. He wrote to Addison on 22 January 1914: "I think that a research worker should have an education comparable to that given to a Jesuit". In his biography of Wright, Colebrook says:

> He would have liked to see established a training school to which those contemplating a career in medical science would automatically go for a course of instruction and preparation. Such instruction, in his view, should include the basic laboratory techniques of which all research workers should know at least the rudiments—for example, elementary glass-blowing, microscopy and microphotography, micro-measurement, electrical technology, staining methods and tissue-culture techniques, and some chemical processes, such as chromatography. And to these he would, of course, add some instruction in the logic of science; the concept of a crucial experiment; the possibilities and the pitfalls of statistical methods. Such a training establishment as he visualised would be virtually the counterpart of the Army's Staff College.

Colebrook adds that Wright "wrote a memorandum embodying these ideas, and submitted it to the Council in 1919, but I do not know if it ever received serious consideration". In fact, the memorandum was only an *aide-mémoire* of views expressed verbally at a special meeting of the Committee on 28 February 1919, which he attended by invitation to discuss this and other questions with the members. The memorandum itself is unfortunately missing from the files, but Fletcher's notes of the discussion and summary prepared for circulation are extant. It appears to have been thought that there were other things to be taught than techniques and logic, and better ways of training than formal instruction.

The Council was, however, slow in adopting the principle of making awards specifically for training graduates in methods of research; and it was not until 1944 that it decided to institute a comprehensive scheme of postgraduate studentships for this purpose. To a small extent, as already mentioned, the need had been met by making grants for scientific assistance to professors and others who had promising graduates available for work in which useful experience could be acquired (Chapter 12).

It could be argued that all participation in directed research provides training, and equally that the work of trainees may add to knowledge. This, although superficially true, tends to confuse two criteria which should preferably be kept distinct—the value of the immediate work for the advancement of knowledge, and the value of the training given to a future investigator. Even if both facets may commonly coexist the motive for making a particular award should be clear. There is an administrative reason for such clarity, in that a personal research grant, or a payment for services under a grant for assistance, ranks as taxable remuneration; on the other hand a payment to enable the holder to continue his education is, subject to certain conditions, free from liability to income tax.

Awards to students-in-training had for long been made by the Department of Scientific and Industrial Research, and latterly also by the Agricultural Research Council. These covered subjects that were likewise basic to medical science—biochemistry bulking largely among them—and a tripartite division of the field, according to the orientation of the particular line of research proposed in each case, might have seemed appropriate. That this view had not been unequivocally accepted earlier by the Council was at least partly due to the fact that the system, on which the Treasury imposed uniformity, was for various reasons less suitable for graduates in medicine than for those who had taken first degrees in science and were proceeding to a doctorate.

Awards in special fields

The Council's first deliberate ventures in the field of training awards were directed towards giving medical graduates further training in branches of research to which it was particularly desired to encourage recruitment. Certain series of awards, each quite small in number, were thus instituted in special subjects.

The first series, instituted in 1935, comprised Junior and Senior Fellowships for Research in Tropical Medicine. The Junior Fellowships were expressly for training in methods of research and were tenable for three years; the Senior Fellowships were perhaps more in the nature of first research appointments, but the motive was still that of training investigators. Each Fellow was placed under a suitable director in a university institution at home; but he could be sent—although not normally during the first two years of a junior award—for periods of work in the tropics, for which expenses were provided under the scheme. Junior Fellows were eligible to be continued as Senior Fellows, for a further three years, and persons who had already acquired the necessary experience could be appointed direct to the latter grade. During the short operation of the scheme, before the Second World War brought it to an end, nine men were appointed to Junior Fellowships and three directly to Senior Fellowships. Some subsequently had careers of distinction in whole-time tropical medical research; others continued to work in the field of tropical medicine, engaging partly in research. Their work is referred to in Volume Two.

In 1936 the Council launched a scheme for the annual award of up to six Postgraduate Studentships for training in methods of research in clinical science or experimental pathology, two fields to which it was thought particularly important to recruit medically qualified investigators. These studentships were awarded to graduates who had already completed the usual 'house' appointments; they were tenable for one year, and were expressly not intended to assist the recipient to study for further examinations. In addition, four Research Fellowships were instituted, in the same fields, for more senior men with some experience in research. These were regarded as probationary research appointments; they were tenable for one year, but could be renewed for a second.

Whereas these two schemes fell into abeyance during the Second World War (and were, in fact, never resumed in the same form), the Council in 1940 instituted studentships for training medical graduates in the methods of experimental psychology. Five awards were made during the short life of the scheme, and three of the recipients subsequently became members of the Council's staff in its Applied Psychology Research Unit at Cambridge (Volume Two).

Studentships or scholarships for training
In the latter part of 1943 the Council, looking to the end of the war, set up a subcommittee to consider the whole question of training awards. Early in 1944 the Council adopted the recommendation of this body that a comprehensive system of Studentships (from 1953 called 'Scholarships') should be set up on the lines of that long operated by the Department of Scientific and Industrial Research. These were to be for "men and women of promise recently graduated in science or qualified in medicine". They were to be for work in subjects of concern to the Council, and were to be awarded for one year in the first instance, renewable for second and third years (not necessarily at the same place of study, although the conditions of eligibility for a higher degree would normally require this). An incidental consequence was that the earlier separate schemes for a few training awards in special subjects became otiose and were allowed to lapse permanently; the pre-war studentships in clinical science and experimental pathology were replaced, at a higher level, by the Fellowships in Clinical Research to be mentioned further below.

In recording the decision to award studentships, the Council made the reservation that it did "not accept general responsibility for training workers for careers in medical research". In other words, the Council would not necessarily operate on a scale dictated by whatever the total demand might prove to be, as distinct from the scale that it might itself consider adequate for the purposes to which it attached major importance; it intended to be selective, making awards to men and women of promise as future research workers and restricting them to subjects of work which it had either chosen itself or specially approved. Nevertheless, in practice the acceptance rate of applications became high. Of the candidates in 1963, 86 per cent were successful, and this proportion included all those with First Class or 'upper' Second Class Honours degrees in science or with medical qualifications. A change of procedure in 1967 is mentioned later.

In 1945 the scheme came into full operation, with 57 awards; the figure on one occasion fell to 36, but in 1970 it reached 262. The number of scholarships in being at any date is, naturally, of the order of three times the annual intake.

From 1957 the ordinary scholarships scheme was supplemented by a series of 'Awards for Further Education in the Medical Sciences'. These were regarded as slightly junior and carried stipends at subsistence level; they were normally tenable for one year. Subsequently the stipends and allowances of these awards were equated with those for Scholarships and the maximum tenure was fixed at two years. The need for such awards arose from a decision that support by the Ministry of Education and local authorities for postgraduate courses should be limited to the Arts Faculty; awards for studies in science and technology became the responsibility of the Department of Scientific and Industrial Research, except in the medical sciences. The awards instituted by the Council in the latter field were intended to enable suitable candidates to take courses of instruction (from 1961 not necessarily formal) at a higher level or in some complementary discipline. The recipients might be aiming at M SC degrees in such subjects as biochemistry, physiology and pharmacology, or at certain diplomas such as those in genetics, statistics, and psychology, or at acquiring knowledge in such specialised fields as microbiology and radiobiology. Candidates were required to have taken a first degree in science (e.g. B SC), or to have passed the '2nd MB' stage in a medical course. Under this scheme, the Council made 8 awards in 1957; by 1970 the number had risen to 94.

The results of the scholarships scheme were surveyed in 1950, 1956 and 1958. On the last occasion the review covered the subsequent histories of the 427 students and scholars who had completed their training under the scheme between 1944 and 1958. Training had been given in 15 different fields, of which biochemistry had taken 30 per cent of the scholars; medically qualified scholars represented 12 per cent of the total.

Of the 427, 3 had died and 28 others had to be omitted from consideration for one reason or another. Of the remainder, 241 had obtained full-time academic or research appointments, fellowships, or grants, in universities or research institutes in the United Kingdom or abroad—one of the earliest had been appointed to a chair of medicine at a London teaching hospital. A further 31 were in the Scientific Civil Service (UK), 5 held governmental posts abroad, and 49 were doing research work in industry; 30 were in the National Health Service (5 with consultant rank; 6 in non-medical posts); 10 were engaged in school teaching, and 6 had adopted 'unexpected' careers (including the Church, the Royal Navy and British Railways). Finally, 24 women (out of 72) had married and given up research. Overall, 10 per cent were working abroad, mainly in the United States, Canada and Australia. On 19 June 1959, with the report of the review before it, the Council "noted with satisfaction that this training scheme was effectively serving the purpose for which it was set up; but that it would be advantageous if means could be found to increase the proportion of medically qualified trainees".

In 1961 the Council decided to extend to medical students of promise who had passed the 2nd MB examination, and to dental students who had passed their BDS examination, eligibility for the Further Education Awards mentioned above, if such students wished to interrupt their professional courses for a year's study of a basic preclinical subject. The response was negligible, however, possibly because support for this purpose was available from Local Education Authorities. But in 1964 full responsibility for making awards to medical and dental students who wished to intercalate B SC courses was taken over by the Council from Local Education Authorities; the value continued to be assessed in conformity with the practice of these authorities for other undergraduate awards. The number of Awards for Intercalated Courses made by the Council increased from 12 in 1964–65 to 101 in 1965–66 and 282 in 1970–71.

The number of candidates for scholarships and further education awards had become so great that in 1967 the Council adopted the practice of allocating blocks of awards to heads of university departments for distribution among suitably qualified candidates. In the Report for 1969–70 a modification of this plan, after two years of experience, was announced in the following terms:

> The basis of the new arrangements is that the Council decides in the light of its own research priorities on the allocation of the available number of awards between broad subject areas, and the Training Awards Committee, in the light of advice from independent referees, allocates quotas to individual departments within the relevant numerical limits set by the Council. The allocations made by the Committee are based on assessment not so much of the particular projects to be undertaken as of a department's capacity to provide good overall research training.

> In the light of the Council's decisions on priority areas for research, preference will be given in 1970 to applications for training in the following subjects: mycology, virology, developmental biology, clinical pharmacology and thera-

peutics, epidemiology and social medicine, psychiatry and clinical psychology, physical anthropology, bioengineering and biomechanics, dentistry, nutrition and parasitology.

The scholarships scheme as a whole continues to be given very high priority by the Council.

Senior awards

The point mentioned above about the small proportion of medically qualified trainees continued to present the Council with its major problem in the particular field; and, when the whole policy in respect of training awards was reviewed in 1961, the Council decided to institute an additional series of awards at first spoken of as 'senior scholarships' but in the event designated Junior Research Fellowships. These were expressly regarded as training awards, although their conditions did not qualify for exemption from income tax on the stipends. They were intended primarily for medically qualified candidates who had completed their obligatory junior hospital appointments; the stipends were in fact equated to the salaries of senior resident posts in the National Health Service. Dental graduates of equivalent standing, and science graduates who had already taken second degrees such as PH D, were also eligible. The first 6 appointments (5 medical) were made for the academic year 1962–63; in the following year the number rose to 22.

Solely in the clinical field, and at a more senior level, the Council already had its Clinical Research Fellowships, instituted in 1950 with the similar intention of attracting men with clinical experience into research. These awards were equated in stipend to registrar posts in the National Health Service, and arrangements were made with the Health Departments for the maintenance of superannuation provision during tenure. They provided for training not only in clinical research but also, if necessary, in the non-clinical subject most relevant to the holder's clinical interests. The awards were for one year in the first instance but renewable. At first an undertaking was in each case required from the academic or hospital department sponsoring the application that, on satisfactory completion, the fellow would be given the choice of returning to employment there; this condition was relaxed in 1965, but the head of department was still expected to take steps to this end.

In establishing these awards, the Council pointed out in its Report for 1950–51 that:

To be equipped to start training in clinical research a man or woman must not merely have graduated in medicine but must have held hospital appointments, of the status of senior house officer, which would give him the necessary clinical experience and which would not normally be held until some eight years after beginning medical study, excluding time spent on military service. Suitable candidates would therefore be of considerable seniority, and the awards would need to be adapted to their age and experience and to take into account the fact that workers of similar seniority in the nonclinical branches of medical research would already be eligible for special research awards or for employment as members of the Council's staff.

In 1963–64 there were 9 Clinical Research Fellowships in being, and in 1964 the Council's Clinical Research Board, in strongly recommending continuation of the scheme, referred to the "notably successful subsequent careers of holders of these awards". In 1970–71 there were 27.

Travelling fellowships

From 1923–24 onwards the Council was entrusted with the award, in the United Kingdom, of Rockefeller Medical Fellowships provided by the Rockefeller Foundation of New York to enable selected graduates to spend a full academic year doing research work in the United States or Canada—later it became permissible to choose an approved centre in a European country on occasion. The arrangement between the Foundation and the Council was made for three years in the first instance and was periodically renewed. The funds covered an average of 5–6 fellowships annually. The general conditions governing the fellowships were similar to those framed by the Foundation for wider use, but the Council was left free to modify them to meet the particular circumstances. The awards and travel arrangements were made by the Council, and arrangements in America by the Foundation.

The Council very warmly welcomed this generous action on the part of the Rockefeller Foundation, because opportunities such as travelling fellowships of this kind could provide were sadly deficient in Great Britain; and at that time the Council was not in a position to set aside money for the purpose from its own general resources. The Council had also reason to think that it was itself well placed, through its ordinary close contacts with universities and medical schools, to administer awards of this type. The fellowships were open to graduates in medicine and related sciences. They were particularly intended for men and women of promise who were expected to proceed to positions in higher teaching and research in the United Kingdom.

Candidates were expected to have already had such training and experience in research work as would enable them to derive maximum benefit from the opportunity of working under the stimulus of a new environment. From the first, accordingly, the Council selected candidates of something more than immediate postgraduate seniority. The standard of qualification was thus high—and in most years, so greatly were these awards sought after, more than the available number of appointments could have been made without sensibly lowering it. When the effect of this policy became known, the Council's fellows were assured of more than ordinarily cordial welcome at centres of research in America.

The success of the scheme was never in doubt, and the record of the subsequent careers of the holders of Rockefeller Medical Fellowships is impressive. A survey of the 214 holders in the period 1923–64, including even the most junior, showed the following occupations: university professors, 82 (including one Nobel Laureate); university readers or senior lecturers, 21; directors of research establishments, 5; other whole-time research or teaching posts, 36; consultant practice, 57; other medical posts, 13.

After the academic year 1935–36 the scheme was interrupted by a change in the general policy of the Foundation, involving concentration on certain special fields. In these fields the Foundation was still prepared to award travelling fellowships to British subjects, but this was to be done directly and not through the Council. The latter was most anxious to fill the gap and in its Report for 1934–35 expressed the hope that finance for the purpose would be forthcoming from other sources. In response, the Leverhulme Trustees generously agreed to award one fellowship annually for five years on the nomination of the Council. For 1936–37 one Leverhulme Travelling Fellowship and two others provided by the Council from its own general funds were awarded. Further building up of a new scheme was rendered unnecessary when the Rockefeller Foundation agreed to renew the old arrangement with effect from 1937–38, thus missing only one year. A longer interruption inevitably resulted from the Second World War; only one of the recipients of awards for 1939–40 was able to take up his appointment, and the next awards were for 1945–46. Thereafter the scheme continued with only the minor modification that, from 1951, the Council itself provided the transatlantic fares and the Fellows were a charge on Rockefeller funds only while in America. Then, with the academic year 1963–64, the Foundation brought its support of the scheme to an end as the result of new decisions regarding its general policy.

By this time the Council was in a position to make provision itself, and for 1964–65 the first six Medical Research Council Travelling Fellowships (apart from two in 1936–37 as mentioned above) were awarded. Meanwhile, the original scheme had come to be supplemented by other more or less similar awards placed at the Council's disposal from various sources: (1) From 1950 Eli Lilly and Company of Indianapolis awarded one or more travelling fellowships each year on the Council's nomination. These were tenable only in the United States; they were at first known as Eli Lilly Research Fellowships, but from 1957 as Lilly Foreign Educational Fellowships. (2) A like arrangement was made in 1955 for an annual Lederle Travelling Fellowship in Medicine, awarded by the Lederle Laboratories Division of the American Cyanamid Company; this arrangement ran for eight years (although in one of them the Council made no nomination). (3) In 1958 the Council was entrusted with the nomination for United States Public Health Service Fellowships, to the number of five or six annually. These were tenable only in the United States; they were open to medical or science graduates, with preference to candidates who had completed a doctoral degree in medical science. (4) To these were added in 1960, by the Wellcome Trustees, an annual group of five Sir Henry Wellcome Travelling Fellowships to be awarded by the Council, with preference to candidates in physiology, biochemistry, pharmacology, and tropical medicine. (5) In 1970 two additional travelling fellowships were made available by the Goldsmiths' Company for award by the Council. Thus by the end of the period of this history the Council had at its effective disposal, for 1970–71, about twenty travelling fellowships with a reasonable prospect of being able to continue on this scale. Although some of these are subject to limiting conditions or preferences, the differences are not of a kind to prevent the whole from being administered as a unified scheme, with a single competitive entry.

The availability of so many awards was most gratifying, as the Council's experience of administering travelling fellowships has certainly led to a very different view of their value from that expressed by Dr Samuel Johnson in 1784:

> It is wonderful how little good Radcliffe's Travelling Fellowships have done. I know of nothing that has been imported by them; yet many additions to our medical knowledge might be got in foreign countries. Inoculation, for instance, has saved more lives than war destroys; and the cures performed by the Peruvian-bark are innumerable. But it is in vain to send our travelling physicians to France, and Italy, and Germany, for all that is known there is known here; I'd send them out of Christendom; I'd send them among barbarous nations.

In 1967 the Council was able, with the agreement of the Treasury, to increase the value of its travelling fellowships by paying the travel and subsistence costs of a Fellow's wife and children when a fellowship runs a year or more. Similar provision was made by the Wellcome Trustees in respect of the Sir Henry Wellcome Travelling Fellowships.

Travel awards of limited scope
'Dorothy Temple Cross Research Travelling Fellowships' in tuberculosis were endowed in 1929 by Mrs Odo Cross in memory of her daughter, with a capital gift of £40 000 to the Council in trust. These were to be awarded to British subjects suitably qualified in medicine or science who intended ultimately "to devote themselves to the advancement, by teaching or research, of the curative or preventive treatment of tuberculosis in all or any of its forms". They were to be "for the express purpose of investigation and study", preferably in some country abroad approved by the Council; and they were to be tenable for one year in the first instance. Two of the first annual group of fellowships were awarded for special investigations of tuberculosis in, respectively, Zanzibar and the Sudan; one in the second group was awarded to a non-medical bacteriologist for work on the subject in laboratories in Berlin and Vienna. Most of the awards, however, went to medical men and women wishing to make

more conventional study visits to outstanding centres of treatment in various European countries or in North America.

After the Second World War it was necessary to raise the rate of stipend and consequently to offer fewer fellowships; by 1953 provision for only a single award could be made. In 1952 the Council obtained the approval of the Charity Commissioners for raising the maximum to which the trust deed had limited any stipend. In 1964, it was decided, with the agreement of the Charity Commissioners, to increase the value of a fellowship still further and also to widen the subject scope (as permitted by the trust deed) to include other diseases of the lungs than tuberculosis; and in 1967 it was necessary to seek the Commissioners' agreement to a further increase in the value of these fellowships to allow for the payment of dependants' travel costs to bring the awards into line with other travelling fellowships at the Council's disposal.

It remains to mention arrangements of a more special kind. Since 1949 the Council has been able to award Travelling Fellowships in Ophthalmology and Otology provided by the Alexander Pigott Wernher Memorial Trust. These are limited to the special subjects and to citizens of the Commonwealth; they can be, and often are, held for periods of less than a year, to facilitate relatively short study visits abroad.

Another arrangement, dating from 1948–49, is for Exchange Scholarships in Medical Science between France and Great Britain. In operating this the Centre National de la Recherche Scientifique collaborates with the Council, each of these governmental agencies annually nominating two scholars to work in the other's country for part or the whole of an academic year, the host country providing stipend and facilities for work. A similar arrangement was agreed in 1965 between the Council and the Institut de la Santé et de la Recherche Médicale to provide four scholarships annually. These enable two British and two French workers, medically qualified and of registrar status, to undertake clinical research in France and Great Britain respectively, normally for one or two years, and in any event not for less than three months.

Chapter 14
Publications and Information Services

Publications policy—Publication in journals—The Special Report Series—
Memoranda and miscellaneous reports—Miscellaneous books—Industrial Health
Reports—Annual Reports—Abstracting journals—Scientific intelligence—Public
information—Editorial work and printing

Publications policy
Responsibility for promoting research, whatever methods be used,
is not discharged until publication of the results is achieved. For a
new agency entering the field, this axiom immediately raises certain
questions of policy. Should the agency establish its own medium of
publication, say a series of official reports, and perhaps even restrict
its research workers to publishing therein? Alternatively, should it
encourage these workers to communicate their findings to the
scientific world through the journals devoted to the particular
subjects, according to normal academic custom? Further, does the
responsibility end even with the publication of original work? If not,
how far should the research agency itself go in promulgating new
knowledge to a wider public, or in maintaining information services
of one kind or another?

This question of the manner of publishing original work has to be
considered in various lights—effectiveness in the advancement of
knowledge; benefit to the agency in its public relations; and fairness
to the scientific workers themselves, in their proper desire for freedom
of expression and for personal recognition. It must be said that this
last aspect has not always ranked as a major consideration in respect
of official scientific publications. The members of the Medical
Research Committee, however, had a clear view of the requirements:
the investigators concerned should be encouraged to publish under
their own names, the intellectual responsibility being theirs and not
that of the sponsoring body; they should publish in appropriate
media, making their results readily available as additions to the
general pool of scientific knowledge; and the conclusions should be
accompanied by descriptions of methods and by details of findings,
sufficient to enable others to check the argument and, if necessary,
to repeat the observations or experiments.

These general precepts properly apply to all scientific research
work undertaken in the public interest and not subject to security
considerations. They concern both the actual staff of an official
research organisation and the independent scientists assisted by its

grants. There is, in science, no official brand of truth; and the imprimatur of a research council or department adds nothing to the value of research results beyond some assurance of the author's qualifications for his task.

The Committee did not regard these principles as self-evident to the public at large, or even in governmental circles, so it included the following statements of policy in the "schemes for research" that it put forward in October 1914:

> It has been the practice of some Government Departments giving grants in aid of scientific research to require that the results shall be published only in the form of a Report to the Head of the Department. In the opinion of the Medical Research Committee this practice is undesirable, and has led to the premature burial in Departmental archives of much valuable scientific work. The Committee propose that liberty shall be given to all the workers aided from the Research Fund who are of such scientific status as to be assigned independent work, to publish their scientific results through the ordinary channels of the technical scientific journals. Those workers who are definitely placed under the direction of a Professor or Head of a laboratory responsible to the Committee will be free to publish only with the consent of their Director.

The important point in the quoted statement is the declared intention to allow the research workers to publish their papers without prior submission for official approval, although relatively junior workers would be expected to obtain the consent of their scientific chiefs. In this way was academic freedom granted to investigators supported from public funds, and there can be no doubt that the decision had far-reaching effects in enhancing the status of the Council's scientific service.

The Report for 1925–26 mentioned a suggestion, arising "in some quarters, perhaps not the best informed", that the Council ought to withhold results from publication until complete certitude had been attained. The Council thought it necessary to counter this and to reaffirm that its policy had always been to leave the scientific workers complete discretion to publish their results:

> This was a natural and proper part of the freedom which all scientific workers rightly claim. But it is much more; it is the only condition under which work can be brought as quickly as possible, both to the bar of scientific opinion for its proper assessment, and also to the knowledge of other workers in the same or other fields who may gain useful information or stimulus from it. No one familiar with the nature of scientific work could suppose that any council of scientific men would be either able or willing to exercise any censorship over scientific results, except by way of assuring themselves that their aid is given only to work honestly performed by men competent to do it. There is no certitude in science except that which is gained by the free and gradual suffrage of general scientific opinion based on repetition at will of the experimental facts reported.

It was, of course, agreed to be against the public interest "that any hopes of some desired practical outcome of research should ever be falsely or prematurely aroused."

Publication in journals

Thus, from the beginning, the great bulk of the findings of the employed or assisted research workers was published in papers contributed by the investigators to appropriate scientific journals, many of them the organs of specialised societies. The Council never seriously considered instituting a periodical medium of its own for this purpose; it would inevitably have been too wide in scope to be, for most items, as effective a channel of publication as one of the journals closely followed by those interested in the relevant branch of medical or related science.

(In its Report for 1932–33 the Council referred to its "position of trusteeship" in respect of the journal *Heart*, founded in 1925 by Sir Thomas Lewis and becoming *Clinical Science* in 1933 under his continuing editorship. The responsibility, assumed at Lewis's request and by agreement with the publishers, was limited to the appointment of future editors and in general to ensuring that the standard of publication was maintained. By agreement among the parties, the trusteeship was in 1939 transferred to the Medical Research Society. Another journal that owed its origin and early policy to a member of the Council's staff, in this case Dr P. G. (later Sir Paul) Fildes, was the *British Journal of Experimental Pathology*. The results of much work supported by the Council were published in these journals.)

The Council did not expect to have to subsidise independent journals for publishing work that it had supported; these journals were deriving much of their best material from this source, to the benefit of their circulations. It is true that economic considerations may weigh heavily against a technical periodical of restricted subject range; but, so far as scientific journals in the United Kingdom are concerned, financial aid can be sought from a government grant administered by the Royal Society—on the very proper basis of the general standard and total requirements of the periodical, not in respect of the merits of individual items. Occasionally the Council has made a grant towards the extra expense of publishing an item of work requiring very costly illustrations or tables for its adequate presentation. More often, in such cases, it has preferred to offer publication in the form of one of its own reports.

In its Report for 1960–61, the last in which all publications appearing during the year were listed, the number of these references approached 2500, of which all but a negligible proportion represented papers contributed to journals.

The Special Report Series

The other side of the picture was that, from the beginning, the Medical Research Committee issued a small proportion of its workers' output in a series of reports published by Her Majesty's Stationery Office. Numbers 1–49 were published for the Committee in the period 1915–20, and No. 50 and its successors for the Council from 1920. These constituted the MRC Special Report Series, commonly known as 'green reports' from the colour of their covers. By the end of 1971 the series had reached No. 310.

For some purposes, separately issued reports have obvious advantages over papers in periodicals—for instance, when a substantial official distribution is advisable, say to the medical branches of the Services; or when a considerable sale to the general public is expected; or when the report is one that the research worker will wish to have always at hand rather than on the library shelf. The first of these circumstances is particularly likely to exist in time of war, and an analysis of the first 50 reports—all published during the First World War or arising from work done in that period—clearly shows this. Of these, 37 reports dealt with subjects of direct importance to the war effort and mostly appropriate to official distribution. Of the second 50 issues, in the post-war period 1920–26, 13 were reports of committees and 7 were of multiple authorship: 6 more were assessments or reviews of the state of knowledge on particular subjects. For reports by single authors giving the results of original research the use of this medium, as contrasted with periodicals, was in fact scarcely significant.

The Special Report Series was, in fact, not at first highly regarded by research workers as a vehicle for publishing their results, except when a monograph too large for a journal was envisaged. The average circulation was—and indeed still is—less than that of a prosperous journal and was also not adapted to particular specialties. Another voiced objection was that authors' names did not appear on the wrapper, and sometimes not even on the title-page, but only in the table of contents or the chapter headings; as a result, reports tended to be listed in bibliographies under the name of the Committee or Council instead of under that of the author. This last point, however, had only to be mentioned to be immediately remedied, and from No. 60 (1922) onwards the authors' names were always shown both on the wrapper and on the title-page. The principle involved was not only one of personal credit, but one of scientific responsibility; and it has happened that reports accepted for publication in the series have differed from each other in their conclusions.

The conditions of the Second World War restricted the issue of green reports, partly in favour of another type of publication presently to be mentioned. After the war, in 1946, the Council formulated its policy in more definite terms than before: "that reports on the results of original research should, whenever suitable, preferably be published in scientific journals". It was at the same time agreed that this series "should be used mainly for the publication of the results of original research, whether sponsored by the Council or not, and for the more extensive type of critical review, such publications being addressed primarily to research workers".

In 1955 it was suggested to the Council, in an office memorandum, that some of the reports accepted for publication during the pre-

Council Publications of Scientific Work*

Numbers in five-year periods

	Special Report Series	War Memoranda and Memoranda	Reports of the IHRB	Emergency Reports, IHRB	Monitoring Report Series	Miscellaneous
1915–19	44		4			
1920–24	45		24			
1925–29	48		28			2
1930–34	52		12			
1935–39	39		14			2
1940–44	12	12	2	5		
1945–49	18	10	5			1
1950–54	21	6				1
1955–59	9	9				3
1960–64	9	4			9	1
1965–69	3	1			7	2

*The table excludes annual reports, abstracting journals, and statements intended for the general public

ceding few years could have been published in journals "if submitted to a not disadvantageous reduction in bulk", although others were necessarily too long for publication except as monographs. This led to a reaffirmation of the general policy, and also to a tightening of the procedure for considering reports proposed for publication. The number accepted has since shown a further decline, as the table shows. It was also decided to prepare a memorandum for the guidance of intending authors, which "should stress the need for brevity, lucidity and readability by more than a specialist public" and "the advisability of relegating technical details and numerical data as far as possible to appendices". This was duly done.

The usual sale of an issue of the Special Report Series is nowadays about 2000–2500 copies, but this may be substantially exceeded. The 'best seller' has been *The Composition of Foods* (No. 297) and its precursor *The Chemical Composition of Foods* (No. 235), with over 15 000 copies. Others selling more than 5000 copies apiece are the *Report of the Committee on Tuberculosis in Wartime* (No. 246, 1942), *Tables of Representative Values of Foods Commonly Used in Tropical Countries* (No. 253, 1945; new edition No. 302, 1962), *The Cultivation of Viruses and Rickettsiae in the Chick Embryo* (No. 256, 1946), and *Hearing Aids and Audiometers* (No. 261, 1947).

These titles exemplify a trend that had been noted in the 1920s, namely that two types of report are apt to be in particularly large and often continuing demand. One is a report containing descriptions of techniques or giving tables of values; copies are required for constant consultation in the laboratory and, moreover, call for replacement as the result of wear and tear. The other is a report making an appeal beyond professional circles, notably if the subject be nutrition. When both factors operate, the result is naturally additive, as for instance, in the case of the first title given above. An early best-seller was the *Report on the Present State of Knowledge Concerning Accessory Food Factors (Vitamins)* (No. 38, 1919; 2nd edition, 1924), which in its third edition became *Vitamins: a Survey of Present Knowledge* (No. 167, 1932).

Memoranda and miscellaneous reports

Early in the Second World War, in view of paper shortage and to meet special needs of the moment, the Council instituted a series of short War Memoranda. Their primary purpose was to convey authoritative practical recommendations, based on existing knowledge, to medical officers in the field or in the civilian emergency services. They were not intended to be the first means of publishing the results of important research work, although reference to the results of recent *ad hoc* investigations was often included. As it was clearly desirable that the recommendations published in this way should be unanimously endorsed by the various authorities concerned, an Inter-Services Medical Editorial Committee was set up, under the chairmanship of the Secretary of the Council and with

G

representatives of the Fighting Services and the Health Departments.

Some of the War Memoranda, of which 17 numbers were published in all, had wide distribution during the war and afterwards. This applies particularly to *Aids to the Investigation of Peripheral Nerve Injuries* (No. 7; still constantly being reprinted), and to *The Medical Use of Sulphonamides* (No. 10), both of which eventually achieved circulations of about 100 000 copies—the former almost reaching that figure on sales alone. *A Guide to the Preservation of Life at Sea after Shipwreck* (No. 8) had a total circulation of the same order, but largely owing to official issue on an unusual scale.

After the war, in 1946, it was decided to continue these 'white memoranda' (latterly given blue covers), omitting 'War' from the title of the series from No. 18 onwards. Their purpose was redefined as being for the publication of "reports of *ad hoc* investigations, short summaries of existing knowledge, and the like, intended for medical practitioners (in general or in some special branch)". By the end of 1971 the series had reached No. 43.

The youngest of the Council's regular series of reports is the Monitoring Report Series (the red reports), published under the general title *Assay of Strontium-90 in Human Bone in the United Kingdom*; these consist basically of the results of analyses, with the minimum of comment. The series was begun in 1960 as a vehicle for publishing the data obtained at the Atomic Energy Research Establishment and elsewhere. From 1956 such data had been issued by the Establishment in multigraphed form, but by 1960 other bone-sampling programmes, notably the Glasgow survey of samples from south-west Scotland, had been initiated and it was thought desirable that the Council should coordinate all the results. These reports appeared twice a year up to No. 15, but have since been issued annually—and are to be discontinued after No. 19.

Out of series have been two reports on human factors in industry issued jointly with the Department of Scientific and Industrial Research; one on feeding antibiotics to farm stock issued jointly with the Agricultural Research Council; and the report of a conference on the application of scientific methods in industrial and Service medicine. A bibliographical curiosity is the Council's Statistical Report Series No. 6, which had no published predecessors (official distribution only) and no successors—as has been said of the mule, "without pride of ancestry or hope of posterity".

Miscellaneous books

One of the earliest acts of the Medical Research Committee was to commission a book on the hygienic relations of milk and to arrange for its issue through a publishing house. The First Annual Report explains that "It appeared to the Committee, in view of the very large and scattered body of researches which have been published upon the subject, that it would be desirable to bring together, for the convenience of workers and for the guidance of future research, the knowledge already available, with a summary of the experimental evidence on which it is based, and a full bibliography". This resulted in the publication of *Milk and its Hygienic Relations* by Dr Janet Lane-Claypon (later Lady Forber). There has been only one closely comparable instance.

Just after the First World War, the Committee nominally sponsored the commercial publication of two books (appearing in 1919 and 1922) on intestinal protozoa by a member of the scientific staff. In 1924 and 1938 the Council took responsibility for the publication of the second and third editions of a little book on *Alcohol and its Action on the Human Organism*, of which the original edition (1918) had been prepared, under the auspices of the wartime Central Control Board (Liquor Traffic), by a distinguished committee which was afterwards reconstituted by the Council.

In 1923 HM Stationery Office published for the Council *Diphtheria: its Bacteriology, Pathology and Immunology*, the preparation of which had been the self-imposed task of the Council's Bacteriological Committee, with Dr P. G. Fildes as its energetic Secretary. From this the Bacteriological Committee proceeded to the more ambitious enterprise of organising the preparation of *A System of Bacteriology in Relation to Medicine*, to which various authors contributed on their special subjects. This was published by the Stationery Office in nine handsome volumes (1929–31) and was a monumental reference book in its day, although naturally in time rendered obsolete by the results of research work which it had helped to stimulate.

An important book more recently produced by the Council was *Mathematics and Computer Science in Biology and Medicine* (1965)—the proceedings of a conference of that title organised by the Council in association with the Health Departments and held at Oxford in July 1964. It consists of twenty-six contributed papers, with summaries of the discussions and an account of a demonstration.

Industrial Health Reports

For many years the Industrial Health (earlier Fatigue) Research Board of the Council (discussed in Volume Two) had its own series of reports. Its First Annual Report was published in 1919 under the joint auspices of the Department of Scientific and Industrial Research and of the Council, the remainder under the auspices of the Council alone; the nineteenth was published in 1939, and there was no resumption after the war. In the period 1919–47 there were ninety 'pink reports' of the Board corresponding to the green reports in the Council's main field. The case here was quite different, in that the bulk of the Board's scientific output was published officially; this was partly because of the lack of suitable scientific journals in the special field, and partly because of the advantage of separate publications for sale in industry.

There were also, in 1940–44, five issues in a series of Emergency

Reports of the Board corresponding to the Council's War Memoranda. The first of these, entitled *Industrial Health in War*, provided "a summary of research findings capable of immediate application in furtherance of the national effort". In addition, there was a wartime enterprise in popular education in the form of three pamphlets entitled, respectively, No. 1: *Ventilation and Heating: Lighting and Seeing*; No. 2: *Absence from Work: Prevention of Fatigue*; and No. 3: *Why is She Away? The problem of sickness among women in industry*. At various dates a few miscellaneous publications of the Board were issued: four unnumbered 'pink reports' on industrial lighting published under the joint auspices of the Board and of the Illumination Research Committee of the Department of Scientific and Industrial Research; and a report of the proceedings of a conference on health research in industry, held in London in 1944.

By 1946 the Board's programme had become more definitely medical in aspect, and the Board itself was being superseded by a group of specialised committees—as recounted elsewhere (Volume Two). The Council accordingly decided that in future (although one pink report did not appear until 1947) the results of research in the Board's field should be published in the usual way—that is, either in journals or in the series of 'green reports' and 'white memoranda', and that the Board's separate series should be discontinued. For administrative purposes, the Council's own annual reports had already been briefly covering the activities of the Board and of the related special committees.

Annual Reports

In a special category are the annual reports which an official body such as the Council is expected to make for the information of Parliament and the public. These are not intended as scientific publications, but aim at giving a general account of the Council's activities. They are nevertheless useful as 'yearbooks' to research workers desiring information about the Council's research establishments, with their staffs and current programmes, and similarly about work indirectly supported by the Council.

Formally, from 1920 to 1965, it was the Committee of Privy Council for Medical Research that was under mandate to report annually on its proceedings to both Houses of Parliament (Chapter 5). In practice this was a short covering statement, addressed to the Sovereign, to the full report that the Medical Research Council made to the Committee. The whole was 'laid' before Parliament as a Command Paper (from the Report for 1926–27), issued to the press and placed on sale. The five annual reports of the original Medical Research Committee were correspondingly addressed to the National Health Insurance Joint Committee and were published as Command Papers. The reports for the six years of the Second World War were amalgamated as one; and, owing to the time that this took to prepare, the same had to be done for the next three, and then for the two after that, before reporting caught up with the march of events.

The earlier annual reports are noteworthy for the distinguished Introductions drafted by Sir Walter Fletcher. The sequence constitutes something of a history in itself, referring to main events and showing the development of a policy, and indeed philosophy, of research promotion. Later Introductions were of composite origin, although including statements and dissertations prepared by successive Secretaries on topics of outstanding importance.

The Report for 1962–63, the first without a covering report by the Committee of Privy Council, covered a period of eighteen months, from October 1963 to March 1965, in order that future reports might deal with a financial rather than an academic year (a minor triumph of the official over the scientific approach!). The report for April 1965–March 1966 had its main title in a new form: *Medical Research Council Annual Report*; it was addressed to the Secretary of State and was laid before Parliament as a House of Commons Paper. It also blossomed into a brightly coloured wrapper. Its selling price was £1. 5. 0, compared with 3*d*. in 1915.

Apart from rearrangement of contents, the principal change in the series was an inevitable growth in size, reflecting the great expansion in the Council's organisation and programme. This increase had to be kept under control by progressive condensation of the subject matter, affecting particularly the summaries of research. In the Report for 1961–62 the step was taken of omitting the lists of published papers; this was a considerable sacrifice from one point of view, as the output displays the fruit of the Council's programme, but bibliographies based on the provenance of research funds served no wider scientific purpose.

Beginning with the Report for 1948–49, a section "Some Aspects of Medical Research" became a special feature and was gradually developed. It consisted of about a dozen articles on research subjects selected as being of special current interest, and not restricted to work that had been promoted by the Council. The general interest of this section led to its being reprinted, from 1955–56, as a separate pamphlet *Current Medical Research*; but after the Report for 1967–68 the section was discontinued.

With the Report for 1969–70 a drastic change was made as an experiment. The document was reduced to less than a hundred pages (from well over three hundred in the preceding year), and consisted of a policy statement, a selective review of recent developments in research supported by the Council, an administrative section and various appendices; the review, intended for the layman, was restricted to half a dozen fields, chosen for the particular year, with a like number of topics in each. The next report included, in addition, some reviews of the general state of research on selected subjects.

Much of the information hitherto included in the annual report was published separately (by the Council itself, not through HMSO) in a *Medical Research Council Handbook*, the first being for 1970–71. In 1970 the Council also published the first of a series of annual scientific reports of the National Institute for Medical Research, and the first of the Clinical Research Centre's scientific reports was published in 1972.

Abstracting journals

In the final stages of the First World War, from January 1918 to April 1919, the Medical Research Committee was responsible for the monthly *Medical Supplement to the Daily Review of the Foreign Press* issued by the War Office. The object was to provide summaries of recent research results for medical officers in the Services, temporarily cut off from seeing the original publications.

This had a peacetime successor in *Medical Science: Abstracts and Reviews*, published monthly by the Oxford University Press for the Council; the issues constituted twelve half-yearly volumes, covering the period 1919–25, and latterly the circulation amounted to about 1200 copies. The journal consisted largely of abstracts of recent scientific papers, grouped by general subjects such as medicine, surgery, pathology and bacteriology, neurology, radiology, and biochemistry. In each of these fields, specialist editorial supervision was provided; but the general editing was undertaken in the Council's small publications department. In addition to the abstracts, each issue was intended to contain one or more review articles, assessing the state of knowledge on some particular topic, with a long list of supporting references. These reviews were probably the most valuable feature of the journal, but they became increasingly difficult to procure; each one was the fruit of much labour of a kind that could be undertaken only by an expert on the subject. It was partly this difficulty that led the Council to abandon the enterprise.

Before taking that decision, the Council sought the advice of representative research workers in different fields, on the basis that the undertaking was a justifiable charge on research funds only if the service to research workers was commensurate with the labour and outlay involved. A typical reply was that the abstracts in his own field were of no use to a research worker—he must see the original publications in any event, and had in fact usually done so before the abstracts of them appeared. On the other hand, it was interesting and convenient for him to have a summary of what was happening in contiguous branches of medical research. Review articles were admittedly valuable in their particular fields, but were too few and becoming fewer. It was clear from this response that the prerequisite condition was not being fulfilled.

A different view was held in Harley Street, among the honorary staff of teaching hospitals. Busy in private practice and (at that date) unpaid for their hospital work, these men had too little time for the constant reading required to keep them effective as teachers. To them abstracts were a boon, and a review article was the substance of a lecture ready-made. Accordingly, resolutions urging the Council to resume publication were passed in 1926 by the Royal College of Physicians of London, the Association of Surgeons, and the Association of Physicians; and a conference with representatives of these bodies was held. The Council was sufficiently impressed by the demand to consider the possibility of an improved scheme under which publication might be resumed. It was concluded, however, that the success of any such scheme would depend on finding a suitable editor, and nobody with the necessary qualifications seemed to be available. Another factor was the appearance of a new abstracting journal, the *Bulletin of Hygiene*, issued by the Bureau of Hygiene and Tropical Diseases. It was agreed to make a survey of the ground covered by the various abstracting journals being published in the United Kingdom; and in the end no action was taken towards the further publication of such a journal by the Council.

In the Second World War the Council again assumed responsibility for an abstracting journal intended especially for medical men deprived of normal access to the original literature. This was the *Bulletin of War Medicine*, published by HM Stationery Office. The preparation of the material was largely undertaken, for the Council, by the staff of the Bureau of Hygiene and Tropical Diseases, and parts were issued two-monthly (Vols. 1 and 2) and later monthly (Vols. 3–6). Some account of the whole venture is contained in two epilogues in the final issue (Vol. 6, No. 12). The period of publication was 1940–46, and at the end of it there was on this occasion— the lesson having been learnt—no question of trying to extend an emergency measure into normal times.

Although, except during the Second World War, no comprehensive abstracting journal has been issued by the Council since 1925, some help has been given to enterprise of this kind in more specialised fields. In 1923, for instance, it had been agreed to provide some editorial assistance to *Physiological Abstracts*, and this arrangement continued for several years. Much later, in 1951, a grant limited to three years was made towards the cost of publishing the annual *Annotated Bibliography of Medical Mycology* (which became the *Review of Medical and Veterinary Mycology*) issued by the Commonwealth Mycology Institute at Kew. From the Report of 1927–28 it appears that the Council regarded the series of monographs that became *A System of Bacteriology*, already mentioned, as falling within the category of "other methods of making readily accessible the ever increasing volume of results achieved in the medical sciences".

From 1931 to 1967 the Council was associated with the Commonwealth (formerly Imperial) Agricultural Bureaux and the Reid Library of the Rowett Research Institute, in the publication of *Nutrition Abstracts and Reviews*, issued quarterly from the Commonwealth Bureau of Animal Nutrition at Aberdeen. Lord Boyd Orr gave an account of its inception in his reminiscences (1966).

Scientific intelligence

The use of abstracting journals is only one aspect of a wider question: to what extent should a research organisation provide a scientific intelligence service, and for what purpose? The answer will, of course, vary from one context to another. The Medical Research Committee had the question in mind from an early date, but without making a comprehensive decision; as in various other matters, a policy gradually took shape in the light of experience.

It is implicit in the earliest references to the subject that there was no thought of providing scientific intelligence except for the assistance of those actually engaged in medical research. This is in accord with the view that the research function ends with the scientific publication of the results of the work that has been promoted. It is for others to apply these results when they reach the requisite stage, whether in professional practice or in public administration; and it is for others to publicise the knowledge, when advisable, in a form suited to the general reader. This policy is indeed almost obligatory for an official agency for medical research, which is obviously inhibited from overlapping the proper functions of the government departments administratively concerned with different aspects of the public health.

As regards scientific intelligence for the Council's research workers, it was eventually concluded that nothing of the kind is necessary. In the normal circumstances of research within the Council's programme, the investigator is free to discuss his current work with scientific colleagues in the widest sense, irrespective of their employment or nationality, whether in private conversation or correspondence or in the public forum provided by meetings of societies and by international congresses. He may properly exercise some reserve in circles where disclosure could lead to anticipation, say in the popular press, of his own scientific publication. His aim, however, is to make publication as soon as his findings justify doing so, even if these represent only a stage in his plans. Once publication has been made the results are generally available; others may apply them or build upon them, or may repeat the work if independent confirmation seems to be desirable.

The consequence is that research workers are usually well informed on what others in their particular field are doing, anywhere in the world; they have often established personal relations with them, as an outcome of visits in one or other direction, or of attendance at international meetings. At the least, they do all they can to keep abreast of publications bearing on their own line of work. It follows that the research workers themselves are the people best informed about relevant activities elsewhere, and that communication is a natural process. In the abnormal circumstances of war, or of isolation in remote areas without personal contacts or good library facilities, there may be a place for central guidance of a kind that would otherwise tend, inevitably, to be tardy and inept in comparison with what the research workers can do for themselves.

This point does not seem to have been fully realised in the days of the Medical Research Committee. In the Report for 1917–18 one reads that:

> The war has almost wholly postponed the practical working out of the plans of the Committee, approved in the first year of their appointment, for establishing a library and some agency for distributing information among workers in medical science. . . . As for the distribution of information or ' intelligence ' service, it will not be possible until the close of the war for the Committee to see the most effective methods by which to serve the convenience and advancement of medical inquiry, and in doing so to coordinate any effort on their part with existing or future private enterprises.

The passages appeared under a new subheading "Library, Bureau of Information and Publications Department" in the section dealing with the National Institute for Medical Research; two years later the words "Bureau of Information" dropped silently out.

Today one can say that current developments in library techniques, in relation to indexing and literature retrieval, reinforce the conclusion that the provision of any other form of information service need not be the concern of a research agency (Chapter 10).

Public information

Although the Council has in general abstained from deliberate public education, not a few of its scientific reports have attracted numerous readers outside the professional circles for which they were primarily intended. This is notably true, for instance, of reports on questions of human nutrition. There was likewise a special lay public for many of the reports and memoranda of the Industrial Health Research Board, as well as for its three frankly educational wartime pamphlets already mentioned. The little book on alcohol served a like purpose. In addition, the Council has from time to time thought it expedient to issue considered statements—either its own or those of specialist committees which it has appointed—on topics of special public interest. In 1957 it issued a statement entitled *Tobacco Smoking and Cancer of the Lung*; this objective appreciation of the scientific evidence appeared first in the medical weeklies and was reissued separately as a Stationery Office publication. The most important instance, however, is that of the reports to the Government, and to the public, on the hazards of nuclear and allied radiations. These have already been mentioned in the discussions of the Council's advisory function (Chapter 9). The more general statements have been supplemented by regular issues of the Monitoring Report Series already mentioned.

In addition to what it publishes, an official agency must always be ready to provide required information to the Minister responsible for its activities, and through him to Parliament. It should also be able to meet reasonable inquiries from the press, and from members of the public, about its work—or about cognate research more generally—provided that this involves no premature disclosure of results not yet published in the proper scientific manner and that it does not call for comment on matters outside the research field. These functions had at first to be exercised only on infrequent occasions, but they have latterly grown so much as to occupy the attention of several members of staff in a section of the headquarters office dealing with, *inter alia*, parliamentary questions, publications, library services and public information (Chapter 17).

Under the last head, the office issues press notices about new developments, regularly arranges press visits to the Council's establishments (about four in a year and well attended), provides material about the Council for works of reference, encourages the directors of establishments to have 'open days' for students and school children, organises participation by the Council in exhibitions, and prepares or edits leaflets, pamphlets and brochures—on occasion in French or Spanish as well as English—on various aspects of the Council. Its press officers provide an information and liaison service to cope with telephone inquiries (commonly 20–30 in a day) and correspondence from the press and public. This service maintains liaison with other information sections in government departments and official organisations; and it circulates news items internally for the information of the staff both in the office and in the research establishments. It also makes arrangements for the reception of scientific visitors from overseas.

Editorial work and printing

From the summer of 1917, the services of Captain E. H. J. Schuster, a Fellow of New College, Oxford, were lent to the Committee by the War Office, primarily for work on the *Medical Supplement to the Daily Review of the Foreign Press* mentioned above. In the following year Schuster was appointed Assistant Secretary (Publications), and in this capacity he remained part-time with the Council until 1938, doing his editorial work at the National Institute for Medical Research. There he also supervised the Library and gave much help to his research colleagues by designing special items of scientific apparatus, which he then made in his private workshop at Oxford for no more than the cost of the metal required. He continued this latter activity after his editorial function had been absorbed by the headquarters office (Chapter 17).

With very few exceptions, the Council's official reports have been published by HM Stationery Office; this applies also to works in periodical and book form (Appendix A). For printing, the Stationery Office has used either its own press or firms under contract; during the period 1917–35 printing was usually assigned to the Oxford University Press.

The earliest reports conformed in typography and layout with the then current practice of the Stationery Office for official publications generally. The type commonly used was a so-called 'modern face' dating from the 18th century and the appearance of the covers was old-fashioned even by the standards of the day, among other things featuring an obscure form of the Royal Arms suggesting one of the drearier products of municipal gardening. In 1920 HM Treasury appointed a committee to select the best faces of type and modes of display for Government printing—and incidentally Sir Walter Fletcher served as a member. The recommendations of the Type Faces Committee, published in 1922, led to the adoption of more pleasing designs, and the Council's reports shared the benefit.

Various modifications of the official style were made by the Stationery Office over the years, but in 1965 the covers of the Council's various non-parliamentary publications were given a 'new look'. This more radical change resulted from a request from the Council to the Stationery Office that these reports should be given a truly contemporary and non-official appearance. The object was partly to make the reports more attractive for display, and partly to remove any misleading implication that such purely scientific publications were in some way officially inspired; for this reason the Royal Arms were omitted. The main feature of the new cover design is that the title is in large white letters on the coloured background, the other lettering being in black; the type-face used is the sans serif Univers, and all the lettering is aligned on the left-hand side.

The first excursion into interesting covers, however, was in 1964 with *The Cytology and Cytochemistry of Acute Leukaemias* (SRS No. 304). This report contained 74 colour plates of blood films, and it was accordingly necessary to have a hard cover—and thus a dust jacket, the design of which was not limited by any strict conventions. It was suggested by the publications section of the Council's office that the jacket might consist basically of a much magnified photograph of leukaemic blood cells, and the Stationery Office produced a striking design with the title of the book overprinted in large black letters from top to bottom. This design won the first prize in the technical books section of *The Scotsman's* International Book Jacket Competition.

Chapter 15
Financial Provision by Parliament

General considerations—The responsibility of the State—The 'penny a head'
phase—The fixed grant in aid phase—Provision for capital expenditure—
The annual estimates phase—The growth phase—Review by Committees
on National Expenditure—Accountability to Parliament: Estimates Committee and Committee of Public Accounts—Characteristics of a grant in aid—The
Council's budget in perspective

General considerations
It is broadly true that lack of money has not been the major limiting
factor in the development of the Council's activities. Restriction has
lain rather in the limited availability of men with first-class ability
and the flair for discovery, and sometimes also in the dearth of new
ideas holding promise of some success with hitherto intractable
problems; or there has been some practical difficulty about staging
an attack under favourable conditions. It is axiomatic, in the
administration of medical research, that the optimum rate of
expenditure depends more on the opportunity for doing fruitful
work than on the gravity of the particular subject in view. The
notion that funds should be allocated on the basis of the relative
importance of various diseases is naïve (Chapter 9).

It is equally true that financial resources have never been lavish
in relation to the demand; annual estimates have been rigorously
scrutinised and margins have usually been small. There has, therefore, been a need for constant economy in expenditure and for
weighing the comparative value of schemes at what have seemed
to be the lower levels of priority. This has on the whole been healthy,
tending to maintain a high standard of quality in the assisted programme; but, especially in the earlier days, the pressure was sometimes unduly severe.

Financial stringency may have a retarding effect that could be
serious. An essential feature of a research programme is that it must
be open to fresh needs and newly arisen opportunity; 'the growing
points of knowledge' deserve to be fostered above all else. This
requirement can be met only by deploying additional resources or
by cutting down on earlier commitments. The latter course is not
easy, beyond the extent of natural wastage in manpower. Men
cannot properly be expected to take up careers in research, or to
devote themselves largely to such work, without reasonable prospects
of personal security. Moreover, research workers are naturally apt to
become highly specialised in their interests and skills, and as a rule
they cannot readily be redeployed to new lines which seem to have

become of more urgent importance. The Council is thus commonly in the position of having its funds heavily committed to the maintenance of existing projects, some of which may be less fruitful than others but cannot be abruptly discarded without laying an axe to the roots of confidence. The result is that, however substantial the Council's funds have been in recent times, there remains a constant difficulty in preserving a sufficient margin for exploiting the new opportunities that arise in unforeseen ways and often with heavy financial implications; yet it is developments of this kind that merit special priority. There is thus a dilemma that can be resolved only by a gradual—and occasionally more than gradual—growth in financial provision for the Council's programme from year to year, apart from meeting inflationary increase in costs.

This does not, of course, imply the omission of regular review of existing expenditure with an eye to the elimination of items of diminishing usefulness. The process is indeed in continuous operation and leads to a classification of projects according to whether they should be further developed, should be stabilised at their existing levels, should be allowed to run down, or can be brought to an early close. The reductions possible in this way, however, do not keep pace with the need for increases; the overall picture is necessarily one of steady growth.

Another factor tending to make the cost of the Council's programme escalate is the increasing 'sophistication', as it has been termed, of the methods of biomedical research. The point was explained in the Report for 1966–67:

> First, the biomedical sciences are at present in a rapidly expanding phase. This is because a number of important discoveries, coupled with the development of a great variety of refined physical and chemical methods, have greatly extended the opportunities for investigation over a wide range of research. Secondly, these methods are themselves becoming increasingly costly. For example, instruments such as automatic amino acid analysers, ultracentrifuges, automatic instruments for analysing the results of radioactive labelling experiments and small special-purpose computers are now quite commonly required. Some of these methods enable entirely new types of measurement to be made, while others make it possible for measurements to be undertaken in sufficient quantity to allow new types of investigation to be carried out. In both cases an increase in technical staff is often needed to run and maintain the equipment, and in many instances the running costs associated with modern techniques are high. Thirdly, these developments in the biomedical sciences have been accompanied by a need for increasing expertise and specialisation and also a demand for scientists whose primary training has been in one of the physical sciences; in consequence, some increase in scientific staffing has also been necessary.

The responsibility of the State

It is worth recalling some words used in 1925 by the Earl of Balfour, then Chairman of the Council but on the occasion referring particularly to a sister organisation threatened with a cut in expenditure in an economy crisis due to industrial depression:

There is one inevitable difficulty in forming a sound judgment on national expenditure for research, namely, that in every research scheme there must be an element of conjecture. Research, by the very meaning of the term, is an attempt to penetrate the unknown: and until the attempt is made there can never be any complete assurance that the resulting knowledge will be adequate to the effort made to attain it. Unfortunately, it is just at the moment when risks of this kind ought most certainly to be run, that the temptation to avoid all risks is most powerful.

It was naturally not easy to obtain official acceptance of a doctrine that steady growth in expenditure on research is not only inevitable but positively desirable. It should be said, however, that the Treasury outlook has greatly changed since the period of the following incident recounted by Sir Henry Tizard. When the National Physical Laboratory was established in 1899, the Royal Society was provided with a Government grant of £4000 per annum towards the running cost. Five years later the Royal Society asked the Treasury for more, and a shocked official minuted: "Like other scientific people they seem incapable of understanding that they must live within their income". Nevertheless, the grant was raised to £7000 per annum, remaining at that level until 1914; it has now increased a hundredfold.

Even after the First World War, something persisted of an official attitude that the State had no total responsibility for supporting research, which was regarded as a kind of extra, or even luxury—a matter primarily for private enterprise or charity, but worthy of partial assistance, of a limited and non-committal kind, by an enlightened Government. This may have been especially true of medical research, which was so largely an object of private benefaction; the view was certainly expressed by a high official of the Treasury, if only in personal conversation, quite late in the period between the wars. By about 1930, nevertheless, there was a wide political acceptance, in all parties, that the support of scientific research was a public responsibility.

The financial provision made for the Council, and for the predecessor Committee, represents the State's direct contribution to the total medical research effort of the country; this is contrasted with its indirect and not easily assessed contributions through its support of the universities and (since 1948) of the hospital services, and through limited programmes sponsored by various government departments for their special purposes. Otherwise there is support of medical research by private benefaction, in these days notably on the part of a few large funds and foundations, and expenditure by the pharmaceutical industry for its particular ends.

Although the Council received valuable augmentations of its official income, as mentioned more fully later (Chapter 16), these have never provided more than a very small percentage of its total annual expenditure. It is thus reasonable to speak broadly about the Council's finances solely in terms of the provision made by Parliament.

The 'penny a head' phase

The provision has developed through several distinct phases. Firstly, there was the phase of the Medical Research Committee, 1913–20, and the 'four pennies' as they were called—one penny per annum for every insured person in, respectively, England, Wales, Scotland and Ireland—which constituted the Medical Research Fund. This provision was fixed by statute (Chapter 2), and its basis was quite arbitrary.

The formula made no provision for major capital expenditure, but in the first two years the inevitable lag in launching research schemes made it possible to finance one large item out of current income. This was the purchase of the building at Hampstead for the future National Institute for Medical Research at a cost of £35 000 (Chapter 10). £11 000 was paid in 1913–14, and the whole of the remainder (although the contract allowed it to be spread over four years) in 1914–15 or out of savings carried forward therefrom. Again, in 1919–20 the Treasury made a supplementary grant of £72 500 (a book transaction) to pay for a quantity of radium transferred to the Medical Research Committee from the Ministry of Munitions.

As regards recurrent expenditure, some £53 000 per annum in 1914 (the equivalent of about £300 000 in 1971) represented riches where there had before been no provision at all. The figure then fell to around £50 000 during the First World War because of the transfer of insured persons to the Forces; but the development of research schemes was in any event inhibited under the conditions prevailing. It rose rather above the original level after hostilities had ceased (and in 1919–20 the Treasury added a special grant of £10 000 for the Industrial Fatigue Research Board); but by then anything of this order was seen to be utterly inadequate, especially as the purchasing power of money had already dropped by nearly half. In its fifth and final Annual Report, the Medical Research Committee forcibly made this point. The report recalls that "a coherent intellectual service" for medical research had been created during the war by the concerted efforts of the Medical Research Committee and of the medical departments in the three Services. (These developments are discussed in Volume Two.) It proceeds to record that since the armistice this had already been widely disintegrated:

> The organisation of research workers during the war has been in large measure already dissolved. Many men fitted for investigation and marked out by distinguished scientific achievements in the war are now demobilised and are either unemployed or are returning to poorly paid teaching posts of which the inadequate stipends can in general be supplemented only by pay for professional work which forbids further effort in research. In this way much active and progressive team work is being broken up and many individual researches are being frustrated. The Committee, as they hope to show in the present Report, have made every effort to preserve and maintain by application of the Medical Research Fund whatever has been most valuable or promising in the work begun

under the stimulus of war. But the Fund, which was never adequate to support more than a small part of the medical research service of the country, has now become insufficient, by fall in the value of money, even to support fully the programme of work the Committee already have in hand.

This is followed by some eloquent paragraphs on the future of medical research in the United Kingdom. These stress the need for a continuing national effort, and especially for the support of research in the sciences contributing to medicine. "Power to prevent or cure a disease must not be expected to come by sudden discovery, nor often as the result of a special campaign, however vigorously prosecuted. Rapid gains, often unforeseen and in unexpected directions, may be confidently expected, however, so long as the area of accurate knowledge is maintained in its growth." It was necessary not only to aid the application of trained workers to specific medical problems, but also to aim consistently at supporting the advance of basic knowledge—"and in so doing to make every effort towards attracting the ablest young brains into this work and towards maintaining them in a national service of research, in which they may be reasonably secure of recognition and a livelihood". And so to the Committee's exordium:

> Our countrymen must decide whether they are to encourage and to maintain this service of research workers or not. The annual loss of life from preventable disease, with its toll of suffering, physical and mental, and its accompaniment of vast economic loss, goes on, but its full appeal is much deadened by familiarity. In times of special plague, as in the recent epidemic of influenza, the cry is raised for the power that only new knowledge can bring, but for which the country has done little indeed to secure the necessary conditions. The vast saving of life and pain and treasure that workers in medical research by their previous studies, or by their improvised work at the time, have actually achieved in the war, is literally beyond reckoning.

The fixed grant in aid phase

With the advent of the new constitution in 1920 (Chapters 4, 5), financial provision became entirely divorced from any such notion as the number of insured persons. It took the form of a grant in aid voted by Parliament for the purposes of the Council's work, the amount being nominally determined on a recommendation of the Committee of Privy Council for Medical Research. The actual process of determination by the Treasury was largely arcane; the views of the Council's officers were received, and after an interval for consideration a verdict was given in the form of a total figure to be submitted to Parliament. In those days, the Treasury officials declined to discuss details; informally they admitted that the claims of medical research were always irresistible, or at least beyond argument by laymen. If the Council thought that some new development was vital, room must be made for it in the budget at the expense of items of lower priority.

To begin with, early in 1920 the Treasury proposed that the

grant in aid for the work of the new Council should be £100 000 in the first year, and thereafter at the rate of £75 000 per annum. The extra £25 000 in the first year apparently represented a naïve idea of the cost of clearing off arrears of research work accumulated during the war, a point with which some play had been made in argument. Apart from that, in real as distinct from money terms, the recurrent provision proposed was substantially less than that with which the Medical Research Committee had started before the war. (In a hand-written postscript to a semi-official letter, a senior Civil Servant in the new Ministry of Health described the whole proposal as a piece of mediaeval obscurantism that made him ashamed of his cloth.) The Treasury's proposal was strongly resisted by the Minister of Health (Dr Addison) and the Lord President of the Council (the Earl of Balfour), as the respective ministers temporarily responsible and about to be responsible for the Council (Chapter 4). Among other things, memoranda on the financial savings directly attributable to medical research had to be produced—a line of argument which at the present time would be taken for granted. Eventually, Their Lordships felt able, "in all the circumstances", to agree to a grant of £125 000 in 1920–21, although saving face by a final minatory remark that "They can hold out no prospect of Their being able to continue the grant at this figure". So the Council at least started no worse off than the predecessor Committee seven years earlier; and the threat of a possible reduction was not taken too seriously.

In the following year, in fact, the amount was increased to £130 000 in respect of the transfer to the Council of certain additional responsibilities. These were for the entire cost of the Industrial Fatigue Research Board (hitherto shared with the Department of Scientific and Industrial Research), and for a grant-aided programme of research into mental disorders hitherto promoted by the Board of Control (England and Wales); a small sum expended by the General Board of Control for Scotland on routine pathological inquiries was also mentioned. All this, however, was a poor bargain imposed on the Council, which received an additional income of £5000 to meet an increase of about £15 000 in expenditure.

The grant was renewed at the same figure, £130 000, in 1922–23 and 1923–24—although in the former year not until a Treasury proposal to cut it by 20 per cent had been successfully resisted. In 1924–25 the grant was increased to £140 000, of which £5000 was a non-recurrent provision to clear off accumulated indebtedness; the rate was £135 000 in each of the next three years. In the last of these an unsuccessful application had been rather belatedly made for an increase of £3000. In the course of discussion about this it was remarked, in a semi-official letter from the Treasury on 21 February 1927, that "the theory of a Grant in Aid service is normally that it goes on from year to year without alteration of the Grant". The writer proceeded to say that "the papers show that we have consistently kept a soft spot for the work of your Council, the value of which to the country we gratefully recognise". Some hope for an application in the following year seemed to be implied.

In 1928–29 the grant was, in fact, increased to £148 000 (£2000 less than had been sought), but the augmentation was coupled with the statement that "My Lords have only been able to agree to so substantial an addition to the amount previously provided on the understanding that the annual grant will be regarded as stabilised, at this figure, in the absence of exceptional emergency, for a period of at least 5 years". In the event, for the fifth year of the quinquennium the Council offered to accept a reduction of £9000 as a contribution towards the general retrenchment made necessary by the financial crisis that had developed in 1931. The Council was able to effect the saving by asking its staff to accept a cut in pay (ranging from £9 to £99) in common with other branches of the public service, by terminating research grants that had been running for some time, and by severely restricting all new commitments. The crisis came at a bad moment for the Council, which was already in need of additional funds to avoid a deficit and was also faced with the withdrawal of certain other sources of support. And so £139 000 was the figure in 1932–33, and in the next two years.

In 1935–36 the cut was restored and more added besides, after an unusually detailed case had been put to the Treasury, urging the claims of specific subjects of research in need of development. The new figure, approved with a restatement of the principle of a quinquennium, was £165 000; and this remained the basic rate until halfway through the Second World War.

From 1937–38 onwards, however, the basic amount was augmented by an earmarked provision of £30 000 per annum for the development of work in the field of chemotherapy, for which a special plea had been made This separate consideration of the claims of a particular subject was a new departure in the Treasury's practice in providing for medical research. The special grant was announced in a speech by the Chancellor of the Exchequer (Mr Neville Chamberlain) at the annual dinner of the Royal Society on 30 November 1936. The subsequent official letter stipulated that the arrangement should be "reviewed at the end of five years, with a view to consideration being given at that time to the possibility of securing some contributions towards the cost, in particular, from industry".

Approval in principle for another special augmentation (of unspecified amount) was sought by the Council two years later, but this time unsuccessfully. The occasion was the Bill that eventually became the Cancer Act 1939, a measure providing (at a time when there was no National Health Service) for expenditure of public funds on making radium therapy more widely available for patients suffering from cancer. The Council, which was not without experience in this field, took the attitude that in the existing state of knowledge the extensive use of the treatment would be wasteful, and sometimes dangerous, unless it were controlled by parallel research work on methods and results. The Health Departments, on the other hand, had assured the Treasury that the requisite knowledge already existed and was ripe for practical application. The Council, although it had not been consulted beforehand, was thus held to be committed to a view that no need for an increase in the research effort was involved. The question was argued at considerable length, and at one stage the Ministry of Health changed its position to the extent of suggesting that research in this field was more appropriate to itself than to the Council and of seeking provision of £15 000 per annum for the purpose; but this found even less favour with the Treasury. The latter suggested that if more research was, in fact, required, this might well be financed by the important voluntary funds specially concerned with cancer. The wrangle engendered more acerbity than is usual in such official discussions, and in recording for the file a conversation with the Deputy Chief Medical Officer (Dr T. Carnwath) of the Ministry on 2 February 1939, the Secretary of the Council ended a long minute with the words: "The discussion then wandered from the point and as we were both tired of cursing each other, we satisfied our minds by cursing everybody else". The dispute went to ministerial level, but the Chancellor remained adamant; and shortly the outbreak of war intervened. It may be said, however, that within a few years the Council had ample opportunity for developing its interest in radiotherapy, as is recounted in Volume Two.

On the other hand, the Treasury did provide an additional £70 000 in 1939–40 "as a special contribution towards the cost of the new buildings for the National Institute for Medical Research" (Chapter 10). This was intended as a first instalment of a sum of £100 000 approved for the purpose, and further reference to the event is made in the next section.

With the advent of the Second World War, finance ceased to be a primary consideration. The quinquennial arrangement quietly expired; and it has never been revived. So many of the Council's normal activities were inhibited that continued provision at the rate of £195 000 per annum was adequate for the first three years; the separate provision for chemotherapy was now merged in this, and the second instalment of the special grant for new buildings was not required at that time. In the later years of the war, the rate was increased as necessary without demur.

An income pegged at a fixed level for five years had never been appropriate, even in normal times, to the support of a programme that was, inevitably and desirably, in a continuous process of development. In the first year or two of a quinquennium, an increased grant allowed some room for manoeuvre; half-way through, the budget could just be balanced; in the last two years the shoe pinched with increasing severity, and at the end there was apt to be an accumulation of forward commitments as an immediate charge on the next grant.

Provision for capital expenditure

Another difficulty about the fixed grant was the absence of provision for capital expenditure on buildings or major items of costly equipment. It has been noted that the site and building at Hampstead were bought by the Medical Research Committee out of the income of the first two years, when the research programme was as yet undeveloped. In 1918–19 an increase in the number of insured persons, consequent on military demobilisation, suddenly raised the Committee's income. A consequent surplus of about £7000 was accordingly set aside, invested in National War Bonds, for the express purpose of acquiring a site for farm laboratories for the National Institute—a procedure permissible at that time, in place of surrender to the Treasury, presumably because the Committee's income was determined on a statutory basis and was regarded as inviolable. This reserve was realised in 1922–23 for the purchase of the site at Mill Hill, at first used as farm laboratories and eventually for a new Institute (Chapter 10).

Other capital projects were made possible only by private benefactions, of which later mention is made (Chapter 16). These included the Ronan Building at Hampstead, the Clark Building at Mill Hill, and the Dunn Nutritional Laboratory at Cambridge (Chapters 10, 11).

It was in fact agreed by the Treasury that at least the first instalment of the extra grant of £30 000 per annum for chemotherapeutic research made from 1937–38 onwards could be applied to the cost of a building for that particular work. The first explicit provision from public funds, however, was the £70 000 in 1939–40 to which reference has been made—that is, if one ignores the notional provision in 1919–20 for the acquisition of radium already owned by the Government. After the Second World War it became the Treasury's regular practice to provide each year for the capital as well as the recurrent purposes of the Council.

The annual estimates phase

From 1946–47 onwards the grant in aid was determined by the Treasury, in each year, on the basis of estimates submitted by the Council for recurrent and capital expenditure respectively. It also became permissible to apply for supplementary provision, during the course of a year, in case of need. Equally, it became understood that any large surplus, in excess of what could be regarded as a reasonable working balance, should not be carried forward on account but should be surrendered to the Exchequer. In some years it was possible to set off a supplement under one head by a surrender under the other. Both the need for supplementary estimates and the occasion for surrenders were due, of course, to the difficulty of estimating expenditure in advance. Latterly, the commonest tendency was for recurrent expenditure to exceed the original estimate—largely because of increasing rates of pay to meet the rising cost of living. In the case of capital expenditure the tendency has been towards a surplus, in any particular year, owing to time-lag in the realisation of building programmes.

The changes in the rate of the grant in aid during the earlier phase have been discussed in some detail because they show a gradual development in the official attitude towards the support of medical research. The same does not apply to this later phase, and the figures in the table may be left to speak for themselves. In brief, they show a progressive increase in the net provision for the Council's work beginning at rather under half a million pounds in 1946–47 and reaching over £23 000 000 for 1971–72. Part of the increase is, of course, illusory, merely off-setting inflationary tendencies. This latter point need not be pursued —as one of Wilde's characters said: "The chapter on the Fall of the Rupee you may omit. It is somewhat too sensational".

The procedure during this phase of financial provision, up to and including the year 1964–65, was based on detailed estimates of committed and proposed expenditure prepared each autumn by the Council's officers, approved by the ministerial chairman of the Committee of the Privy Council, and submitted to HM Treasury. There then followed a period of discussion between officers of the Council and of the Treasury, ending with a decision on the total figures to be included in the Civil Estimates to be laid before the House of Commons with a view to 'supply' in the financial year beginning on 1 April.

The annual discussions at official level led to greater understanding on both sides, with resulting good relations. The Council's proposals were received sympathetically by the Treasury, and with a sense of responsibility for the support of medical research that was not fully accepted in earlier days. The Council's staff, for their part, aimed to establish a reputation for economical administration and for submitting estimates that were realistic, not inflated in anticipation of cuts.

The growth phase
Towards the close of the period covered here, the situation was altered by the constitutional changes to which reference has earlier been made (Chapter 6). Not only was the Committee of the Privy Council replaced by the Secretary of State for Education and Science, but the staff of his Department was interposed between the Council and the Treasury. At the same time, with the financial year 1965–66, a new estimating procedure was introduced. The Treasury notifies the Department of Education and Science of the total sum available for civil scientific research in the forthcoming financial year and the Secretary of State, after taking the advice of the Council on

Scientific Policy, apportions this sum among the research councils; each of the latter is then invited to submit estimates for a grant in aid equal to its allocation.

The original sum and its fractions were, of course, closely related to the existing budgets of the several agencies. Future increases, on the other hand, are being considered in a context of theoretical 'growth rates' (recently become fashionable in economic planning) by percentages of an arbitrary and diminishing scale fixed in advance. These financial brakes on research were applied as a policy of forward planning, and their introduction coincided with an economic situation which was thought to require diminishing growth rates for the next few years. In consequence, to quote an office paper of 1966, "the councils are faced with a vista of predetermined ceilings which are fixed at such levels as will undoubtedly reduce their ability to respond to applications".

The requirements involve elaborate methods of framing forecast estimates for future years. Apart from the uncertainty of such calculations, the Council is constantly faced with the dilemma between planning for the development of its own establishments and meeting the demand for grant aid. The latter, moreover, is always difficult to estimate, because it varies so greatly (and to some extent in relation to external influences of unexpected kinds). Above everything there is the difficulty of preserving some margin of resources for the pursuit of those new ideas that are the life blood of research.

Review by Committees on National Expenditure

In the Council's early days its grant in aid twice came under review by a Committee on National Expenditure specially set up by the Government, on each occasion, to make recommendations with a view to retrenchment. The published report of such a body makes a big impact, and the effect may be immediate where the Government quickly decides to act on a recommendation.

In 1921 the Government appointed a Committee on National Expenditure under the chairmanship of Sir Eric Geddes to review the expenditure of public funds and to make proposals for retrenchment. The famous (or notorious) 'Geddes axe' was wielded in a truly drastic manner in various directions, but it was turned aside from the Council. Of the latter, the Committee reported as follows:

> We are assured that the work of this Council in preventive medical research produces very substantial economies in administrative services falling on other Departments, and at a time when the prevention and combating of disease and the alleviation of physical disability is a matter of such vital concern from an economic as well as from a humanitarian point of view, we do not feel justified in recommending any reduction of a grant in aid of medical research conducted by a body of selected specialists.

In 1931, in relation to the financial crisis in the autumn of that year, the Government again appointed a Committee on National

Expenditure, this time under the chairmanship of Sir George May. The report of this body proposed some restrictions on the expenditure of sister organisations but exempted the Council from these; it also recommended retention of the existing form of financial provision:

> We do not extend these recommendations to the third Research Council (viz. the Medical Research Council) for the reasons that the element of economic benefit in this field is not as a rule capable of assessment and that the Government contribution represents but a small part of the total effort now being made in the field of medical research. The State at present makes an inclusive grant to the work of the Council, leaving the Council entirely free as to the disposal of the money, and we think that this arrangement should continue.

Accountability to Parliament: Estimates Committee and Committee of Public Accounts

Although the amount of the provision made by Parliament in any year is in effect a matter of Government decision, the House of Commons does retain two forms of control in its own hands. One of these is exercised by the Select Committee on Estimates (now simply Committee on Estimates), appointed on a non-party basis in each Session "to examine such of the Estimates presented to this House as may seem fit to the Committee, and to suggest the form in which the Estimates shall be presented for examination, and to report what, if any, economies consistent with the policy implied in those Estimates, may be effected therein". The Committee, which appoints subcommittees to hear evidence, is thus concerned with the form of estimates and with economy in method rather than in policy. In each Session it chooses certain fields of public expenditure for thorough study, without too close regard to the estimates for the particular year. Its reports, and the verbatim minutes of evidence on which these are based, are published as Parliamentary papers and must obviously command respect.

The other and more formidable body similarly appointed by the House is the Committee of Public Accounts. This receives the reports of the Comptroller and Auditor General, who is an official independent of the Treasury and with a staff of auditors under his own direction. Criticisms and questions contained in these reports are considered by the Committee, which calls the departmental accounting officers for interrogation. The Committee is concerned with questions of financial propriety, and especially with deviations from the estimates originally approved. Its findings are likewise published and submitted to the House, as are also the comments of the Treasury upon them. The Council's affairs have been before each of these Committees more than once.

In the Parliamentary Session 1946–47 the Select Committee on Estimates concerned itself with, among other things, expenditure on research and development; and this formed the subject of its Third Report for that period. Appendix 3 to that document gives the text of a memorandum submitted by the Council briefly explaining its status and functions. To this, one annex gave an outline of current research schemes, in much the same form as that used in the annual reports, and drew attention to some recent trends and developments. A second annex gave a detailed account of assistance given by the Council to Government departments (Chapter 7). Also appended to the report were verbatim minutes of the oral evidence given before subcommittee B on 26 February 1947 by the Secretary (Sir Edward Mellanby) and Under-Secretary (Dr A. Landsborough Thomson) of the Council. The interrogation of these witnesses by seven Members of Parliament resolved itself into a very amicable and useful discussion of the Council's work, with special reference to relations with other departments and agencies of Government, such as the Ministry of Supply, the Ministry of Food, and the University Grants Committee. The risk of overlapping or uncoordinated activities was clearly much in mind, and questions were also asked from this point of view about relations with research work in the Dominions. Other subjects touched upon included colonial research, industrial research, personnel research, hearing aids, chemotherapy, and animal experiments; finally, there was some discussion of the practical application of the results of research. In the body of the report, which dealt mainly with general questions, the five paragraphs devoted specially to the Council were purely factual statements based on the written and oral evidence submitted.

In the parliamentary Session 1948–49, the Committee of Public Accounts considered the general question whether the grant in aid system was appropriate to such bodies as the Medical Research Council, which derived almost the whole of their income from moneys voted by Parliament and had their accounts audited by the Comptroller and Auditor General. In the Third Report for the Session it is stated that:

> Your Committee cannot help wondering whether the time has not come to consider converting bodies of this sort into ordinary departments subject to normal Parliamentary and Ministerial control. If, however, it is desired for the time being to maintain their independence and to continue financial support by way of grant in aid, Your Committee recommend that certain changes should be made with a view to giving Parliament fuller information about the way in which these large sums are being used. In particular, the Committee of Public Accounts should be able to compare the estimate for each main item of expenditure on which the provision for the grant in aid is based with the figures in the account.

Neither the Treasury nor the Council saw any difficulty in meeting this latter condition.

The same Report referred to unexpended balances carried forward, as may be permitted in the case of a grant in aid although not in that of a normal departmental vote. It was recommended that the size of such balances should be restricted, any excess being in effect surrendered to the Exchequer (technically, 'short-issued') before the end of the fiscal year; this had, in fact, already been done by the

Council on occasion and has since become normal practice, a reasonable working balance being now defined as £250 000. The Council was not heard directly on the particular occasion, although one of its officers was present in case he was required; the witness before the Committee was the Treasury official who had been nominated as accounting officer for the grant in aid.

On the next occasion the Council's representative, in addition to the Treasury accounting officer, was interrogated. This was in the Session 1950–51, and the findings were published in the Fourth Report for that period. The Comptroller and Auditor General had drawn attention to the great excess of the actual cost of the new buildings at Mill Hill (Chapter 10), and their equipment, over the Council's original estimates. The building was still incomplete on the outbreak of the Second World War, and was wholly unequipped. When work on the project could be resumed after the war, costs had of course risen enormously; moreover, they continued to rise while the work of completion and equipment was slowly progressing under difficult conditions, so that forecasts were repeatedly erroneous. The Committee of Public Accounts, although agreeing that the increases had been inevitable in the circumstances, were "far from convinced, however, that the resulting requirements were subjected currently to the rigorous financial scrutiny they deserved". This was a criticism of the Treasury rather than of the Council, and it was accepted as such; but the Committee also considered "that the absence of specific authority in the Council's minutes for some of the additional items was unfortunate", and regarded "formal submission to, and approval by, the Council of all but minor services as an important factor in ensuring that the financial aspects of all proposals are fully considered".

This brought the Committee, following the lead of the Comptroller and Auditor General, to further discussion of the question of Treasury control of expenditure under a grant in aid. As a result, the Council's grant in aid was included in the Civil Estimates (Class IV) for 1952–53 under eight main sub-heads, with a more detailed breakdown appended for information. Before then there had been merely two sub-heads, providing for current and capital expenditure respectively; earlier still there had been just a single amount.

The Civil Appropriation Accounts are published in the same form, so that a direct comparison can be made. Under the grant in aid system, however, transference ('virement') is generally permitted at the Council's discretion between sub-heads; the main exceptions are transfers to or from major capital sub-heads (buildings and equipment costing £10 000 or more, for which Treasury authority must be obtained). Treasury authority is also required for expenditure on projects costing £50 000 or more and other expenditure of a special nature.

In the Session 1953–54, the Select Committee on Estimates turned its attention to the general question of grants in aid, with special regard to the adequacy of parliamentary control over the expenditure of public funds in that form; the record is in the Committee's Second Report for the period. The grant in aid to the Council was among those reviewed by way of example. This was done on the basis of a memorandum (No. 13 in the Report) drafted in the Council's office and submitted by the Treasury, an official of the latter being examined on the subject by Subcommittee C on 22 February 1954. To some extent the examination traversed ground that had already been covered by the Committee of Public Accounts as described, as there had not yet been time for the changes in procedure recommended by that body to become fully apparent. The main reference made to the Council in the Select Committee's own report referred to differences between one grant in aid and another:

> For instance, the intention of Parliament has always been that the Medical Research Council should have freedom in all matters of scientific policy, complete discretion in deciding how the grant in aid should be spent and the flexibility necessary for any research organisation. They are not bound to spend their grant in aid exactly in accordance with the sub-heads set out in the appendix to their vote, which is only explanatory.

In the examination of the Treasury witness, Mr R. W. B. (later Sir Richard) Clarke, reference was made to a suggestion by the Committee of Public Accounts that a representative of the Treasury should serve on the Council. Explaining why this had not been acted upon, the witness said:

> We did not quite like the policy implication of that. We felt it would be a mistake to put on the Council someone who might become a sort of lightning conductor for financial matters. We felt that the Members of the Council ought to have the financial responsibilities squarely on their own shoulders, and not have a Treasury official who could take the load of responsibility away from them. I would say on this that the Medical Research Council is a very economical body. They believe that the real bottleneck in medical research is the number of people of really good quality whom they can get. The limitation is brains rather than money. As a matter of doctrine they are opposed to the view that if you spend enough on something you can always get results. This doctrine is, of course, a welcome one for the Treasury.

Again, in the Session 1960–61 the Estimates Committee (as it had come to be called) was considering the general question of variations in estimates as recorded in its Fourth Report for the period. The estimates of the Council were among those that received some attention; desired information about them was included in a memorandum submitted by the Treasury, and two officers of the latter, together with the Council's Deputy Chief Medical Officer (Dr R. H. L. Cohen), were heard by Subcommittee G on 8 May 1961. The Committee's brief reference to the Council dealt mainly, and in a factual manner, with capital expenditure on new buildings. The Report did, however, include the following sentence: "While your Committee agree with the Treasury that 'it is very generally felt that medical research occupies a high priority in its call on expenditure', they consider that the Estimates of the Medical Research Council should be regularly subjected to the normal scrutiny"—a view at which nobody would cavil.

Characteristics of a grant in aid

A grant in aid contrasts with an ordinary vote for the expenditure of a government department. The receiving body or institution may be a governmental agency such as the Council, or it may be an unofficial organisation. The subvention may meet only a fraction of the total expenditure or, as in the Council's case, almost the whole of it. According to these and other factors, there are different degrees of accountability for the expenditure; in the Council's case detailed accounts are subject to scrutiny by the Comptroller and Auditor General and reported by him to the Committee of Public Accounts.

The grant in aid system allows the recipient body considerable discretionary freedom and administrative flexibility. Reasonably, however, Treasury control tends to increase with the size of the grant, with the proportion of total expenditure that it represents, and with the extent to which the amount of the grant is open to review from year to year. The grant to the Council has evolved through successive stages, from the time when it was small and approved simply as a total sum, the Council's allocations of the money being virtually unquestioned. Eventually, the estimating and accounting procedures approached those for an ordinary departmental vote; but the Council still retained a degree of power to make transfers from one sub-head to another within the total, and substantial liberty to decide details of allocation at its own discretion.

A characteristic of any grant in aid is that it is not supplemented indirectly by services borne on other votes. Thus, the cost of the Council's buildings and their maintenance is met from the grant in aid itself, the Council pays the postage on its own outgoing mail, and it does not have the services of the Paymaster General's Office but makes payments from its own account with the Bank of England. Where, exceptionally, a free service is in fact given, the cost of this has nowadays to be mentioned in notes accompanying the estimate; examples are work done by HM Exchequer and Audit Department and by the Publications Division of HM Stationery Office.

Technically, until 1965, money was voted by Parliament to the Treasury to enable it to make the grant to the Council; the latter was answerable to the Treasury, a senior official of which was the accounting officer to Parliament. This arrangement was discontinued, among other changes, in pursuance of the Science and Technology Act 1965 (Chapter 6). The financial provision for the Council and sister organisations was from 1965–66 voted to the Department of Education and Science, and the Permanent Under-Secretary of State had a general responsibility as accounting officer for the several grants in aid. At the same time the Secretary of the

Council became accounting officer, with more detailed responsibilities, for the Council's own grant in aid—with, of course, the assistance of appropriate members of his staff.

The Council's budget in perspective

For 1971–72 the Council's share of the 'civil science budget' amounted to £23 015 000. Some other figures help to place this sum in perspective. Thus, the following breakdown (based on figures for 1970–71 prepared by the Office of Health Economics) has been given of the total national expenditure on medical research in the United Kingdom:

	£m	%
Medical Research Council	21	26·9
University Grants Committee	27	34·6
Other UK government expenditure ..	2	2·6
Pharmaceutical industry (incl. development)	22	28.2
Charitable bodies	6	7·7
	78	100·0

Another calculation expressed the total expenditure of the Council in recent years as a percentage of the 'gross national product'. The figure had risen steadily from 0·0133 in 1954–55 to 0·0456 in 1969–70. This was the equivalent of a cumulative growth rate of almost 10 per cent per annum; and there was evidence that the corresponding rate for other governmental expenditure on medical research was about 6 per cent.

A comparison with the United States of America was also interesting. Federal agencies provided a total of $1180 m (£240 m) for medical and health research in 1965, according to a publication of the US Department of Health, Education and Welfare. This was 18 or 19 times the corresponding figure for governmental expenditure in the United Kingdom, or at least 5 times the amount per head of population and about double when expressed as a percentage of gross national product. In both countries the governmental expenditure represented roughly 63 per cent of the total outlay for the purpose.

THE GRANT IN AID*

(adjusted in respect of supplementary estimates and unissued surpluses)

Year	Recurrent	Buildings, etc.	Total
1913–14	(1)		£
1914–15	53 229		53 229
1915–16	49 783		49 783
1916–17	49 203		49 203
1917–18	50 000		50 000
1918–19	54 600		54 600
1919–20	76 000	72 500[2]	148 500
1920–21	125 000		125 000
1921–22	130 000		130 000
1922–23	130 000		130 000
1923–24	130 000		130 000
1924–25	140 000		140 000
1925–26	135 000		135 000
1926–27	135 000		135 000
1927–28	135 000		135 000
1928–29	148 000		148 000
1929–30	148 000		148 000
1930–31	148 000		148 000
1931–32	148 000		148 000
1932–33	139 000		139 000
1933–34	139 000		139 000
1934–35	140 500		140 500
1935–36	165 000		165 000
1936–37	165 000		165 000
1937–38	195 000[3]		195 000
1938–39	195 000		195 000
1939–40	195 000	70 000[4]	265 000
1940–41	195 000		195 000
1941–42	195 000		195 000
1942–43	195 000		195 000
1943–44	215 000		215 000
1944–45	250 000		250 000
1945–46	295 000		295 000
1946–47	415 000	50 000	465 000
1947–48	618 000	130 000	748 000
1948–49	770 000	365 000	1 135 000
1949–50	1 216 000	319 000	1 535 000
1950–51	1 363 671	290 750	1 659 421
1951–52	1 616 500	176 050	1 792 550
1952–53	1 505 917	181 000	1 686 917
1953–54	1 671 146	134 700	1 805 846
1954–55	1 877 441	97 428	1 974 869
1955–56	2 097 000	88 100	2 185 100
1956–57	2 229 500	49 500	2 349 000
1957–58	2 775 500	37 500	2 813 000
1958–59	3 056 600	80 500	3 137 100
1959–60	3 445 050	81 200	3 526 250
1960–61	4 113 060	355 500	4 468 560
1961–62	4 861 950	808 550	5 571 950
1962–63	5 489 000	370 000	5 859 000
1963–64	6 524 000	509 000	7 033 000
1964–65	8 151 000	602 000	8 753 000

* For the first seven years this was a statutory payment under the National Insurance Act 1911.

Year	Recurrent	Buildings etc.	Total £
1965–66	9 637 536	450 000	10,087 536
1966–67	11 203 488	621 488	11 824 788
1967–62	12 542 896	1 215 108	13 758 004
1968–69	13 358 203	1 872 288	15 230 491
1969–70	16 393 189	1 197 434	17 590 623
1970–71	19 486 837	1 567 731	21 054 568
1971–72	22 260 521	1 200 016	23 464 537

NOTES

(1) The first year's finances were handled by the National Health Insurance Joint Committee. The main item of expenditure was £11 000 as a first instalment of the purchase price (£35 000) of the building at Hampstead for a 'central institute'.

(2) To finance transfer of radium from Ministry of Munitions.

(3) Includes first instalment of special provision of £30 000 per annum for the development of research in chemotherapy.

(4) First provision specifically for capital expenditure on new buildings (National Institute for Medical Research, Mill Hill).

Chapter 16
Additional Financial Support

Augmentation of the grant in aid—Additional payments from public funds—
International and foreign government aid—Grants by foundations and
trusts—Cooperation with appeal funds—Contributions from industry—
Private benefactions—Testamentary bequests—Personal donations—Investment of capital funds

Augmentation of the grant in aid
The grant in aid voted by Parliament has always provided the bulk
of the Council's income (Chapter 15). The proportion has probably
never been below 90 per cent of the total on any reckoning; and in
recent years it has been more than 95 per cent, leaving out of
account repayments for technical services, not primarily of the
nature of research, which have been rendered to government
departments. Nevertheless, the augmentations of the grant from
other sources have been extremely valuable, sometimes out of proportion to their actual amount. In the days when the grant in aid
was both small and fixed, certain important new projects could not
have been undertaken without external help. Even in the days of a
more generous and flexible grant, the estimates for any particular
year are apt to be so tight that it might often not be practicable to
make immediate use of some unexpected opportunity unless a
reserve source of funds were available. As the vitality of a research
programme depends so much on attention to 'the growing points of
knowledge', these are important considerations.

There are also projects, from time to time, that may seem valuable
to the Council but are somewhat peripheral to its main objective.
The Council might hesitate to accord them a high priority, or
indeed to use general revenue for them at all; but when income can
be separately provided for such special purposes the embarrassment
is removed. Some valuable schemes have been made possible in this
way.

The main sources of supplementary income are: (*a*) additional
payments from public funds; (*b*) grants from foundations, trusts, or
industrial companies; and (*c*) private benefactions. Income in the
first and second categories is naturally earmarked for specified purposes additional to the existing programme. In the third, the donor
may or may not restrict the benefaction to some particular field of
medical research, but in any event the money would not be applied
simply to ease the burden of an existing expenditure commitment;

and in some instances the benefaction is in the form of a capital endowment, of which only the interest can be spent. In the financial year 1970–71, the total of extra income available to the Council from all these sources was about £1 684 000; but of this about £856 000 represented repayments for technical services.

Additional payments from public funds

There are government departments or agencies which may aid the Council's programme, either indirectly or directly, as shown below. There have also been contributions from international funds partly of British origin; and there are instances of direct help from the public funds of a foreign country.

The Council's work has sometimes been indirectly aided in joint undertakings with government departments in fields of common interest, notably with the Department of Scientific and Industrial Research and with the Ministry of Health (now the Department of Health and Social Security). In such cases, each party has usually been responsible for its appropriate share of the total enterprise.

As regards direct contributions, from time to time various government departments, and notably the Services (latterly through the Ministry of Defence), ask for investigations to be made for their own special purposes and, with Treasury approval, agree to reimburse the Council for the cost. Special investigations have in this way been undertaken for the Department of Health and Social Security, the Department of Employment, the Post Office and others. This procedure is considered to be appropriate where the Council has the required experts and methodology at call, but where the investigation is not one that the Council would spontaneously undertake or would regard as likely to contribute substantially to general knowledge in the medical field. (As a matter of principle, also, this is the only formula under which the Council would normally promote an investigation if there were any security inhibition on the free publication of the results—and even then with some reluctance, except under conditions of national emergency.) More usually, the Council accepts it as one of its functions to undertake special investigations of a suitable kind at the request of government departments (Chapter 9), the cost being met from its own grant in aid and, if substantial, included in its estimates. Much work has been done in this way, often by informal arrangement, particularly for the Health Departments.

Technical services undertaken for government departments on a repayment basis are intended to meet some practical need, rather than to increase knowledge; but that new knowledge may sometimes emerge is natural enough. Anyhow, it is proper for the Council to help the Government in applications of the results of research and continued use of the same technical methods.

The Department of Health and Social Security is the principal user of such services. On its behalf the Council administers Divisions of Biological Standards and Immunological Products Control (Chapter 10), a Blood Group Reference Laboratory and a Blood Products Laboratory; there are also various minor or temporary projects. There was also the Radiological Protection Service, but this has latterly been transferred to the control of a new National Radiological Protection Board (Volume Two). These may all be regarded as technical adjuncts to the National Health Service. The largest scheme of the kind ever undertaken for the Ministry, from 1939 to 1961, was the Public Health Laboratory Service (discussed in Volume Two). An item of outstanding importance has been the provision of money by Parliament, originally as the Colonial Development and Welfare Fund (1940) and latterly through the Ministry of Overseas Development (now the Overseas Development Administration of the Foreign and Commonwealth Office), for purposes that include research in tropical medicine. Substantial grants have been made for projects administered directly by the Council, as well as for other schemes of interest to it and coming within the purview of the Tropical Medicine Research Board (discussed in Volume Two).

Two official agencies expending public funds, in one case raised under statute and in the other provided by the Exchequer, contributed substantially to the resources of the Council in the period between the two World Wars—each, of course, for a special purpose. The Dental Board of the United Kingdom (later called the General Dental Council) was established by the Dentists Act 1921 to perform functions analogous to those of the General Medical Council. It had the statutory privilege of being able to raise a levy for research on the members of the profession that it regulated, and from the money thus available, the Board offered to provide the Medical Research Council with up to £3000 per annum for the support of an expanded programme of research in dental science. This proposal was gladly accepted, early in 1923, and it was agreed that the Council should be advised in the matter by a special committee on which the Board would be directly represented. The Council in fact already had such a Committee, consisting partly of dentists and partly of representatives of relevant branches of medical science. The arrangement, which continued until 1939, was parallel with one between the Board and the Department of Scientific and Industrial Research in respect of the more technological aspects of dentistry.

The other body was the one-time Empire Marketing Board (1926–33), of which mention has already been made (Chapter 7). From the public funds at the Board's disposal the Council for some years received grants for programmes of research on the vitamin contents of fruit, on dairy products, and on bovine tuberculosis.

On a smaller scale were subventions for particular purposes from the Miners' Welfare Fund (dietaries of coal-miners), from various industrial Research Associations sponsored by the Department of Scientific and Industrial Research, and from the Foot-and-Mouth

H

Disease Research Committee under the Ministry of Agriculture and Fisheries.

International and foreign government aid
Grants from international funds have been made to the Council from time to time, first by the Health Committee of the League of Nations and later by the World Health Organisation of the United Nations; the purposes included international biological standards and the maintenance of international reference laboratories for the subspecific identification of various microorganisms. Grants have also been received, for specific projects, from the International Atomic Energy Agency and the International Agency for Research on Cancer.

In the category of public funds of foreign origin, the US Public Health Service and National Institutes of Health (under the Department of Health, Education and Welfare, USA) have given substantial grants to the Council for several purposes since the time of the Second World War. The provision of travelling fellowships for British workers to visit America has already been mentioned (Chapter 13). Other grants have been in aid of particular investigations that were thought to be more readily capable of promotion in Britain. A grant of £11 614 for the Council's Biophysics Research Unit in 1963 is also notable. And grants have likewise been made to the Institute of Cancer Research, of which the Council is the main supporter (Chapter 12). Shortly after the Second World War, some special investigations into industrial productivity, undertaken by the Council together with the Department of Scientific and Industrial Research, were financed under the 'Conditional Aid' agreement.

The expenditure of public funds for medical research in a foreign country is not without parallel in British experience. The Council was able to secure the Treasury's approval for promoting investigations on bilharzia in Egypt and on trachoma in Jordan and Iran, on the principle that research should be done where the best opportunities lie, and that the benefit of the results is in any event universal.

Grants by foundations and trusts
The Council has been indebted to a number of foundations and trusts for cooperation or direct support, and in some instances for both. The Rockefeller Foundation (New York) has given the Council most aid and over the longest period. For many years it provided the Council with funds for travelling fellowships (Chapter 13). It has on occasion made grants to the Council for special purposes—thus $38 000 in 1952 for the purchase of scientific apparatus in America during the difficult post-war period in Britain; and $121 000 in 1957 in aid of the Council's work on the X-ray crystallography of proteins. Many generous grants by the Foundation to British institutions have been in the Council's line of interest; and the endowment of a post on the Council's pay-roll, at University

College Hospital Medical School, released money for expenditure on other objects (Chapter 11).

The Nuffield Foundation has made important grants in the Council's sphere, sometimes in explicit collaboration. In recent years the Wellcome Trust (Trustees of the late Sir Henry Wellcome) has been closely associated with the Council in various enterprises at home and overseas. It has directly helped by providing the Council with money for travelling fellowships (Chapter 13), for work on trachoma in Africa, and for various smaller projects. In 1957 the Trust made a valuable gift in kind, a motor-cruiser and floating laboratory costing some £26 000, for the Council's use on the River Gambia.

In 1923 the Carnegie Trust of the United Kingdom gave the Council £2000—a substantial sum in those early days—for an extension of its investigations in child life. On various occasions the Leverhulme Trust has been most helpful in providing research or travelling fellowships to be awarded by the Council in furtherance of its programme; certain projects were possible in times of financial stringency only because remuneration for staff was provided in this form (Chapter 11). In 1963 the Knickerbocker Foundation Inc., of New York, gave the Council $10 000 in aid of its Blood Group Research Unit; and in 1966 the Ford Foundation of America gave $148 000 for the Council's Clinical Endocrinology Research Unit.

The Council has been similarly helped by a number of smaller trusts, some of them self-extinguishing. In the 1920s, the Trustees of the late Sir William Dunn gave the Council £10 000 for general purposes (allocated by the Council to the development of the Applied Optics Department of the National Institute), and £6000 for the cost of the Dunn Nutritional Laboratory at Cambridge (Chapter 11). The Trustees were also largely guided by the Secretary of the Council in making benefactions in the Universities of Oxford, Cambridge and London. Also between the wars, the trust set up by Sir Halley Stewart assisted in staffing some of the Council's projects by means of research fellowships (Chapter 11). More recently, the trust set up by the first Lord Dulverton has assisted the Council with grants for work on coronary thrombosis, and the Eleanor Dowager Countess Peel Memorial Trust with a grant for work on arterial hypertension. The trust created by the will of Lord Nathan provided a non-recurrent fellowship for research on cancer (Chapter 12).

From 1949 onwards, the Council has been glad to administer funds provided by the Alexander Piggott Wernher Memorial Trust in the special fields of ophthalmology and otology (Chapter 12).

Cooperation with appeal funds
In the main, it is indirect assistance that the Council has had from the governing bodies of funds raised by public subscription for the support of medical research in special fields. Of these, that from the Cancer Research Campaign (formerly the British Empire Cancer

Campaign) has been the most substantial. The Council has for long had a special relationship with this organisation, as mentioned elsewhere, and it has combined with it in the support of programmes of research on malignant disease (discussed in Volume Two). The Council has, more recently, received both cooperation and direct financial help from the National Fund for Research into Poliomyelitis and Other Crippling Diseases. It has received grants from the Association for the Aid of Crippled Children for investigations of the effects of institutional life on normal children and for studies of growth and development in childhood. The Council has also had the cooperation of what is now the Arthritis and Rheumatism Council (formerly Empire Rheumatism Council) and other voluntary bodies with specialised interests.

An association of an unusual kind was that with the *Field* Distemper Council (1923–32). This body was responsible for a fund, raised through the well known sporting and country newspaper (then edited by Sir Theodore Cook), for research on dog distemper. The circumstances in which the Medical Research Council undertook the scientific work are recounted in Volume Two. Here it need be said only that the fund provided, in all, £37 000 for research work that yielded very valuable results for both veterinary and human medicine.

Contributions from industry

Industry, and particularly the pharmaceutical industry, plays a major part of its own in medical research, although this is normally subject to commercial secrecy until resulting products come on the market. Firms of pharmaceutical manufacturers, or even consortia of such firms, do nevertheless sometimes enter into definite agreements with the Council for cooperation in particular research projects (Chapter 9). There is also, from time to time, some mutual assistance of a less formal kind; the Council have on many occasions been indebted to pharmaceutical manufacturers for valuable gifts of material, or for help in large-scale chemical operations.

Some firms have also made occasional cash donations to the Council in aid of investigations of particular interest to them. For example, in 1932 the Nitrate Corporation of Chile presented £1000 for work on iodine in medicine.

Two American pharmaceutical firms have been substantial benefactors. Both Eli Lilly and Company of Indianapolis and the Lederle Laboratories Division of the American Cyanamid Company have provided funds for travelling fellowships, as already stated (Chapter 13). The former also made a generous gift of $20 000 to the Council in 1952 for the purchase of scientific apparatus in the United States, when dollars for purchasing equipment, of types not available at home, were particularly scarce.

The largest single contribution from industry has been a subvention of £250 000 by a group of British tobacco manufacturers in aid of research on cancer of the lung. This was made to the Council in 1954, payment being spread over seven years.

It could be claimed that industry makes an eventual larger financial contribution to medical and other research in that great charitable foundations such as those already mentioned owe their origin to the personal fortunes of industrialists. Among these, the Wellcome Trust is especially noteworthy because its funds are derived from the pharmaceutical industry; moreover, it continues to draw revenue therefrom, as the Trustees of the late Sir Henry Wellcome in effect own the commercial organisation known (by a somewhat confusing switch in nomenclature) as the Wellcome Foundation Ltd, in which the old pharmaceutical firm of Burroughs, Wellcome & Co. is now merged.

Private benefactions
The Council has gratefully received many benefactions from private individuals, either by testamentary bequest or by gift during the donor's lifetime. Some of the more substantial of these have been made expressly as permanent endowments, of which only the interest can be applied by the Council, but in most cases the latter can expend the principal at its discretion and occasionally a preference for rapid use of the whole amount has been stated by the benefactor. Some benefactions are earmarked for research on a particular subject, and in respect of others a preference is expressed without imposing any legal obligation.

By the terms of its original Charter, the Council was explicitly empowered to acquire, hold and dispose of property of any kind and to accept trusts (Appendix E); and it performs this function independently of ministerial control. As a corporation, the Council is able to act as a trustee of its own endowments, and is in fact authorised by the Lord High Chancellor to act as a trust corporation, but it is not invariably put in this position. As a body established for charitable purposes, the Council is exempt from United Kingdom income tax on the revenue from its investments, and from 1972 a legacy to the Council or recent gift *inter vivos* is not subject to estate duty. It is the Council's practice, whenever feasible, to associate the name of the benefactor with any use of the gift or bequest, unless he has expressed some different wish.

As a matter of principle, private benefactions are used to augment and not to relieve the public funds, the money being set aside in one of a series of special accounts. The Council is able to apply benefactions solely to the cost of research work without deduction of any overhead charges, other than audit fees, as the administrative machinery is already provided. It is well placed to apply benefactions to the best advantage, because it is at any time necessarily aware of the chief needs and best opportunities for developing new research. Indeed, the Council is always happy to advise intending benefactors, or executors with discretionary powers, who wish to place their money in other hands.

In the Council's early days, knowledgeable benefactors were in no doubt that it was a body needing and deserving their help; and this was in line with the view then held by the Treasury that there was only a limited public obligation to support medical research (Chapter 15). After the passage of the National Health Service Act 1946, doubts were raised both in Parliament and in the press about the need for private support of medical research, not particularly through the Council but rather through the independent organisations making wide appeals for funds. It is a fact, however, that the philanthropically inclined derive satisfaction from giving or leaving their money in aid of good causes; and as many such people see in medical research one of the most fruitful forms of expenditure, this charitable outlet should not be closed to them. For another, the public purse is not inexhaustible and there is always something more that can usefully be done beyond what it can afford in the particular field. Again, the availability of additional funds that can be deployed at short notice is most helpful in meeting unexpected scientific developments.

Nevertheless, although it welcomes support from private sources, the Council does not publicly appeal for benefactions in competition with independent research institutions or fund-raising organisations. It is gratified by all help given to the common cause.

The Council has printed several editions of a pamphlet entitled *Benefactions for Medical Research by Gift or Bequest*, issued free to inquirers. This is intended for the assistance of prospective benefactors and their professional advisers, and of trustees exercising discretionary powers. Two warnings given in the pamphlet have been fully justified by experience. One is that a benefactor wishing to earmark funds for a specific subject should define that as broadly as possible or perhaps merely express a preference; too rigid a definition may diminish the value of the gift or bequest as the state of knowledge changes. It is likewise important that any administrative or financial conditions attached to a benefaction should allow latitude for variation to meet changes in circumstances or in the value of money. The other point is that the title of the intended beneficiary should be carefully checked before a will is executed. Too often has money been left to the 'Cancer Research Society' or the 'Medical Research Association' because of the testator's belief that this is the name of the body he has in mind; this has led to various complications, and sometimes even to litigation (usually at the cost of the estate).

In 1967 the Council agreed to accept trusteeship of the Fleming Memorial Fund for Medical Research (raised by subscription in honour of the late Sir Alexander Fleming) from the original trustees. The amount available up to that date had been expended, but various legacies in its favour were due to take effect in course of time and the assignment was arranged by a scheme made by the Charity Commissioners of England and Wales.

Testamentary bequests

The Council received its first substantial bequest under the will of Miss Olivia Hamilton Stubber, who died in 1922 leaving her residuary estate, amounting to more than £6000, "unto and to the use of the Medical Scientific Research Society". There was in fact no body bearing that or any closely similar name, but it seemed probable that the testatrix had the Council in mind. This view was contested by the Medical Society of London, and a reference to the Chancery Division of the High Court was necessary; to avoid depletion of the sum at stake by an action between the two parties the judge agreed to a division by which the Council received two-thirds and the Society one-third. For many years the Council's moiety usefully provided a 'cushion' against over-spending on a tight budget, being repeatedly pledged but never spent.

The Rt Hon. Stephen Ronan, KC, formerly a Lord Justice of Appeal in Ireland, died on 3 October 1925, and by his will left his residuary estate in the following terms: "I leave the residue of my property and Estate to the Medical Research Council incorporated by Royal Charter to be applied in assisting and promoting scientific research as they think best, and without limiting their discretion I would wish that special attention should be given to the relief, cure and prevention of physical pain by physical means." About £13 000 became available to the Council immediately, and a further £33 000 on the expiry of a life interest not long afterwards. Fortunately, the expressed preference was not mandatory, as it might have been difficult to interpret; it was believed that the desire was to exclude psychological aspects. Some personal information about Stephen Ronan has been given by Maurice Healy (1939).

The Ronan Bequest was a very substantial one relatively to the Council's normal resources in those days; and it was the more valuable in that it could be applied to capital purposes for which no special provision by the Treasury had so far been contemplated. It was in fact used to cover expenditure on buildings for the National Institute for Medical Research, beginning with £18 000 in 1929 for an extension of the Hampstead premises; this was called the Ronan Building. Other additions at Hampstead and Mill Hill were later financed by the Council from the Ronan Bequest Fund; and in 1953 £14 000 of the remainder was used for the purchase and adaptation of a residential property at Mill Hill, for the accommodation of visiting workers; this was a useful purpose for which Exchequer funds were not appropriate.

Another early bequest was by Alexander Clark of Yokohama, who died in 1931 and under a will executed in 1923 left the whole of his property to be divided equally among six charities in England and Scotland. One of these was named as "the Medical Research

Society, London, England", but the view that this was intended to designate the Council passed unchallenged. (There is in London a Medical Research Society of more recent date, as well as a Medical Research Club, which exists for purposes of scientific discussion.) The Council's share eventually amounted to £11 209, and a major part of this was used to erect the Clark Building at Mill Hill (Chapter 10).

The personal circumstances of the Clark bequest were intriguing. The testator was a British subject who had lived in Japan for about sixty years, paying only rare visits to his native Scotland. He was a bachelor and apparently without near relatives. He had clearly prospered in his business, but was described as leading the life of the proverbial miser, in a poorly furnished house with his overcoat as an extra blanket in winter. The Japanese woman who had looked after him for many years made a claim against the estate, and a man purporting to be her husband created "quite a little unpleasantness" (in which an old revolver of the deceased's figured) for the executor; a settlement of her claim was reached. There was also a German medical practitioner who demanded substantial recompense for professional services over several years; but this claim was rejected. A lengthy correspondence exemplified the difficulties inherent in testamentary dispositions involving the laws and customs of different countries.

This last point was even more strikingly evident in another instance, not eventually producing any very substantial sum for the Council. The residuary estate of Alfred Leonard Lawley, who died in 1935, was under his will to be divided equally among seven medical charities in Great Britain; of these the Medical Research Council was one, with research on tropical diseases as the specific object. The testator died leaving property in many parts of the world (although the estate in England was actually insolvent); there was, inter alia, a liability for estate duty in the United Kingdom and for succession duty in (as it then was) Southern Rhodesia. Pecuniary legacies amounted to a large sum, and another substantial sum was to be temporarily set aside from the residue to yield life rents for five relatively young women—a provision likely to postpone a final settlement for many years. The annuitants were graded to receive eight-, nine- or twelve-fiftieths of the total, but as one of them had predeceased the testator this became thirty-eighths of a proportionately reduced sum. The complications became really international when a Madame Proussakoff claimed that her son, then under age, was an illegitimate child of the testator. She was originally of Russian nationality but was living in Norway when her child was born; and she had meanwhile become a French subject. And although the testator died in London, his legal domicile at that time was Portuguese East Africa; and under Portuguese law an illegitimate child had a right, if sole, to one-half of the entire estate, wherever situated, notwithstanding any provisions of the will. In these circumstances, the Council and six other residuary legatees were advised to accept a compromise with the mother (confirmed by the son on coming of age) whereby "the Infant Proussakoff" should receive half the net residue of the estate. The principle of grading was thus reintroduced—in terms of fourteenths, of which the charities received one each. The residue includes the capital falling in on further deaths of beneficiaries for life, two of whom are still with us.

Among other substantial bequests received by the Council at later dates mention must be made of the largest single private benefaction ever received by the Council, amounting to about £160 000. This was the residuary estate of Lady (Julia) Wadia, who died in 1957 leaving it to form a fund named after her late husband, Sir Cusrow Wadia, a Parsee who had been a prominent millowner and philanthropist of Bombay. There was no restriction on the expenditure of capital, and no limitation to a particular subject; but the money was to be applied "for the benefit of medical or scientific research in the University of Cambridge". This local restriction offered no difficulty, as the Council is at any time supporting numerous projects at Cambridge. The bequest included portraits of Sir Cusrow and Lady Wadia, and the testatrix wished that these should be hung in some appropriate place; this was arranged at Cambridge.

Personal donations

The earliest substantial benefaction received by the Council from a private individual was a gift during life. This was the Tropical Medical Research Fund established in 1926 by Major-General Sir Leonard Rogers, late of the Indian Medical Service, who then transferred certain investments to the Council and added others at later dates. It was a condition that the capital should be conserved as a permanent endowment. The original investments, retained by his wish, were largely in rubber companies in Burma, and these suffered a heavy depreciation a few years later; but the position was more than restored by the donor's subsequent generosity, and at the time of his death in 1962, aged 94, the value of the fund stood at about £95 000. The benefactor remained anonymous to the public until 1946, when he agreed that his surname be added to the title of the Fund. The use of the income was restricted to the support of "research in British territories in the Tropics where the medical departments are under the direct control of British Officials". In 1953 the donor consented to a variation whereby work done under the direction of the Council was exempted from the restriction relating to medical departments. The term 'British territories' is construed as covering all Commonwealth countries.

Of the other major donations received by the Council, two were made by parents in memory of daughters who had died young from the conditions specified as the subjects of research. One of these, the generous benefaction of £40 000 made by Mrs Odo Cross (Florence Temple Cross), for travelling fellowships in tuberculosis (Chapter

H*

13), had a curious history. Mrs Cross was a widow and had transferred £80 000 of her fortune to her young daughter. The latter,
not realising that she was the legal owner of any substantial means,
had made a will in favour of a friend, an older woman. When the
daughter died, the friend was indisputably entitled to this large sum
of money; but appreciating that this was due to a mistake, she
agreed to return half to Mrs Cross. This half was the source of the
benefaction to the Council; and, by the donor's wish, the public
announcement of the gift included a statement that the amount
represented the only benefit that she had derived from her late
daughter's estate. The establishment of the Kathleen Schlesinger
Research Fellowships has already been mentioned (Chapter 13).

Two other donations were strictly anonymous, being transmitted
through a solicitor and a Canadian bank respectively; in one of these
cases, no explanation was offered, but the other gift was designated
as in memory of Princesse Edmond de Polignac. This lady was
American by birth, Winaretta Eugenie Singer, daughter of the
inventor of the Singer sewing-machine. She had married first a
French count and then Prince Edmond, and she was described by
the *New York Times* as "one of Europe's leading patronesses of art and
music". She had been a widow for many years when she died in her
London flat on 26 November 1943, aged 78. In another instance, the
London Stock Exchange Dramatic and Operatic Society honoured
the services of its secretary.

There have been donations (as well as bequests) of moderate
amount, sometimes running into four figures, in addition to those
mentioned above. A special case is that of the fund subscribed in
memory of Sir Walter Fletcher, when he died in office as Secretary
of the Council in 1933; this was used to meet the cost of a portrait
bust, and the larger part remaining was then contributed towards
the cost of the Fletcher Memorial Hall at Mill Hill (Chapter 10).

There have also been many smaller donations, and it is interesting
that the number of minor donations has greatly increased over the
years although no appeal has been made. These small donations
are often in memory of someone recently dead and sometimes, when
this has been suggested in place of sending flowers, they come from
individuals, from relatives and friends collectively, or from groups of
fellow-workers. Other donations represent special church collections,
or the proceeds of social functions such as concerts, dances, or whist
drives. Others again come, without mention of special occasion,
from school forms, church societies, women's institutes, clubs, firms,
and so on—or simply from individuals or families. Some are repeated
annually. A few have come from overseas, including one from the
NCOs of an Infantry Brigade that was serving in East Africa. In the
majority of cases no particular subject is mentioned; in others the
contribution is specifically earmarked—for the common cold, or
rheumatism, or poliomyelitis, perhaps. Occasionally, the reason for
the choice is apparent, as when a gift is *in memoriam* or, for instance,

when an Over 60's Club designates diseases of the heart and chest as the subject of research.

The circumstances of donations have occasionally been bizarre, as in the fund-raising project of Miss Gloria Minoprio (the late Mrs Stefan Caroll). When a girl in 1933, glamorous in appearance as in name, she had caught the public eye by playing in the English Women's Golf Championships with only one club (plus identical spare) and wearing an all-black outfit of turban, blouse and tight trousers that was regarded as highly newsworthy by the press of those days. She was also, it later appeared, a very talented amateur conjuror; and in 1936 she offered to make a tour of India, at her own charge, to give a series of entertainments at the courts of ruling princes to raise money for medical research. The Council was naturally unable to sponsor the enterprise, although open to accept any benefits that might emerge. These might have been quite substantial, but again Miss Minoprio was not destined to survive her first round; the dust of India almost immediately induced severe tonsillitis, so that she lost her voice and had to return home. The only rabbit she produced, through a performance on the liner outward bound, was a cheque for £150 for the Council from His Highness the Maharaja Gaekwar of Baroda.

Investment of capital funds

The capital of private funds is invested in consultation with a firm of brokers regularly advising the Council, and the portfolio is kept under constant review. The market value of all stocks and shares held for the Council's private funds on 31 March 1971 was £1 216 790. Property and cash add about £200 000 to this figure.

The original Charter allowed all property vested in the Council to be held in such manner as the Committee of Privy Council might approve, and a Pooled Fund was established in 1958 for the investment of funds which were not permanent endowments or unsuitable for other reasons. Up to two-thirds of the Pooled Fund could be invested in equities and each account was allotted a number (reassessed as necessary) of shares in the pool. The other funds were invested separately in accordance with the Trustee Act 1925, and later the Trustee Investments Act 1961.

The new Charter granted in 1966 (Chapter 6) was silent on investment powers; but in the light of a subsequent decision of the Courts amendments were approved by an Order in Council in April 1971. These virtually give the Council full investment powers for funds other than those set up by formal trust deeds, which are invested separately in accordance with the Act in a second Pooled Fund similar to the 1958 scheme but without restriction on investment in equities.

Chapter 17
The Council and its Administration

Principles of administration—Relations with Ministers—The Council in session—The role of the Chairman—The Treasurer—The position of Secretary—Sir Walter Fletcher—Sir Edward Mellanby—Sir Harold Himsworth—Sir John Gray—Second Secretary—Other headquarters staff—Administrative organisation—Investigation by 'O & M' Division of the Treasury—Office premises

Principles of administration
It has been said that one of the highest capacities of Man is his power to create institutions. Each of these is an organisation of human beings that transcends the qualities of any or all of them and so becomes greater than the sum of its parts; it likewise transcends the span of human life, as by a constant replacement of individuals it is potentially immortal.

Administration has been called the art of institutional relations. There are the relations of an institution with other institutions or organisations; and there are the relations of an institution with the public at large and with individual members of the community, including its own employees. In each kind of relationship an institution such as the Council must determine an attitude appropriate to its special functions; and in doing so it will evolve a characteristic type of administration. This process is, of necessity, largely in the hands of the headquarters staff.

Some look upon administration as a special art which, once acquired, may be applied to any subject matter. There are not wanting examples of the disastrous results of acting upon that view in its extreme form, so that administrative theory has made havoc because its application has not been guided by any real understanding of the matters concerned. Others hold that administration is not a separate entity, being no more than a capacity developed by those conducting affairs of which they have technical understanding. This also is an extreme view, in that it ignores the existence of certain principles and methods that are applicable to all administration, whatever its particular purpose.

The Council's staff has sought the middle course. On the one hand, it has wished to be free from the errors of doctrinaire administration applied in ignorance of the subject matter, the assumption that skill can be a substitute for understanding, and the transference of inappropriate precedents from different fields of activity. On the other hand, it has sought to avoid the amateurism of wholly opportunist methods, the dangers of disregarding general principles established in wider experience, and action based on knowledge without wisdom. The aim has thus been a form of administration that has due regard to the best practice elsewhere but is at the same time specially adapted to the Council's particular needs; and one that is sufficiently flexible to conform with changes in these needs or with the lessons of the Council's own special experience.

All administration has an inherent tendency to become rigid, because in the handling of a large volume of detailed work delegation is facilitated by rules for guidance and safeguarded by observance of precedent. There are also, of course, certain administrative considerations of wide application that cannot be ignored except at peril, because they are strictly imposed by higher authority or are clearly inherent in general principles of conduct in public affairs. Nevertheless, in the experience of the Council's office there is a wide range of questions in which rules and precedents should not be accepted as immutable, but in which the final decision must be based on primary objectives; the exception may be more important than the rule. It is thus essential for such a body as the Council to secure the greatest obtainable freedom from external regulation of a kind inevitably implying conformity with decisions taken in a different context and with rules designed to standardise practice throughout a wide field. The Council's administrators have thus to defend its freedom of action against inappropriate measures of external control, while also checking any encroachment upon this freedom by too zealous regimentation from within.

Relations with Ministers

The Medical Research Committee, from 1913 to 1919, was responsible to the National Health Insurance Joint Committee, with a junior Treasury or other minister at its head (Chapter 3; and Appendix G); for a few months during the period of reconstruction, 1919–20, the Committee was responsible to the Minister of Health as successor to the Insurance Commissioners (Chapter 4). There was an obligation, under the statutory regulations, to submit the annual research schemes to the Joint Committee; and for the latter to consult the Advisory Council that formed part of this early machinery. Very few other matters, after the initial phase, concerned higher authority at all; financial provision was automatic on a basis fixed by statute (Chapter 15).

From 1920 to 1965, the Medical Research Council was responsible to the Committee of Privy Council for Medical Research (Chapter 5). The wise provision that the same Secretary served both bodies ensured that the relations between them involved a minimum of formality; and also that the Council had immediate access to the ministerial Chairman of the superior body. It also meant that the officers of the Council dealt directly with those of the Treasury. The relations with that department were at first almost confined to the annual, or less frequent, determination of the grant in aid (Chapter

15). Later, as the Council's affairs increased in scale, the occasions became more frequent and extended to other than financial matters, especially conditions of service for staff. This phase was marked by a sympathetic understanding, on the part of the Treasury, that left the Council the greatest practicable freedom of action in its special field.

In 1965 the Council became responsible to the Secretary of State for Education and Science (Chapter 6); in consequence, the officers of the Council thereafter dealt with those of his Department, and the direct link with the Treasury was lost.

The Council has always been free to deal directly with government departments and agencies on scientific questions and on arrangements for research projects.

The Council in session
The Council, as has been seen, is no mere advisory body but controls its own executive; and most of its decisions require no ratification at a higher level. Members can thus engage in their deliberations in a thoroughly realistic frame of mind, knowing that these will usually result in immediate or early action. This is much appreciated by members, who may have had too much experience of service on bodies that merely report to others. It was Sir Geoffrey Jefferson who said, in valedictory remarks at a Council meeting: "What I like about this body is that one afternoon we decide to give a grant to someone—and, by God, he gets it!"

A minute recording a decision of Council is, for most purposes, the ultimate authority for action; and it has already been noted that the Public Accounts Committee has regarded it as important that projects involving expenditure should be formally approved in this way (Chapter 15). There are, of course, many secondary decisions that have to be taken by officers in pursuance of policies laid down by the Council; but when these are important they are subsequently reported to Council and recorded in its minutes.

As noted elsewhere, there are about a dozen members; there have in earlier periods been one or two fewer, and now—under the 1966 Charter—there may be rather more (Chapters 5, 6). Of these, three have hitherto been 'laymen', in the scientific sense, and one of the latter has always been Chairman. The other members are appointed on scientific grounds and are in most cases members of the medical profession; most of them are university professors, and the others have some equivalent status. The meetings have always been attended by the Secretary and at least his immediate deputy—nowadays, usually, by several other officers of the headquarters staff. There are also certain assessors, of whom mention has already been made (Chapter 6); and on occasion other persons are invited to be present for particular items.

Ordinary meetings are held once a month except at vacation seasons, and special meetings when occasion demands. Much work is done by subcommittees appointed for particular purposes. The scientific members of Council also serve on one or other of the Boards by which much of the preparatory and detailed business is nowadays done—the Clinical Research Board and the Biological Research Board (Chapter 9), each of which is assisted by two Grants Committees; and there is also the Tropical Medicine Research Board (discussed in Volume Two). The Council devotes one special meeting in each year to considering the whole of its research programme and to deciding which fields need to be reviewed in detail in the coming year. There are also regular visits to establishments by subcommittees of the Council; and to the National Institute for Medical Research—and now to the Clinical Research Centre (see Volume Two)—by the Council itself.

The proceedings at Council meetings are both confidential and informal. The members, although drawn from various scientific fields and different parts of the country, are not appointed as representatives of particular interests; they are thus quite free to express their individual views and can speak very frankly. It is not customary to have resolutions in set terms or to put questions to a formal vote; a consensus of opinion usually becomes apparent, and the wording of the decision to be recorded is left to the staff.

A chronological list of members, stating what scientific fields they represented, is given later (Appendix H). From among so many men of high distinction one may particularly mention here six who were elected Presidents of the Royal Society and received the Order of Merit: Sir Frederick Hopkins, Sir Charles Sherrington, Lord Adrian, Sir Henry Dale, Lord Florey and Sir Alan Hodgkin. Some members have been recalled to serve for a second full term; a few served for three.

The role of the Chairman
The Chairman presides over meetings of the Council and is available between times for consultation by the Secretary on urgent matters. He has seldom any external role and is not ordinarily the Council's spokesman to ministers.

The Chairman has nearly always been a member of the House of Lords; for two short periods he was a member of the House of Commons, but there is no formal requirement that he should be either. It was, however, considered desirable to have a member other than a scientist in the position, and a person of standing in public life. The Council adhered to this view when constitutional changes were under discussion in 1965 and there was a question of having a whole-time scientific Chairman—the former Secretary writ large (Chapter 6).

A complete list of Chairmen, with dates, is given elsewhere (Appendix H); and as such men have obviously had notable public careers only a little need be said about them here. Those who presided over the old Medical Research Committee have already been mentioned (Chapter 3).

Lord Goschen was the first Chairman of the Council as such; he left after four years on appointment as Governor of Madras (eventually for a few months acting as Viceroy and Governor-General of India). One recollects him especially as a man of great, if somewhat inscrutable, urbanity; and as frock-coated and top-hatted in the everyday manner of the House of Lords of an era that was already passing. Next, for a few months the position was held by the Rt Hon. Edward Wood, MP, who then had to resign on appointment as Minister of Agriculture and Fisheries; shortly afterwards he became Viceroy and Governor-General of India, as Lord Irwin, and he eventually succeeded to the title of Viscount (later Earl of) Halifax and held many high appointments.

For the next five years, 1924–29, the distinguished occupant was the Earl of Balfour (Arthur James Balfour). At 76, he brought to the position, as well as great charm of manner and a wide experience of public affairs, a keen interest in the scientific side of the work. As a philosopher, he was concerned more with general principles than with technical detail, and often he would ask to have the bearing of some particular scientific point explained to him. It was at first usually Dr (later Sir) Henry Head who provided a few moments of lucid exposition; fortunately the list of agenda was in those days much shorter than it has since become, and these sparkling interludes were welcome. In 1925 Lord Balfour was appointed Lord President; he thus became Chairman of the Committee of Privy Council for Medical Research, but he saw no reason to resign on that account from his chairmanship of the Medical Research Council, remarking that he believed himself to have enough sense of humour to be his own Minister! In referring to this, after Lord Balfour's retirement, the Report for 1928–29 says: "In this way there came about an anomalous position warmly welcomed by the Council—anomalous perhaps, but as a precedent it is hardly in danger of imitation unless indeed there should ever recur personal circumstances so rare and so desirable." As will be seen, they did in fact recur.

From 1929 to 1934 the Chairman was the first Viscount d'Abernon (earlier Sir Edgar Vincent), who had had a varied and distinguished career, largely in the spheres of public finance and diplomacy; other interests were as diverse as the national art collections and the turf. As Chairman, he had the amiable habit of inviting a few senior members of the Council's staff to dine with him at the Ritz Hotel. He also frequently asked either the Secretary or someone else from the office, at short notice, to lunch with him alone at his house. Latterly, owing to a neurological affection, he became rather slow of speech and was content to leave to the Secretary a large part in the conduct of meetings.

Very different was the Marquess of Linlithgow, who served for two years, 1934–36, before leaving to become Viceroy and Governor-General of India. A man of commanding presence and dynamic manner, he pushed business through at top speed—leaving forever unheard the thought of any members whose latent periods were longer than he was prepared to allow. It is a remarkable coincidence that three former Chairmen of the Council should have occupied, in one case as a deputy, the seat of the Viceroy—one of the highest positions in the British Empire of that day.

Lord Balfour of Burleigh (11th Baron), who as George Bruce had been a personal friend of the first Secretary, had the longest tenure of office. He was Chairman for twelve years, 1936–48, including the whole period of the Second World War and the particularly difficult years that immediately followed. His firm hand was most helpful in times of stress.

He was succeeded by the Viscount Addison, who as Dr Christopher Addison had been a member of the Medical Research Committee and in a ministerial capacity had played a big part in the origins of the Council (Chapter 4). He was unique, among the Chairmen, in being a member of the medical profession, and he had been a Professor of Anatomy; but he was too wise, after half a lifetime in politics, to rate himself as an expert. On the other hand, his shrewdness and knowledge of affairs was a great asset to the Council. When he came to it as Chairman in 1948 at the age of 79 he showed unaffected pleasure in renewing his old association—although only the present writer (habitually addressed as "old boy" on the strength of it) remained from the actual persons who had attended meetings almost thirty years before. He nearly resigned in 1951 on being appointed Lord President, deeming the two positions to be incompatible; but on being told the anecdote about the Earl of Balfour in like circumstances, he decided that he also could fill the dual role. He did not do so for long, however, as he died in office towards the end of the same year.

Thereafter, the fifth Earl of Limerick (1888–1967) was Chairman for eight years. He took a close interest in the affairs of the Council; and he visited many of its research establishments, including even the tropical station in The Gambia. The more recent Chairmen have been the Viscount Amory, who resigned after a year on being appointed High Commissioner for the United Kingdom in Canada; Lord Shawcross (1961–65); the Viscount Amory again from 1965; and the Duke of Northumberland from 1969.

The Treasurer
Before 1966 there was no formally designated post of Deputy Chairman; but until that date there was a Treasurer, who was the natural substitute. The financial functions of the Treasurer were rather nebulous, as has been noticed (Chapter 5). The post was usually held by the third of the three non-scientific members of Council prescribed by the Charter of 1920. One of these members had to be a member of the House of Lords and was usually Chairman of the Council; another had to be a member of the House of Com-

mons; for the third no qualification was defined, and from 1937 onwards it became customary to choose someone in public life outside the purely political field.

The Treasurers of the Medical Research Committee have been mentioned (Chapter 3). The first Treasurer of the Council was the Hon. Edward Wood, MP, who later became Chairman as noted above. He was succeeded in the following year by the Rt Hon. F. B. Mildmay, MP, who in 1922 became Lord Mildmay of Flete and continued as Treasurer until 1937. He was an old parliamentary hand, who had won wide respect and been made a Privy Councillor —a most courteous, helpful man of patent integrity. His pheasant shooting in Devon was renowned; and once or twice in a season the office mail would include a brace of birds apiece for the Secretary and the Assistant Secretary. Lord Mildmay's useful role as intermediary between foxhunters and scientists over dog distemper is mentioned later (Volume Two).

From 1937 the Treasurers were Sir William Goodenough, a banker; Sir George Schuster, who had been "Chancellor of the Exchequer in two countries" (Sudan and India); Sir Geoffrey Vickers, a solicitor; and Sir Edward Collingwood, mathematician, former naval officer, and—like the others—a frequent chairman of public bodies. The office was allowed to lapse in 1966 (Chapter 6)

The position of Secretary

The Secretary was the only member of the Council's staff whose post was specifically mentioned in the Charter of 1920; it was there laid down that he was to be appointed by the Council, and no formal stipulation was made about consulting anyone else or obtaining approval from higher authority (Chapter 5). In the Charter of 1966 it is laid down that he is to be appointed by the Council with the approval of the Secretary of State. More significant is that the new instrument is so flexible that the Secretary could be also Chairman or Deputy Chairman and a member of Council, or could still be Secretary and nothing besides (Chapter 6). This leaves open a number of possible permutations for the future; but the immediate choice was to give the Secretary then in office, Sir Harold Himsworth, the additional status of Deputy Chairman and member of Council.

The Secretary is the Council's principal informant on matters which it should consider, and is the channel through which all submissions to it should be made. He is its chief spokesman, and is the director of administrative action taken on its behalf; it is he who presents the Council's view to Ministers. He has always been not only the servant of the Council but also its guide and a leader in framing its policy.

The post can be adequately filled only by a gifted man of appropriate scientific qualifications and experience. By practical necessity, although not by any formal requirement, he must be a member of the medical profession. It is likewise essential that he should be a man with much experience in research and of high standing in the scientific world. Obviously, he must also have skill in handling people and affairs, and be able to carry a heavy load of responsibility. In short, he has to be capable of dealing on level terms with leading men in the scientific world, the medical profession, and administrative departments.

All this has been obvious for many years, but the need was not envisaged in such high terms at the outset. In appointing a Secretary in 1914, the Medical Research Committee thought first in terms of medical men of high standing whose experience lay in public health administration rather than in scientific research; it even seriously considered a hospital administrator without either medical or scientific qualifications (Chapter 3). One therefore feels that it was as much by good fortune as by prescience that the Committee was led to make the choice that it then did.

Even as late as 1919 there was the dissentient voice of Sir Almroth Wright, who persisted in his contention that the Secretary should be a 'lay' administrator—which can scarcely have endeared him to Sir Walter Fletcher, already five years in post and steadily enhancing its prestige. Wright's view was doubtless derived from his own earlier concept of an organisation consisting mainly of a central institute, with the Committee as its governing body and himself as its director. This serves to remind one how small were the beginnings and how limited the vision of future development. There was then no thought of an organisation of the present dimensions, with a widespread periphery of 'external' establishments; nor of the addition of important new functions to the original programme of a central institute and a system of grants. Yet by the end of the First World War there was indeed some vision of a greater role, as shown by Fletcher's stirring Introduction to the Report for 1918–19 and by the ideals reflected in the Royal Charter of 1920.

It is inconceivable that the subsequent great development could have occurred had there not been a man, with all the requisite qualities, free to give his best thought and whole endeavour to framing the policy and guiding its execution. Four men have in turn performed this task, which has become progressively heavier by dint of its own success. Two of these have passed into history, and particularly of them some account must be given.

Sir Walter Fletcher
Dr Walter Morley Fletcher became Secretary of the Medical Research Committee early in 1914, when nearly 41 years of age; he was then an MD, SC D of Cambridge, was elected FRS in the following year, and was knighted (KBE) in 1918. He automatically continued as Secretary of the Council under the new constitution of 1920; and he died in office in 1933 when he was just approaching his 60th

birthday and had recently had his term of service extended to age 65. Summaries of his career as a research worker and scientific administrator have been given, notably by Elliott; and a more personal account of his life in a book by Lady Fletcher.

He brought with him the experience and reputation gained by work in the Physiological Laboratory at Cambridge, where in a series of researches (latterly with Hopkins) he had achieved a 'classical' elucidation of the chemical exchanges of contracting muscle; he brought also the skill derived from his participation in the affairs of the University and particularly of Trinity College, of which he had been a Fellow since 1897 and Tutor from 1905. He had a veneration for truth and an intense belief in the value of science in the service of humanity; and no better opportunity could have been offered him for advancing this cause. Wide cultural, social and athletic interests had given him a host of friends; and his administration was marked by the extent of his personal contact with the research workers, and by his abhorrence of bureaucratic methods. His was a vivid personality—spectacular physique, striking features, dynamic energy, quickness of thought, and an elegance in the spoken and written word—but with a "hovering stutter", as Elliott called it, when excited. With these gifts, although he had warm human qualities as well, it would have been difficult for him to avoid being masterful, and he could be vehement in controversy if principles that he valued were assailed.

Although excellent foundations had been laid before he came on the scene, Fletcher was undoubtedly the principal architect of the structure that stood after twenty years. He was also influential in a wider context, among other things in being personally consulted by potential benefactors of medical education and research wishing to apply funds directly to particular objects. In the middle 1920s much of his time was taken up by committee work in planning the future London School of Hygiene and Tropical Medicine. Some of his activities were remote from medical research; it was characteristic, for instance, that the Achilles Club should have been founded in his office room, at a meeting of athletes recently down from the universities.

At his death, following a sudden turn in a recurring illness, there was wide evidence of the great esteem in which he was held. The Presidents and Councils of the Royal College of Physicians of London and the Royal College of Surgeons of England paid him the signal honour of attending in state the memorial service in the Church of St Martin-in-the-Fields. The Council itself minuted, and published in its next Report, this tribute drafted by Wilfrid Trotter:

> Walter Fletcher brought to the service of the Council a unique assemblage of gifts. He had had a highly distinguished career in experimental research; he was an influential teacher of science; he possessed a culture in which scientific and humane studies were well and fruitfully balanced; and he was a master of practical affairs. Even this equipment would, however, hardly have given to his

management of the work of the Council its extraordinary success if it had not been animated by one of the most vigorous spirits of his time. He was always and even painfully aware of the suffering and disorder of mankind and profoundly convinced that their root lay in ignorance. The zeal and the unmistakeable honesty with which he held this conviction were the foundation of his singular power.

His deference for conscientious work, his understanding of the difficulties peculiar to original research, his eye for ability of all kinds, and his immense knowledge of the medical sciences, made him a perfect intermediary between the Council and its workers, and the inspiring helper of both.

The gifts and character which were so influential in determining the policy of the Council in its early days, and which imparted so strong a momentum to the work of its maturity, will find in the continuing progress of that policy and that work their best and most lasting memorial.

Sir Edward Mellanby

The choice of a successor to Fletcher was virtually settled by the scientific members in private meetings, and fell on one of their own number who had been closely involved in the Council's programme from the beginning. So, after an interregnum of a few months, Professor Edward Mellanby, MD, FRS, became Secretary in the latter part of 1933, at the age of 49; he was made KCB in 1937 and GBE in 1948, also receiving several foreign honours. He retired from office in 1949 after reaching the age of 65 and thereafter devoted himself to his personal research work; but he died very suddenly in 1955, in his 71st year, during a stroll outside his laboratory. An account of his career has been given by Dale.

Like Fletcher, Mellanby was a product of Cambridge (Emmanuel College) and its Physiological Laboratory, where he came under the influence of Gowland Hopkins. He was before all else a research worker, and his investigations were throughout largely supported by the Council and its predecessor Committee; something is said in Volume Two about, in particular, his discovery of the cause of rickets. He did his earlier work while holding academic appointments, becoming a Professor of Physiology in the University of London (King's College for Women, now Queen Elizabeth College) and afterwards Professor of Pharmacology in the University of Sheffield; the latter appointment was coupled with that of Honorary Physician to the Sheffield Royal Infirmary, where for thirteen years he had charge of beds. When he accepted appointment as Secretary it was on the understanding that the Council would provide facilities for him to continue his own research work in his spare time, particularly at weekends, and so the Nutrition Building at Mill Hill was constructed (Chapter 10). This arrangement was effective only because he was able to bring with him an experienced assistant staff and, more especially, because he had the devoted collaboration of Lady Mellanby (née May Tweedy, herself a Cambridge physiologist), who throughout their married life worked alongside him on cognate problems of her own. And after his retirement the Nutrition Building enabled them both to continue their investigations.

Mellanby had a wider knowledge of clinical medicine than his predecessor; he was a voracious reader of the literature and had a most retentive memory; he possessed an undoubted flair for seeing what was important in scientific ideas. On the other hand, he lacked Fletcher's interest in the techniques of administration and tactful skill in handling people. He, too, had great force, but it was concentrated more closely; had it been otherwise he could scarcely have done justice both to his official duties and to his personal scientific work, even if the latter did afford him a form of relaxation. In a remarkable way he retained his originality of thought, and his ability to make scientific discoveries, to the end of his life.

Mellanby was a large man physically, and he had shone at athletics and games as a schoolboy; except during his last few years in office he had excellent health. Yet he displayed no restless energy, striking one as massive and curiously immobile—as if conserving his powers; he was once disrespectfully described in the office as "the great white chief Sitting Bull". But he could be dynamic when he wished.

It was Elliott who said that neither Fletcher nor Mellanby could have done the other's job. Mellanby took over a well established organisation, with a momentum for further evolution. The critical battles had been won, and his task was to consolidate what had been gained, to expand gradually by judicious selection from the plenitude of possibilities now presented, and to entrench the scientific control ever more deeply. He left the Council in a strong position.

Sir Harold Himsworth

In 1949 the appointment of a new Secretary could be considered in advance, and the Chairman gave an active lead. The retiring Secretary himself took part in the discussions, and in fact put forward the name of a distinguished medical scientist overseas; but the nominee did not wish to be considered—nor did one or two others who were sounded. Two members of the Council were understood to be interested, and the eventual choice fell on one of them, who was immediately available to step into the vacancy in the autumn. Professor Harold Percival Himsworth, MD, FRCP, was then 44 years old; he was knighted (KCB) in 1952 and elected FRS in 1955. He had graduated in the University of London from University College Hospital Medical School; and he had been Professor of Medicine there for ten years. His personal research work had been largely on diabetes and disorders of the liver.

Any attempt here at a personal assessment of Sir Harold Himsworth would be unfitting. It must suffice to say that his period of office was one of very great development in the Council's resources, programme and prestige—as other chapters in this work should show. With his background, it was understandable that Himsworth should be particularly anxious to increase the opportunities for clinical research, and in this much success has been achieved; psychological medicine, too, has taken a greater place in the Council's programme. He was also notably active, making many visits abroad, in promoting research in tropical medicine at a very difficult time. The emphasis on clinical science was by no means incompatible with a noteworthy further development of 'biomedical' research on basic problems. The development of all these fields is discussed in Volume Two. The writer may be allowed to say how specially agreeable were his eight years of close collaboration with Harry Himsworth; and to make warm acknowledgement of the generous appreciation which his own part in that always received.

At the end of September 1968 Sir Harold Himsworth retired from the Council's service, after having been Secretary for nineteen years and latterly also a member and Deputy Chairman of Council. The event was the occasion for a tribute in the Report for 1968–69, which said that "like each of his distinguished predecessors he has added new dimensions and fresh lustre to the post from his own particular genius and experience"; and also that "In all things he has brought wise guidance to the Council in its deliberations and skill in the direction of its affairs". After reviewing at some length the main developments during his period of office, the Report concludes the tribute as follows:

All this Sir Harold could not have achieved had he not possessed great powers of vision and leadership and great administrative ability; but the matter does not end there. The success of his service to the Council owed much also to the personal relationships that he established with the scientific staff of the Council's establishments both in this country and overseas. This he did by seizing every opportunity that the preoccupations of his official work allowed to visit the Council's laboratories, and in the course of these visits he was at pains to meet individual members of the staff at all levels and to discuss their work with them. These visits brought and maintained a realisation throughout the whole of the Council's organisation of the genuine enthusiasm for scientific investigation that Sir Harold himself felt and a sense of his keen interest in the efforts of individuals; this was a source of great encouragement. That part of his work was indeed by no means the least of Sir Harold's contributions as Secretary of the Council, and it is one for which he will be remembered with gratitude and affection by many.

Sir John Gray

When Sir Harold Himsworth retired in 1968 he was succeeded (as Secretary and a member of Council) by Dr John A. B. Gray, then aged 50, who had come to the office two years earlier as Second Secretary after being Professor of Physiology at University College London, and also serving for a time as Dean of the Faculty of Science in the University. Earlier he had been a member of the Council's scientific staff at the National Institute for Medical Research. He had before that, during the Second World War, done research on service problems for the Council and as Surgeon Lieutenant, RNVR. He was knighted in 1973.

Second Secretary

The title attached to the second post on the Council's headquarters staff has changed so often that, in a historical context, a generic term is lacking. The title 'Second Secretary', first used in 1949–57 and revived early in 1965, has now become established for an officer able to act as the Secretary's second-in-command and deputy in the conduct of both scientific and administrative affairs. This chief of staff is the deputy for the Secretary in all matters; and he has a special responsibility for coordinating action where necessary.

For the first few years the Secretary had no regular assistance above clerical level. In October 1919 Lieutenant-Colonel A. L. (later Sir Landsborough) Thomson joined the headquarters staff as Assistant Secretary; he had a degree in zoology and physiology, and during the latter part of his service in France he had gained administrative experience on the staff, eventually as an Assistant Quartermaster General at GHQ. He continued to be deputy to successive secretaries until his retirement in 1957. His post was upgraded to Principal Assistant Secretary in 1936 and to Under Secretary in 1946; and in 1949 its title was changed to Second Secretary when a new Secretary took office. To this new title was attached the formula that the particular holder of the post was directly responsible to the Council in matters which the Secretary agreed to be of a purely administrative nature. As mentioned in the Report for 1956–57, Thomson retired from whole-time work in 1957.

In 1957, Dr R. H. L. Cohen was promoted to be chief of staff with the title of 'Deputy Chief Medical Officer' (regarding the Secretary as Chief Medical Officer). As before, both scientific and administrative business passed through his hands. On his secondment to the Ministry of Health in 1963, however, a different arrangement was made; Mr C. Y. Carstairs was seconded from the Civil Service (Colonial Office) for two years to be Deputy Secretary. This made the post a purely administrative one, and the Secretary had to make a more regular practice of dealing directly with the medical side of the office. This represented the extreme swing towards having a wholly administrative chief of staff; and it was made possible only by another appointment intended to relieve the Secretary, personally, of some of the work calling for high scientific qualifications. The opportunities of filling such a post are at any time limited by largely fortuitous circumstances; but on his retirement as Director of the National Institute for Medical Research, Sir Charles Harington joined the headquarters staff as a 'Consultant Adviser', a title not implying any place in the official chain of command.

Early in 1965, Treasury approval was obtained for up-grading the post of chief of staff to make it possible to attract a scientific man of professorial standing; and the title 'Second Secretary' was revived.

Sir Charles Harington agreed to act temporarily in this capacity, until Professor Gray became free to take up the appointment in the spring of 1966. Meanwhile, in place of Mr Carstairs, Mr D. A. Smith was temporarily seconded from the Civil Service (Board of Inland Revenue) to fill a new post of Administrative Secretary, standing third in the hierarchy; and when he returned to his normal duty at the end of 1967, Mr J. G. Duncan was promoted to the position. On the arrival of Professor Gray, Sir Charles Harington reverted for a final year to his position as Consultant Adviser; a similar but part-time post on the clinical side was for a short time held by Emeritus Professor Sir Robert Platt (from 1967, Lord Platt). After Dr Gray moved up to be Secretary in 1968, his place as Second Secretary was taken by Dr S. G. Owen, who had been Reader in Medicine and Clinical Sub-Dean in the University of Newcastle upon Tyne, and a Consultant Physician at the Royal Victoria Infirmary there; the choice of a clinician as colleague of a physiologist was deliberate.

Other headquarters staff

Around 1930, the senior staff still consisted only of the Secretary and two others—Dr A. L. Thomson (scientific) and Dr F. H. K. Green (medical); the next in rank was an Accountant of higher clerical status. It was, however, becoming obvious that more staff would soon be needed, and the question was whether there should be a dichotomy between staff with scientific or medical qualifications and administrative officers without special knowledge in these fields. At that time the volume of purely administrative work, apart from financial routine, was so small that it could be handled by officers who were giving most of their time to scientific business—nor was this wholly without advantage.

Eventually it became clear that it would be an abuse of man-power to expand on the basis of employing scientific and medical men on duties for which their special qualifications were not required; and also that increasingly complex demands of adminis-tration made it desirable to import men with other special skills. In 1934 the retiring Accountant was replaced by a Finance Officer (D. V. T. Fairrie) of administrative rank, a university graduate professionally qualified as an accountant. The next appointment was that of another Medical Officer (Dr F. J. C. Herrald), but in 1945 an Establishment Officer (J. G. Duncan) with a legal qualification was appointed for personnel administration; and in the following year a Supplies Officer (J. D. Whittaker) with technical experience was added (Appendix J). These three administrative officers were recruited for particular posts; but they were all eventually assigned to different duties and further recruitment was on a more general basis.

It was, however, not easy to recruit able young men to a small and isolated administrative service, in the absence of a wholly satisfactory career structure. The highest posts were barred, and the chances of finding advancement elsewhere did not seem bright. In the 1960s, accordingly, the expedient was adopted of introducing a few men from the Civil Service to fill new senior posts. Such officers were, of course, already experienced in official administration; and in most cases they were only on temporary secondment and would return to the Civil Service later on. Although this met the needs of a sudden expansion, it did not provide a lasting solution.

Another step taken, beginning in the 1950s, was the creation of an 'executive' staff—using the term not in its business sense but with its Civil Service connotation of a category between the administrative and the clerical. Although in the junior ranks of this staff the work may be largely routine, the more senior members have substantial responsibilities. Many of the executive officers are women; some of them, especially those engaged in publications work or assisting in medical sections, are university graduates. There is no barrier to promotion from the executive to the administrative staff; and the salary scales overlap.

The recruitment of both men and women for medical administrative work has, in the long run, proved to be less difficult than might have been expected. They enter, at various levels of professional experience, in a grade of Medical Officer, with eligibility for promotion to be Senior and Principal Medical Officers. Moreover, the medical side of the office has shown itself to be by no means a dead-end employment. Dr F. H. K. Green left to be Scientific Secretary of the Wellcome Trust, where he was later joined and eventually succeeded by Dr P. O. Williams; Dr R. S. F. Schilling left for an academic post and is now Professor of Occupational Health in the London School of Hygiene and Tropical Medicine; Dr J. M. Rogan went to be Chief Medical Officer of the National Coal Board; Dr Martin Ware became an Assistant Editor of the *British Medical Journal* and is now its Editor; and Dr R. H. L. Cohen was seconded to the Ministry of Health as a Principal Medical Officer (with duties relating to research, including liaison with the Council), and was later made a Deputy Chief Medical Officer and eventually Chief Scientist.

Administrative organisation

Below the level of the 'chief of staff', work begins to be divided according to its nature. Obviously, any large volume of detail must be broken down, on some logical scheme, into progressively smaller fields; this produces the familiar pyramid, at successive levels of which there are diminishing degrees of delegated authority and increasing specialisation in subject matter.

The detailed arrangement of headquarters staff is variable from time to time to fit changing circumstances, but at the close of the period under review it is as follows. The Secretary and Second Secretary take the lead in assisting the Council in the formulation of policy, and have an overall responsibility for the management of the Council's activities; in addition, the Second Secretary is formally the 'executive head' of the headquarters office. Below that level there are four divisions, one coming under the Administrative Secretary ranking third in the office hierarchy, and each of the others headed by a Principal Medical Officer. The Administrative Division is subdivided into three functional sections, each under an Assistant Secretary, dealing respectively with personnel, with finance, accounts and supplies, and with accommodation. A new division deals with relations with the universities and with grants and training awards. The two older 'medical' divisions (now known as Research Programme Divisions) deal with different parts of the field and they are subdivided by subjects. According to the predominant subject interest, every research establishment and advisory committee in the Council's organisation is a special concern of one of these divisions (or of the Tropical Medicine Section). A feature of the last few years has been the increasing number of scientifically qualified staff in addition to the medical staff in the headquarters office.

Outside the divisions there are three special groups severally responsible directly to the Second Secretary. One is the Secretariat, formerly known as the General Department, in charge of an Assistant Secretary. It assists in or deals with certain types of business not easily classified as either scientific or administrative and often carrying a high degree of priority; examples are Council and Board agenda, ministerial requirements, parliamentary questions, information services and the library, and the Council's publications. Another is the Headquarters Establishment Section, with obvious functions. The third is the section, already mentioned, dealing with the research programme in tropical medicine.

Recent additions to the headquarters machinery are a Policy and Planning Committee and a Management Committee (concerned with day-to-day management issues); the former is under the chairmanship of the Secretary and the latter under that of the Second Secretary. Both committees are served by the Secretariat.

Regular administrative procedures are of course necessary; but it has been laid down in the office that on occasions of special urgency a senior officer should make it his affair to see that the stages are telescoped into immediate action—and the knots in the red tape left for tying afterwards. Correct administrative practice should likewise not preclude good personal relations between headquarters staff and the research workers. The maintenance of personal contacts was a notable feature of the Council's administration in the early days; it becomes less easy with the increasing size of the organisation.

Administration has been discussed here as a function of the headquarters office, because the deliberate policy has been to maintain a high degree of centralisation. The object is to lighten the burden of routine falling on directors who are actively engaged in scientific work and commonly have no more than secretarial help for other purposes; only the larger establishments carry administrative officers on their staffs. Action is naturally taken, subject to any overriding considerations, on the recommendations or reports of directors.

Investigation by 'O & M' Division of the Treasury

In 1955, the Council was offered, and gladly accepted, the services of the Organisation and Methods Division of HM Treasury to examine its administration. The Division undertook several detailed investigations in 1955–57, presenting the Council with a series of helpful reports on organisation and procedure. Only a few of the recommendations were felt to be unacceptable, for reasons that were duly given and recorded. Action was taken at once on many of the proposals, while others were kept in view for implementation when circumstances might permit.

Internal reviews of headquarters administrative machinery were made in 1962–63 and 1969, on the second occasion with the help of two management consultants selected after talks with the Department of Education and Science and with the Civil Service Department.

Office premises

In August 1914 rooms for a temporary office were taken at St Stephen's House, Westminster, at a rent of £25 per annum; meetings of the Committee continued to be held at the Chairman's house—or, later, in his room in the Ministry of Munitions. In referring to this office, the First Annual Report added: "The question whether the offices of the Secretary to the Committee should ultimately be within the Central Institute or be provided separately and nearer to the official districts of London has been left for later settlement". It was in the event realised that a headquarters office in the Institute would have been inappropriate.

In February 1916 the office moved to the ground floor of 15 Buckingham Street, off the Strand, alongside the Duke of Buckingham's watergate by Inigo Jones; of the five habitable rooms, that used by the Secretary was large enough for meetings. Then in 1922 the Council's office moved to an upper floor in the next street, at 15 York Buildings, backing on the Adelphi. Here there were eight rooms, one of them spacious and with an outlook across the Thames towards the old Shot Tower on the south bank (near where the Festival Hall now stands). Before another complete move had to be faced, a couple of extra rooms were taken on the opposite side of the street for the Accounts Branch.

In October 1928 the office again moved, this time into the upper half of 36–38 Old Queen Street, Westminster. This building was a combination of two houses of the Queen Anne period, to which an extra storey had later been added. The best rooms faced north across Birdcage Walk to St James's Park; and down the side of the building ran the steps named after the cockpit situated there in the time of Charles II. For office purposes it was an awkward building in various ways; and as a structure it left much to be desired—the whole block was said to be "gradually sinking towards the west" and there were quaint slopes on the floors, but it was a shock to discover later that the owner of the overlease had taken out a 'collapse policy'! Nevertheless, the office had attractions, and the three floors provided sixteen rooms at a short distance from Whitehall. Earlier, the building had been in official occupation as the Irish Office; this circumstance brought back recollections of the dynamitards to the Chairman of the Council, the Earl of Balfour, who had been Chief Secretary for Ireland at the time of those troubles.

The prospect of much greater explosions led to the decision that the building would be unsafe for occupation in time of war. In September 1939, in accordance with a prearranged plan, the office was temporarily evacuated to the modern building of the London School of Hygiene and Tropical Medicine in Bloomsbury, where the normal function of postgraduate teaching was in abeyance. As it chanced, however, it was this building that suffered some bomb damage, and not (apart from windows) the house that had been left empty in Old Queen Street.

At the beginning of 1946 the School was resuming its activities, and the office returned to Old Queen Street after the premises there had been restored to order. Now, however, the Council had the whole building, subject to the expiry of a subtenancy of one floor. When all six floors were available, the Council at last had control of its own front door (No. 38); and it could also set aside a large room solely for meetings. The other front door (No. 36) was converted into a window, and its hall into a room; and as time went on some of the larger rooms were partitioned. Such expedients, however, could not keep pace with the growing needs of the headquarters of a greatly expanding organisation.

In 1948 the Council was able to purchase the freehold of No. 26 Old Queen Street from the Chinese Maritime Customs (an at last expiring relic of the Boxer Rising) and to transfer part of the office to it. In 1956 a floor at No. 32 Old Queen Street was rented for the Publications Section; and in 1957 the Accounts Branch had to be moved to premises half a mile away. The headquarters office was thus divided between four different locations, or five including a separate storeroom; this was a severe handicap to internal efficiency.

With Treasury approval, search was accordingly made for a building designed for use as an office and sufficiently large to accommodate the whole headquarters under the one roof, with some margin for further expansion. The requirement was eventually met by a new building constructed on a site where several large houses had been destroyed by bomb damage in the war and not yet replaced. This was in Park Crescent (the main door is No. 20), in the W.1 district of London and not far from Regent's Park. The building was put up as a commercial undertaking, under a concession from the Crown Estate as owners of the land, with a view to tenancy by the Council on a long lease.

The Council had a say in the internal layout and division of the building; but the front elevation, including the fenestration and the levels of the various floors, had to conform with the general design of the Crescent. The latter was a key part of Nash's famous plan, executed in 1812, where the long avenue of Portland Place first opens out into the area of Regent's Park embraced by his famous terraces. The original Georgian façade was faithfully reproduced, as also in another new building in the Crescent; and since then all those that had survived the war have been demolished and rebuilt to the same external pattern. The setting thus still retains its dignity; and internally the building is very conveniently arranged, notwithstanding a somewhat uneconomical excess of height in the rooms on the ground and first floors. The Council moved to Park Crescent in September 1961, while giving other bodies short subtenancies of parts of the building not immediately required. The whole office building has a frontage of about 255 feet, with a depth of just over 42 feet. The lower ground, ground and four other floors provide a total area of approximately 65 000 square feet. The rent is £57 500 per annum. Incidentally, the telegraphic address MEDRESCO has been unaffected by the successive moves.

The Council's administration has indeed come a long way, meta-phorically, from the original tiny office of the predecessor Committee, near the Houses of Parliament, at the outset of the First World War. The writer of this history can personally recall, with some nostalgia, all the subsequent stages—the modest suite close to the old Water-gate; the third-floor flat looking out over the Thames from beside the Adelphi; the double Queen Anne house by the Cockpit Steps, over-looking Birdcage Walk and St James's Park; the period of exile in Bloomsbury during the Second World War. And now there is the building, in Nash's stately layout, that more amply accommodates the headquarters of an organisation that has so greatly developed during the half-century or so now under review. This last seems likely to remain the Council's home for some time to come.

Appendices

Appendix A
Sources and references

General

Unpublished

Minutes and papers of the Medical Research Committee and Council

Minutes and papers of Boards and Committees of the Council

Correspondence and documents in the files of the Council's headquarters office

Annual Reports to Parliament

(All published by Her Majesty's Stationery Office, London, and all as Command Papers except those for the period 1920–26 and from 1965–66 onwards.)

National Health Insurance [1915]. First Annual Report of the Medical Research Committee, 1914–1915. Cd. 8101. And four subsequent annual reports)

Committee of the Privy Council for Medical Research. 1920. Report of the Medical Research Council for the Year 1919–1920. Cmd. 1088. And nineteen subsequent annual reports

Committee of the Privy Council for Medical Research. 1947. Medical Research in War: Report of the Medical Research Council for the Years 1939–45. Cmd. 7335

Committee of the Privy Council for Medical Research. 1949. Report of the Medical Research Council for the Years 1945–1948. Cmd. 7846. And report covering 1948–50, followed by thirteen annual reports

Report of the Medical Research Council, October 1963–March 1965. 1965. Cmnd. 2787

Medical Research Council Annual Report, April 1965–March 1966. 1966. And subsequent annual reports

Handbooks

Medical Research Council Handbook 1970–71. 1970. MRC, London. Subsequently published annually

NIMR and CRC Scientific Reports

National Institute for Medical Research: scientific report for 1968–69. 1970. MRC, London. Subsequently published annually

Clinical Research Centre: scientific report for 1970–71. 1972. MRC, London

Statutes and Instruments relating to MRC

Acts of Parliament. See Appendix B

Statutory Regulations. See Appendix C

Orders in Council. See Appendix D

Royal Charters. See Appendix E

Chapter 1

Advisory Committee appointed by the Secretary of State for India, the Royal Society, and the Lister Institute, 1906. Reports on Plague Investigations in India. *Journal of Hygiene* 6: 421–536. And subsequent reports

Brockington, C. F., 1965. *Public health in the nineteenth century*. Edinburgh and London

Charles, J., 1961. *Research and public health (Heath Clark lectures)*. London

Chick, H., Hume, M., and Macfarlane, M., 1971. *War on disease: a history of the Lister Institute*. London

D'A[rcy] P[ower]. 1901. Sir George Buchanan, FRS. *Dictionary of national biography*, Supplement Vol. 1

Debuch, H., and Dawson, R. M. C., 1965. Prof. J. L. W. Thudichum (1829–1901). *Nature* 207: 814

Drabkin, D. L., 1958. *Thudichum, chemist of the brain*. Philadelphia and London

Drury, A. N., 1948. The Lister Institute of Preventive Medicine. *Proceedings of the Royal Society*, B, 135: 405–418

Fosdick, R. B., 1956. *John D. Rockefeller, Jr: a portrait*. New York

Lambert, R., 1963. *Sir John Simon, 1816–1904, and English social administration*. London

MacLeod, R. M. 1971. The support of Victorian science: the endowment of research movement in Great Britain. *Minerva* 9: 197–230

MacNalty, A. S., 1948. *The history of state medicine in England (Fitzpatrick lectures)*. London. (Contains numerous references to the original sources; see also Brockington 1965, above, and Newman 1939, below)

Miles, A., 1966. The Lister Institute of Preventive Medicine 1891–1966. *Nature* 212: 559–562

Newman, G., 1939. *The building of the nation's health*. London

Royal Commission appointed to inquire into the Relations of Human and Animal Tuberculosis, 1904. *Interim report*. London (Cd. 2092). (Final report published in 1911, with appendices appearing up to 1915)

Chapter 2

Addison, C. 1924. *Politics from within, 1911–1918*. 2 vols. London

Braithwaite, W. J. (ed Bunbury, H. N.). 1957. *Lloyd George's Ambulance Wagon*. London

Departmental Committee on Tuberculosis, Final Report of the. 1913. Vols. I and II (Appendix). HMSO (Cd. 6641 and 6654)

Gilbert, B. B. 1966. *The evolution of National Insurance in Great Britain: the origins of the Welfare State.* London

Hansard (House of Commons). 1911. *The parliamentary debates (official report).* Fifth Series, vols. 25–33

Hansard (House of Lords). 1911. *The parliamentary debates (official report).* Fifth Series, vol. 10

National Health Insurance Commissioners, 1914. *Report for 1913–1914 on the administration of National Health Insurance.* HMSO (Cd. 6641). (The relevant section is quoted almost in full in the MRC Report for 1914–15. In the NHI Report for 1912–13 the paragraph on research merely summarises, without comment, the recommendations of the Departmental Committee on Tuberculosis.) *National Insurance Act 1911.* See Appendix B

Thomson, A. L., 1973. Origin of the British legislative provision for medical research. *Journal of Social Policy* **2** (1): 41–54

Chapter 3

Albutt, C. 1916. Work of the National Medical Research Committee. *British Medical Journal* 1916, ii: 785–788

Hopkins, F. G., with Trevelyan. See under Chapter 17

Moulton, H. Fletcher. 1922. *Life of Lord Moulton.* London

National Health Insurance: Minute of appointment of Medical Research Committee, made by the Chancellor of the Exchequer 20 June 1913

National Health Insurance: Minute of appointment of Advisory Council for Research, made by the Chancellor of the Exchequer, 20 June 1913

National Health Insurance: Scheme for research. (A contemporary circular embodying the substance of the foregoing Minutes of Appointment)

HM Treasury. *National Insurance (Joint Committee) amendment regulations.* Provisional Regulations, 7th August 1913 (eventually definitive in effect). See Appendix C

National Insurance Act (1911) Amendment Act 1913. See Appendix B

National Health Insurance Joint Committee. *National Insurance (National Health Insurance): provisional regulations,* 20th August 1913. See Appendix C

National Health Insurance Joint Committee. *National Health Insurance (Medical Research Fund) regulations,* 1914, 21st March 1914—Statutory Rules and Orders, 1914, No. 418. Reproduced in full in Appendix C

National Health Insurance: Scheme of medical research. November 1913. (Correspondence submitting and embodying the proposals of the Medical Research Committee and consulting the Advisory Council)

National Health Insurance: Medical research. Letter of 15th December 1913, from the Chairman of the National Health Insurance Joint Committee approving the Scheme of Research

National Health Insurance: Schemes for research proposed by the Medical Research Committee. 31 October 1914

* Printed for official circulation.
I*

Chapter 4

Addison, C. See under Ch. 2

Agricultural Research Council Act 1956. 4 & 5 Eliz. 2. Ch. 28

Allen, B. M. 1934. *Sir Robert Morant, a great public servant.* London

Bridges, Lord. 1957. Haldane and the machinery of Government. *Public Administration* 35: 254–264

Brock, L. Unpublished statement quoted by Markham

Cole, M. (ed.). 1952. *Beatrice Webb's diaries 1912–1924*

Daalder, H. 1963. The Haldane Committee and the Cabinet. *Public Administration* 41: 117–135

Department of Scientific and Industrial Research Act 1956. 4 & 5 Eliz. 2. Ch. 58

Gilbert, B. B. 1966. See under Ch. 2

Haldane of Cloan, Viscount. 1929. *Richard Burdon Haldane: an autobiography.* London

Local Government Board. 1919. *Memorandum on the provisions of the Ministry of Health Bill, 1919, as to the work of the Medical Research Committee.* HMSO (Cmd. 69).

MacLeod, R. M., and Andrews, E. K. 1970. The origins of the DSIR: reflections on ideas and men 1915–1916. *Public administration* 48: 23–48

Markham, V. 1956. *Friendship's harvest.* London

Maurice, F. 1939. *Haldane 1915–28.* London

Ministry of Health Act 1919. See Appendix B

Ministry of Reconstruction. 1918. *Report of the Machinery of Government Committee.* HMSO (Cd. 9230). Reprinted 1962

Newman, G. 1939. See under Chapter 1

Newman, G., Fletcher, W. M., *et al.* 1920. Contributions to obituary notice of Sir Robert Morant. *British Medical Journal* 1920, 1: 419–421

Nicolson, H. 1952. *Life of George V.* London

Salter, Lord. 1961. *Memoirs of a public servant.* London

Selby-Bigge, L. A. 1927. Sir Robert Laurie Morant (1863–1920). *Dictionary of national biography, 1912–1921.* London

Somer, D. 1960. *Haldane of Cloan: his life and times, 1856–1928.* London

Tizard, H. 1955. A scientist in and out of the Civil Service. *22nd Haldane Memorial Lecture.* London

Chapter 5

Ministry of Health Act 1919. See Appendix B

Orders in Council. See Appendix D

Charter of the Medical Research Council. See Appendix E

Chapter 6

Hansard (House of Commons). 1919. *The parliamentary debates (official report).* Fifth Series, vol. 114: col. 2085

Himsworth, H. 1969. Administration and the structure of scientific knowledge. *British Medical Journal* 1969, 4: 517–522

Himsworth, H. 1970. *The development of scientific knowledge.* London
Pickering, G. 1970. Science and government. *Lancet* 1970, 2: 1297–1300
Prime Minister. 1963. *Committee of Inquiry into the Organisation of Civil Science.* (Trend Report) HMSO (Cmnd. 2171)
Public Health Laboratory Service Act 1960. See Appendix B
Radiological Protection Act 1970. See Appendix B
Zuckerman, S. 1970. *Beyond the ivory tower.* London

Chapter 7

Agricultural Research Act 1956. 4 & 5 Eliz. 2. Ch. 28
Atomic Energy Authority Act 1954. 2 & 3 Eliz. 2. Ch. 32
Development and Road Improvement Funds Act 1909. 9 Edw. 7. c. 47. Ch. 47
Melville, H. 1962. *The Department of Scientific and Industrial Research.* (The New Whitehall Series, No. 9) London and New York
National Parks and Access to the Countryside Act 1949. 12, 13 & 14. Geo. 6. Ch. 97

Chapter 8

Caldwell, D. S. L. 1957. *The organisation of science in England.* London
House of Commons papers. 1926. *Vol. VI: Second report from the Select Committee on Estimates*
House of Commons. 1972. *First report from the Select Committee on Science and Technology.* Session 1971–72. Research and Development. HMSO
Imperial Conference 1926. *Summary of proceedings XI: Report of the Research Special Sub-Committee.* HMSO (Cmnd. 2769)
Jones, T. (ed. Middlemass, K.). 1969. *Whitehall diary,* vol. II. 1926–30
Layton, D. 1968. Lord Wrottesley, FRS, pioneer statesman of science. *Notes and records of the Royal Society of London* 23: 230–246
Lord President of the Council. 1944. *Scientific research and development.* HMSO (Cmd. 6514)
Lord President of the Council. 1946. *Scientific man-power: Report of a Committee appointed by the Lord President of the Council.* HMSO (Cmd. 6824)
Lord President of the Council. 1946. *First Report of the Committee on Future Scientific Policy.* HMSO (Cmd. 6824)
Lord President of the Council. 1948. *First Annual Report of the Advisory Council on Scientific Policy (1947–1948).* HMSO (Cmd. 7465); and subsequent annual reports
Lord Privy Seal. 1971. *A framework for Government research and development.* HMSO (Cmnd. 4814)
Lord Privy Seal. 1972. *Framework for Government research and development.* HMSO (Cmnd. 5046)
MacLeod, R. M., and Andrews, E. K. 1969. The Committee of Civil Research: scientific advice for economic development. *Minerva* 7: 680–705
Ministry of Reconstruction. 1918. *Report of the Machinery of Government Committee* (Haldane Committee). HMSO (Cd. 9230)
Office of the Minister for Science. 1961. *Report of the Committee on the Management and Control of Research and Development.* HMSO
Prime Minister. 1963. *Report of the Committee on Higher Education* (Robbins Committee, 1961–63). HMSO (Cmnd. 2154)

Prime Minister. 1963. (Trend Report). See under Chapter 6

Royal Commission on Scientific Instruction and the Advancement of Science. 1875. *Eighth report.* (C. 1298)

Strange, A. 1871. On the necessity for a permanent commission on state scientific questions. *Journal of the Royal United Services Institution* 15: 537–566

HM Treasury. 1928. *Committee of Civil Research: report of the Research Co-ordination Sub-Committee.* HMSO

HM Treasury. 1945. *The Scientific Civil Service: reorganisation and recruitment during the reconstruction period.* (Annexe: Report of the Barlow Committee on Scientific Staff). HMSO (Cmd. 6679)

HM Treasury. 1965. *Report of a Committee appointed to review the Organisation of the Scientific Civil Service* (Tennant Committee). HMSO

Chapter 9

Cruelty to Animals Act 1876. 39 & 40 Vict. Ch. 77

Home Office. 1965. *Report of the Departmental Committee on Experiments on Animals* (Chairman: Sir Sydney Littlewood). HMSO (Cmnd. 2641)

Lane-Petter, W., and Pearson, A. E. G. 1971. *The laboratory animal—principles and practice.* London and New York

Medical Research Committee. 1919. *Memorandum upon the Dogs Protection Bill.* HMSO (Cmd. 161)

Medical Research Council. 1927. *Memorandum upon the Dogs Protection Bill.* HMSO (Cmd. 2880). (Revised version of 1919 Memorandum)

Medical Research Council. 1956. *The hazards to man of nuclear and allied radiations.* HMSO (Cmd. 9780); and further reports

Prime Minister. 1963. *Higher education: report of the Committee* (Robbins Committee). HMSO (Cmnd. 2154)

Royal Commission on Experiments on Animals. 1912. *Final Report of the Royal Commission on Vivisection.* HMSO (Cd. 6114)

Short, D. J., and Woodnott, D. P. (eds.). 1963, 1969. *The IAT manual of laboratory animal practice and techniques.* (Institute of Animal Technicians; first and second editions) London

Starling, E. H. 1918. The law of the heart. *Linacre Lecture at Cambridge, 1915.* London

University Grants Committee. 1964. *University development 1957–1962.* HMSO (Cmnd. 2267)

Chapter 10

Andrewes, C. H. 1953. William Ewart Gye, 1884–1952. *Obituary notices of Fellows of the Royal Society* 8: 419–430

Anon. 1952. Design coordination at Mill Hill. *Art and Industry* 52: 44–49 (illus.)

Bullard, E. 1965. What makes a good research establishment? Chapter 15 in Cockcroft, J. (ed.). *The organization of research establishments.* Cambridge

Chick, H., *et al.*, 1971. See under Chapter 1

Colebrook, L. 1948. Almroth Edward Wright, 1861–1947. *Obituary notices of Fellows of the Royal Society* 6: 297–314

Colebrook, L. 1954. *Almroth Wright: provocative doctor and thinker.* London

Cope, Z. 1966. *Almroth Wright, founder of modern vaccine-therapy.* London

Corner, G. W. 1964. *The history of the Rockefeller Institute, 1901–1953: origins and growth.* New York

Dale, H. H. 1935. Harold Ward Dudley, 1887–1935. *Obituary notices of Fellows of the Royal Society* 1: 595–606

Dale, H. H. 1941. Patrick Playfair Laidlaw, 1881–1940. *Obituary notices of Fellows of the Royal Society* 3: 427–447

Dale, H. 1963. Fifty years of medical research. *British Medical Journal* 1963, ii: 1287–1290

Douglas, C. G. 1953. Leonard Erskine Hill, 1866–1952. *Obituary notices of Fellows of the Royal Society* 8: 431–443

Feldberg, W. S. 1970. Henry Hallett Dale 1875–1968. *Biographical memoirs of Fellows of the Royal Society* 16: 77–174

Edwards, A. T. 1950. The Institute of Medical Research. *Building* 25: 258–265 (illus.)

Harington, C. R. 1956. Harold King 1887–1956. *Biographical memoirs of Fellows of the Royal Society* 2, 157–171

Harington, C. [R.]. 1965. The National Institute for Medical Research. Chapter 5 in Cockcroft, J. (ed.). *The organization of research establishments.* Cambridge

Harington, C. [R.] 1949. The work of the National Institute for Medical Research. *Proceedings of the Royal Society,* B, 136: 333–348

Harington, C. R. 1958. The place of the research institute in the advance of medicine. *Lancet* 1958, 1: 1345–1351

Hogben, L. 1950. Major Greenwood 1880–1949. *Obituary notices of Fellows of the the Royal Society* 7: 139–154

Laidlaw, P. [P.] 1936. Stewart Ranken Douglas 1871–1936. *Obituary notices of Fellows of the Royal Society* 2: 175–182

Medical Research Committee. 1915. *First Annual Report, 1914–1915*

Medical Research Council. 1970. *National Institute for Medical Research: scientific report for 1968–69.* London

Murray, J. A. 1950. Joseph Edwin Barnard 1870–1949. *Obituary notices of Fellows of the Royal Society* 1950–1951, 7 (19): 3–8

Chapter 11

Lewis, A. 1965. The Medical Research Council Social Psychiatry Research Unit. Chapter 6 in Cockcroft, J. (ed.). *The organization of research establishments.* Cambridge

Chapter 12

Anon. n.d. (ca. 1963). *History of the Strangeways Research Laboratory (formerly Cambridge Research Hospital) 1912–1962.* Privately printed at Cambridge

Brunning, D.A., and Dukes, C. E. 1965. The origin and early history of the Institute of Cancer Research of the Royal Cancer Hospital. *Proceedings of the Royal Society of Medicine* 58: 33–36

Haddow, A. 1961. The Chester Beatty Research Institute (of the Institute of Cancer Research: Royal Cancer Hospital). *Nature* 191: 430–432

World Health Organisation, 1969. *International Agency for Research on Cancer: Annual report 1968.* Lyon; and subsequent reports

Chapter 13

Boswell, James. 1799. *The life of Samuel Johnson, LL D.* Third edition. London

Colebrook, L. 1954. See under Chapter 10

Chapter 14

(For MRC Annual Reports, see under 'General')

MRC Serial and Periodical Publications:

Medical Research Committee Special Report Series, Nos. 1–49 (1915–20); Medical Research Council Special Report Series, Nos. 50 *et seq.* 1920 *et seq.* HMSO (Known as 'green reports'. The title of the series and the numbering were in fact not instituted until No. 3, and appeared only on the wrapper until No. 100—except on the title pages of Nos. 3 and 10 and some revised editions of others. By the end of 1971 the numbers had reached 310)

Medical Research Council Statistical Report Series, No. 6. 1920. HMSO (Nos. 1–5 were issued for official use during the First World War, but not published, and the series ended with No. 6)

Medical Research Council War Memoranda, Nos. 1–17. 1940–46; Medical Research Council Memoranda, Nos. 18 *et seq.* 1948 *et seq.* HMSO (Known as 'white memoranda'. By the end of 1969 the numbers had reached 43)

Medical Research Council Monitoring Report Series, No. 1 *et seq.* 1960 *et seq.* Assay of Strontium-90 in human bone in the United Kingdom. HMSO

Medical Supplement to the Daily Review of the Foreign Press. January 1918–April 1919 (monthly). War Office

Medical Science: Abstracts and Reviews, Vols. 1–12. 1919–25. Oxford University Press (for MRC)

Bulletin of War Medicine, Vols. 1–6 (two-monthly at first, monthly from Vol. 3). 1940–46. HMSO

Current Medical Research. Reprint of the articles in the Annual Report of the Medical Research Council, 1955–56 (and annually thereafter until 1968–69). HMSO

First Annual Report of the Industrial Fatigue Research Board, Medical Research Council and Department of Scientific and Industrial Research. Second to Eighth Annual Reports of the Industrial Fatigue Research Board, Medical Research Council. 1921–28; Ninth to Nineteenth Annual Reports of the Industrial Health Research Board, Medical Research Council. 1929–39. HMSO

Reports of the Industrial Fatigue Research Board, Nos. 1–54. 1919–29; Reports of the Industrial Health Research Board, Nos. 55–90. 1929–47. HMSO (Known as 'pink reports'; discontinued as a separate series since 1947)

Emergency Reports of the Industrial Health Research Board, Nos. 1–5. 1940–44. HMSO

Conditions for Industrial Health and Efficiency: Pamphlets (Industrial Health Research Board) Nos. 1–3. 1943–45. HMSO

Joint Reports of the Industrial Health Research Board and the Illumination Research Committee of the Department of Scientific and Industrial Research (four unnumbered reports on lighting in industry). 1926–35. HMSO

MRC occasional publications:

National Health Insurance: Medical Research Committee. 1915. *Interim report on the work in connection with the war at present undertaken by the Medical Research Committee.* HMSO (Cd. 7922)

The hazards to man of nuclear and allied radiations. A report to the Medical Research Council. 1956. HMSO (Cmd. 9780); and second report 1960 (Cmnd. 1225).

Statement on the Report of the United Nations Scientific Committee on the Effects of Atomic Radiation. A Report to the Medical Research Council. 1958. (Cmnd. 508)

The assessment of the possible radiation risks to the population from environmental contamination. A report to the Medical Research Council. 1966. HMSO

Alcohol: its action on the human organism. By a Committee originally appointed by the Central Control Board (Liquor Traffic) and later reconstituted by the Medical Research Council. Third edition, revised, 1938. HMSO

Tobacco smoking and cancer of the lung. Statement by the Medical Research Council. 1957. *British Medical Journal* and *Lancet*: re-issued separately by HMSO

Health research in industry: proceedings of a conference (IHRB). 1945. HMSO

The application of scientific methods to industrial and service medicine: proceedings of a conference (MRC). 1951. HMSO

Department of Scientific and Industrial Research and Medical Research Council. 1958. *First report of the Joint Committee on Human Relations in Industry,* March 1953 to March 1954. 1954. *Final report of the Joint Committee on Human Relations in Industry, 1954–57,* and *Report of the Joint Committee on Individual Efficiency in Industry, 1953–57.* HMSO

Agricultural Research Council and Medical Research Council. 1962. *Report of the Joint Committee on Antibiotics in Animal Feeding.* HMSO

Mathematics and computer science in biology and medicine. 1965. Proceedings of a conference held by the Medical Research Council in association with the Health Departments. HMSO

Books published for, or sponsored by, MRC:

Lane-Claypon, Janet E. 1916. *Milk and its hygienic relations.* London: Longmans, Green & Co. (for MRC)

Dobel, Clifford. 1919. *The amoebae living in man.* London: Bale, Sons and Danielsson. (Sponsored publication)

Dobel, Clifford and O'Connor, F. W. 1921. *The intestinal protozoa of man.* London: Bale, Sons and Danielsson. (Sponsored publication)

Diphtheria: its bacteriology, pathology and immunology. By the Bacteriological Committee of the Medical Research Council. 1923. HMSO

A system of bacteriology in relation to medicine, Vols. 1–9. 1929–31. HMSO

Other references:

Boyd Orr, Lord. 1966. *As I recall*

HM Treasury. 1922. *Report of the Committee Appointed to Select the Best Faces of Type and Modes of Display for Government Printing.* HMSO

Chapter 15

House of Commons 1947. *Third report from the Select Committee on Estimates, Session 1946–47.* Expenditure on Research and Development
House of Commons 1954. *Second report from the Select Committee on Estimates, Session 1953–54.* Grants in Aid
House of Commons 1961. *Fourth report from the Estimates Committee, Session 1960–61.* Variations in estimates

Chapter 16

Dentists Act 1921. 11 & 12 Geo. 5. c. 21
Healy, M. 1939. *The Old Munster Circuit.* (Information about Stephen Ronan in Chapter VIII)
Newton, D. 1968. *Sir Halley Stewart.* London
US Department of Health, Education and Welfare. 1965. Resource analysis. *Menco* No. 7

Chapter 17

Dale, H. H. 1955. Edward Mellanby 1884–1955. *Obituary notices of Fellows of the Royal Society,* 193–221
Dugdale, B. E. C. 1936. *Arthur James Balfour: First Earl of Balfour,* KG, OM, FRS vol. 2: 371–372. London
E(lliott), T. R. 1933. Sir Walter Morley Fletcher KBE, MD, FRS. *Nature* 132: 17–20.
E(lliott), T. R. 1933. Sir Walter Morley Fletcher. *Obituary notices of Fellows of the Royal Society,* No. 2, 153–163
Elliott, T. R. 1949. Fletcher, Sir Walter Morley. *Dictionary of National Biography, 1931–1940:* 284–285
Fletcher, M. 1957. *The bright countenance—a personal biography of Walter Morley Fletcher.* (With supplementary chapters by Sir Arthur MacNalty on the subject's scientific and official work.) London
Fletcher, W. M. 1930. Lord Balfour and the progress of medicine. *British Medical Journal* 1930, 1: 660–661
Hopkins, F. G. See below under Trevelyan
Medical Research Council. 1961. *Conditions of service on the staff of the Medical Research Council.* Revised edition. London (printed for official use)
Thomson, L. 1963. *Medical Research Council: administrative handbook for headquarters staff.* London (printed for official use)
HM Treasury. 1965. *Report of a Committee appointed to review the organisation of the Scientific Civil Service* ('Tennant Committee'). HMSO, London
HM Treasury. 1945. *The Scientific Civil Service: reorganisation and recruitment during the reconstruction period.* (Annexe: *Report of the Barlow Committee on Scientific Staff*). HMSO (Cmd. 6679)

Medical Research Council. 1967. *The services of MRC Central Store: an explanatory booklet.* (Printed by the Council, at the Store, for official use)

Trevelyan, G. M., and Hopkins, F. G. 1936. *Memorial to the late Sir Walter Morley Fletcher.* (Addresses at the ceremonial installation of the posthumous portrait-bust by Dora Clarke at the National Institute for Medical Research). Oxford (printed for private issue)

Appendix B
Acts of Parliament

Item 1 represents the statutory background of the constitution of the Medical Research Committee (see further in Appendix C). Item 4 similarly represents the statutory background of the constitution of the Committee of Privy Council for Medical Research and of the Medical Research Council, and there is an express reservation of the powers and duties of the Committee of Privy Council in Item 7 (see further in Appendices D and E). Item 15 provides the basis of a revised constitution for the Medical Research Council.

Items 5, 6, 10, 11, 12, 13 and 16 incidentally placed certain specific obligations on the Medical Research Council. Items 9 and 14 provide the statutory backgound of the Public Health Laboratory Service, for which the Council was for long responsible. Items 3, 4, 7, 8 and 9 conferred powers to promote or undertake medical research on certain departments and bodies other than the Medical Research Council.

(1) **National Insurance Act, 1911** (1 & 2 Geo. 5. Ch. 55)

Section 16 laid down *inter alia* that:

> "(2) The sums available for defraying the expenses of sanatorium benefit in each year shall be:
>
> (a) one shilling and threepence in respect of each insured person resident in the county or county borough, payable out of the funds out of which benefits are payable under this Part of this Act;
>
> (b) one penny in respect of each person payable out of moneys provided by Parliament;
>
> Provided that the Insurance Commissioners may retain the whole or any part of the sums so payable out of moneys provided by Parliament to be applied, in accordance with regulations made by the Commissioners, for the purposes of research."

Sanatorium benefit was defined in Section 8(1)(b) and further dealt with in Sections 16(1), (3) and (4) and 17. The bodies of Commissioners and their Joint Committee were established under Sections 57, 80, 81, 82 and 83. The date for the Act to come into operation, save as otherwise expressly provided, was named in Section 115 as 15 July 1912, with power of limited variation by Order in Council. The Act was subsequently repealed by amending legislation.

In the Financial Resolution of 6 July 1911 relating to the Act the following words occur: "(1) To authorise payment out of the moneys provided by Parliament . . . as respects sanatorium benefit, including research work in connection therewith, a sum not exceeding one penny a year for every insured person."

(2) **National Insurance Act (1911) Amendment Act, 1913** (3 & 4 Geo. 5. Ch. 37)

Section 29 (1) empowered the Treasury to make Regulations incorporating the Joint Committee constituted under Section 83 of the principal Act. Section 29 (2) validated documents issued by the Joint Committee before the commencement of this Act (which became law on 15 August 1913).

(3) **Scottish Board of Health Act, 1919** (9 & 10 Geo. 5. Ch. 20)

Section provided that "It shall be the duty of the Board . . . to take all such steps as may be desirable to secure the effective carrying out and co-ordination of measures conducive to the health of the people, including measures for . . . the initiation and direction of research, . . .". And Section 4 (1) that "There shall be transferred to the Board . . . (b) all the powers and duties of the Scottish Insurance Commissioners;"

(4) **Ministry of Health Act, 1919** (9 & 10 Geo. 5. Ch. 21)

This provided *inter alia* that:

"2. It shall be the duty of the Minister . . . to take all such steps as may be desirable to secure the preparation, effective carrying out and co-ordination of measures conducive to the health of the people, including measures for . . . the initiation and direction of research, . . .".

"3. (1) There shall be transferred to the Minister:
(a) all the powers and duties of the Local Government Board;
(b) all the powers and duties of the Insurance Commissioners and the Welsh Insurance Commissioners; . . .".

Provided that:

(i) the power conferred on the Insurance Commissioners by the proviso to subsection (2) of section 16 of the National Insurance Act, 1911, of retaining and applying for the purposes of research such sums as are therein mentioned shall not be transferred to the Minister, but the duties heretofore performed by the Medical Research Committee shall after the date of the commencement of this Act be carried on by or under the direction of a Committee of the Privy Council appointed by His Majesty for that purpose, and any property held for the purposes of the former Committee shall after that date be transferred to and vested in such persons as the body by whom such duties as aforesaid are carried on may appoint, and be held by them for the purposes of that body;"

Sections 9 (1) and 10 (1) dealt with the transfer of powers in Ireland, including those relating to research. Section 11 (1) dealt with dates for the Act to come into operation. Section 11 (2), together with the Second Schedule, repealed *inter alia* the proviso to subsection (2) of Section 16 of the National Insurance Act 1911.

The Act became law on 3 June 1919. An Order in Council of 25 June 1919 (S.R. & O. 1919, No. 850) brought parts of the Act into operation, Section 1 from 25 June 1919, and amongst others Section 3 (1) (b), except proviso (i) of the subsection, from 1 July 1919. An Order in Council of 9 February 1920 (S.R. & O. 1920, No. 252) brought into operation the parts relevant to the

Committee of Privy Council for Medical Research from 1 April 1920 (see Appendix D, No. 1).

(5) **Therapeutic Substances Act, 1925** (15 & 16 Geo. 5. Ch. 60)

This was "an Act to provide for the regulation of the manufacture, sale and importation of vaccines, sera and other therapeutic substances . . . being substances the purity or potency of which cannot be adequately tested by chemical means". By Section 4 (1) the framing of regulations under the Act was put in the hands of a joint committee consisting of the Minister of Health as chairman, the Secretary for Scotland and the Minister of Home Affairs for Northern Ireland. Section 4 (2) provided that the joint committee should be assisted by an advisory committee consisting of members of whom one was to be appointed by each of the following: the Minister of Health, the Scottish Board of Health, the Minister of Home Affairs for Northern Ireland, the Medical Research Council, the British Medical Association, the Council of the Pharmaceutical Society of Great Britain, and the Council of the Institute of Chemistry of Great Britain and Ireland."

Various further references to the Medical Research Council, and in particular to the National Institute for Medical Research, were made in the series of Regulations made under the Act. The measure was eventually repealed by the consolidating Act of 1956 (see No. 12 below).

(6) **London Gas Undertakings (Regulations) Act, 1939** (2 & 3 Geo. 6. Ch. 99)

The Act provided "for the making of regulations with respect to the installation of supplies of gas and of gas-fire appliances to and in premises in the county of London". The gas companies were required to submit draft regulations for approval of the Board of Trade, which was by Sections 6 (1) (a) and 17 (2) required to refer the proposed regulations to a Committee consisting of representatives of various bodies. Section 6 (3) named the Medical Research Council —and also the Royal College of Physicians—among the bodies to be so represented. Owing to the Second World War, the provision did not operate until 1946.

(7) **National Health Service Act, 1946** (9 & 10 Geo. 6. Ch. 81)

Section 16 is concerned with powers relating to research:

"(1) Without prejudice to the general powers and duties conferred or imposed on the Minister under the Ministry of Health Act, 1919, and the duties imposed on the Committee of the Privy Council for Medical Research under the said Act, the Minister may conduct, or assist by grants or otherwise any person to conduct, research into any matters relating to the causation, prevention, diagnosis or treatment of illness or mental defectiveness.

"(2) The Board of Governors of a teaching hospital and a Regional Hospital Board and a Hospital Management Committee shall have power to conduct research into any of the matters aforesaid."

Section 17 is the legislative background for the eventual Public Health Laboratory Service:

"The Minister may provide a bacteriological service, which may include the provision of laboratories, for the control of the spread of infectious diseases, and the Minister may allow persons to make use of services provided at such laboratories on such terms, including terms as to the payment of charges, as the Minister thinks fit."

(8) **National Insurance (Industrial Injuries) Act, 1946** (9 & 10 Geo. 6. Ch. 62)

The general purpose of this Act, applicable to the whole of Great Britain, was to substitute for the Workmen's Compensation Acts, 1925 to 1945, a system of insurance against injuries and diseases arising out of a person's employment. Section 73 (1) conferred on the Minister of National Insurance, later Minister of Pensions and National Insurance, certain powers relating to research: "The Minister may promote research into the causes and incidence of, and methods of prevention of, accidents, injuries and diseases against which persons are insured under this Act or which it is contemplated might be prescribed for the purpose of Part IV of this Act, either by himself employing persons to conduct such research or by contributing to the expenses of, or otherwise assisting, other persons engaged in such research."

(9) **National Health Service (Scotland) Act, 1947** (10 & 11 Geo. 6. Ch. 27)

Section 17 gives powers in relation to research:

"(1) Without prejudice to the general powers and duties conferred or imposed on the Secretary of State under the Scottish Board of Health Act, 1919, the Secretary of State may conduct, or assist by grants or otherwise any person to conduct, research into any matters relating to the causation, prevention, diagnosis or treatment of illness or mental deficiency, or to the development of medical or surgical appliances including hearing aids.

(2) A Regional Hospital Board and a Board of Management shall have power to conduct or assist by grants or otherwise any person to conduct research into any of the aforesaid matters."

Section 18 relates to the provision of a bacteriological service:

"(1) The Secretary of State may provide or secure the provision "of a bacteriological service, which may include the provision of laboratories, for the control of the spread of infectious diseases, and the Secretary of State may allow persons to make use of services provided at such laboratories on such terms, including terms as to the payment of charges, and on such conditions as the Secretary of State may determine.

(2) Regulations and schemes under section 12 of this Act may provide for the administration of the services under the last foregoing subsection as if those services formed part of the hospital and specialist services."

(10) **Penicillin Act, 1947** (10 & 11 Geo. 6. Ch. 29)

The purpose of the Act was "to control the sale and supply of penicillin and certain other substances". The main provision (Section 1) was to prohibit, with certain necessary provisos, the supply of penicillin except by (a) a duly qualified medical practitioner, registered dental practitioner or registered veterinary surgeon, or (b) a registered pharmacist or authorised seller of poisons under the authority of a prescription signed and dated by any such practitioner or surgeon. Section 2 (1) defines the substances:

"The substances to which this Act applies are penicillin and such other anti-microbial organic substances produced by living organisms as may be prescribed by regulations made by the Minister of Health, the Secretary of State for Scotland and the Minister of Health and Local Government for Northern Ireland, jointly, after consultation with the Medical Research Council. . . ."

Various other antibiotics were subsequently brought under the Act by regulations made after consultation with the Council. The Act was amended by the Act of 1953 and repealed by the consolidating Act of 1956.

(11) **Income Tax Act, 1952** (15 & 16 Geo. 6 & 1 Eliz. 2 Ch. 10). Section 335 (*b*) and (*c*) provided that the approval of "the appropriate Research Council or Committee" (the Medical Research Council being among those specified in the definition in Section 340 (4)) should be obtained for allowances against tax where a person carrying on a trade makes a payment to a scientific research association or a university (or similar institution) to be used for scientific research related to the particular class of trade. The provision in that form remained effective until 1965 (see under 15).

(12) **Therapeutic Substances (Prevention of Misuse) Act, 1953** (1 & 2 Eliz. 2. Ch. 32)

Section 1 (1) amended Section 2 (1) of the Penicillin Act 1947 to read as follows:
"The substances to which this Act applies are penicillin and such other therapeutic substances as may be prescribed by regulations made by the Minister of Health, the Secretary of State [for Scotland] and the Minister of Health and Local Government for Northern Ireland, jointly, after consultation with the Medical Research Council, being substances appearing to those Ministers to be capable of causing danger to the health of the community if used without proper safeguards."

Section 2 (2) provided that:
"The power of making regulations under this section shall be exercisable by the Minister of Health, the Secretary of State [for Scotland] and the Minister of Health and Local Government for Northern Ireland, jointly, after consultation with the Medical Research Council and, in the case of regulations appearing to those Ministers to concern agricultural matters, with the Agricultural Research Council."

(13) **Therapeutic Substances Act, 1956** (4 & 5 Eliz. 2. Ch. 25)

This was a consolidating measure which repealed and replaced the Acts of 1925, 1947, 1951 and 1953; the Act of 1951 was the Penicillin (Merchant Ships) Act, which did not involve the Council. Section 4 (2) re-enacted the provisions of Section 4 (2) of the 1925 Act. Section 8 (1) re-enacted the provisions of Section 2 (1) of the 1947 Act as amended by Section 1 (1) of the 1953 Act. Section 9 (2) re-enacted the provisions of Section 2 (2) of the 1953 Act. The First Schedule listed, with slight variations in definition, the substances listed in the Schedule to the 1925 Act.

(14) **Public Health Laboratory Service Act, 1960** (8 & 9 Eliz. 2. Ch. 49)

The purpose of this Act was "to established a Public Health Laboratory Service Board for the exercise of functions with respect to the administration of the bacteriological service provided by the Minister of Health under Section 17 of the National Health Service Act, 1946".

Section 1 (1) provided that:
"For the purpose of exercising such functions with respect to the administration of the public health laboratory service as the Minister may determine there shall be constituted, in accordance with the Schedule to this Act, a board by the name of the Public Health Laboratory Service Board (in this Act referred to as the Board)."

Section 2 (1) regulated the transfer of staff from Council to Board:

"Any officer or servant of the Medical Research Council who, immediately before the commencement of this Act, was employed for the purposes of any laboratory provided as part of the public health laboratory service, or was employed as the medical director of that service, shall, if his employment as such an officer or servant would be continued but for this section, be transferred to and become an officer or servant of the Board at the commencement of this Act, and his employment immediately after the transfer shall be on the same terms as to remuneration and conditions of service as immediately before the transfer."

Section 3 (1) regulated the transfer of property:

"There shall be transferred to and vested in the Minister by virtue of this Act all property, whether real or personal, which immediately before the commencement of this Act was vested in the Medical Research Council and used by them solely for the purposes of the public health laboratory service, and all rights acquired and liabilities incurred by the Council solely for those purposes, other than rights and liabilities arising out of any contract of employment."

The Schedule constituted the Board as a body corporate, with power to hold property on trust. It provided that the Board shall consist of a chairman and other members appointed by the Minister, the other members to include not less than two persons appointed after consultation with the Medical Research Council; not less than two persons with experience as bacteriologists, appointed after consultation with such organisations as the Minister thinks appropriate; and not less than two persons holding office as medical officer of health of a local authority; at least one person appointed after consultation with such organisations as appear to the Minister to represent the Hospital Service; and at least one fully registered medical practitioner engaged in general medical practice, appointed after consultation with such organisations as the Minister may recognise as representative of practitioners so engaged.

Under the powers given by Section 5 (3), the Minister appointed 1 August 1961 as the day on which the Act was to come into force.

(15) **Science and Technology Act 1965** (Eliz. 2. 1965. Ch. 4)

The purpose of this Act was "to make further provision with respect to the responsibility and powers in relation to scientific research and related matters of the Secretary of State for Education and Science, the Minister of Technology and certain chartered bodies and other organisations, and for purposes connected therewith". The following extracts are relevant:

"1. (1) The following bodies established or to be established by Royal Charter shall be Research Councils for the purposes of this Act, that is to say,

(a) the Agricultural Research Council and the Medical Research Council; and . . ."

"2. (1) The Secretary of State may, out of moneys provided by Parliament, pay to any of the Research Councils such sums in respect of the expenses of the Council as he may with the consent of the Treasury determine, and so far as relates to the use and expenditure of sums so paid the Council shall act in accordance with such directions as may from time to time be given to it by the Secretary of State.

(2) The provisions of Schedule 1 to this Act shall have effect with respect

to the making of returns and reports by the Research Councils to the Secretary of State, with respect to the keeping and auditing of their accounts and with respect to related matters.

(3) Land occupied in the United Kingdom by any of the Research Councils shall be deemed, for the purposes of any rate on property, to be property occupied by or on behalf of the Crown for public purposes.

(4) The obligations of the Medical Research Council and the Agricultural Research Council under this section in relation to the Secretary of State shall be in place of any corresponding obligations imposed on either Council by its charter or otherwise . . .; and subject to the foregoing provisions of this sub-section anything which under the charter of either of those Councils is to be done by or to a committee of the Privy Council shall instead be done by or to the Secretary of State.

(5) Nothing in this Act or in any other enactment relating to the general functions of any of the Research Councils shall be taken as restricting the activities of a Research Council to the United Kingdom or any part thereof, nor shall the expenses in respect of which payments may be made under subsection (1) above be restricted to expenses incurred in the United Kingdom; . . ."

"5. (1) The Secretary of State and the Minister of Technology may defray out of moneys provided by Parliament any expenses which, with the consent of the Treasury, they may respectively incur:

(a) in carrying on or supporting scientific research or the dissemination of the results of scientific research; . . .

(c) in making payments in respect of remuneration, allowances or pension benefits payable to or in respect of members of any advisory body established for the purpose of assisting the Secretary of State or Minister, as the case may be, in matters connected with scientific research."

'6. (1) In this Act 'scientific research' means research and development in any of the sciences (including the social sciences) or in technology.

(2) Nothing in this Act shall prejudice or affect any power to amend or revoke the charters of any Research Council, or any power of Her Majesty to grant new charters, or affect the operation of any amendment made or charter granted after the passing of this Act.

(3) The enactments mentioned in Schedule 4 to this Act are hereby repealed to the extent specified in the third column of that Schedule, with effect in each case from such day as Her Majesty may by Order in Council appoint."

"SCHEDULE 1. Reports, Accounts, etc., of Research Councils

1. Each of the Research Councils shall furnish the Secretary of State with such returns, accounts and other information with respect to its property and activities as he may from time to time require, and shall prepare programmes and estimates of expenditure in such form and at such times as he may require.

2. (1) Each of the Research Councils shall as soon as possible after the end of each financial year make to the Secretary of State a report on the exercise and performance by the Council of its functions during that year.

(2) The Secretary of State shall lay a copy of any report under this paragraph before each House of Parliament, together with such comments as he may think fit to make.

3. (1) Each of the Research Councils shall keep proper accounts and other records, and shall prepare for each financial year statements of account in such form as the Secretary of State with the approval of the Treasury may direct

and submit those statements of account to the Secretary of State at such time as he may direct.

(2) The Secretary of State shall, on or before the 30th November in any year, transmit to the Comptroller and Auditor General the statements of account of each Council for the financial year last ended.

(3) The Comptroller and Auditor General shall examine and certify the statements of account transmitted to him under this paragraph, and lay copies of them together with his report thereon before each House of Parliament."

Schedule 2 amends Section 335 (b) and (c) and Section 340 (4) of the Income Tax Act 1952 by substituting the Secretary of State or Minister of Technology for the appropriate Research Council or Committee.

Schedule 4 repeals from "but" onwards in Section 3 (1) proviso (i) of the Ministry of Health Act 1919; and also repeals the definition of the appropriate Research Council or Committee in Section 340 (1) of the Income Tax Act 1952.

(16) **Radiological Protection Act 1970** (Eliz. 2. 1970. Ch. 46)

Section 1 sets up a National Radiological Protection Board, supported by an Advisory Committee, in order (subsection 1):

"(a) by means of research and otherwise, to advance the acquisition of knowledge about the protection of mankind from radiation hazards; and (b) to provide information and advice to persons (including government departments) with responsibilities in the United Kingdom in relation to the protection from radiation hazards either of the community as a whole or of particular sections of the community." Also (Subsection 3) *inter alia*, to "assume responsibility for the Radiological Protection Service heretofore provided by the Medical Research Council"; and to carry on relevant activities of the U.K. Atomic Energy Authority.

Section 1 (6) empowers the Secretary of State for Education and Science to vary the functions of the Board after consultation with the Atomic Energy Authority and the Medical Research Council.

Under Section 1 (7) the Health Ministers are to give directions to the Board, and under Section 2 (1) to appoint members of the Board, after similar consultation.

Appendix C
Statutory Regulations Relating to the Medical Research Committee

The following Regulations were all made under the National Insurance Act, 1911 (Appendix B). Those in Item 1 below were made by the Treasury and gave powers in respect of moneys for research to the National Health Insurance Joint Committee. Those in Items 2 and 3 were made by the Joint Committee by virtue of these powers. Those in Item 2 were provisional and were replaced by the definitive version in Item 3, which did not differ substantially except that clauses 9 and 10 were new. The definitive Regulations were in effect the constitution of the Medical Research Committee and are given below at length.

(The Provisional Regulations had been in part anticipated by two Minutes of Appointment of 20 June 1913 in which the Minister responsible for National Health Insurance purported to appoint the members of the Medical Research Committee and of the Advisory Council, respectively, and to determine the functions of these bodies. The Committee in fact met twice in July 1913, before the Regulations had been promulgated.)

(1) **National Insurance (Joint Committee) Amendment Regulations, 1913**

These were Provisional Regulations, dated 7 August 1913, made by the Treasury under Section 83 of the National Insurance Act, 1911. Not needing any amendment, they eventually acquired definitive force. The operative clause read as follows:

"2. For the purposes of the proviso to subsection 2 of Section 16 of the Act relating to the retention by the Insurance Commissioners of the whole or any part of the sum payable out of moneys provided by Parliament under that subsection for defraying the expenses of sanatorium benefit the Joint Committee alone shall exercise the following powers, namely:

(*a*) the power, so far as the terms of the grant may place such sums under the administrative control of the Joint Committee, of retaining the whole or any part thereof for purposes of research;

(*b*) the power to make regulations as to the manner in which any sums which may be retained either by the Joint Committee or by any of the several bodies of Commissioners shall be applied for such purposes."

(2) **National Insurance (National Health Insurance): Provisional Regulations, 20 August 1913**

These were made by the Joint Committee established under the National Insurance

Act, 1911, as to the application of moneys made available for the purposes of research by subsection (2) of Section 16 of the Act and were replaced in 1914 (next item).

(3) **The National Health Insurance (Medical Research Fund) Regulations, 1914** (Statutory Rules and Orders, 1914. No. 418. National Insurance— National Health Insurance)

These were made by the National Health Insurance Joint Committee under the powers conferred by subsection (2) of Section 16 of the National Insurance Act, 1911, and by the National Insurance (Joint Committee) Amendment Regulations, 1913 (above). Clauses 1 and 2 were formal (definitions, etc.); Clause 3 read, in part, as follows:

"All sums which may be retained for the purposes of research . . . either by the Joint Committee or by any of the several bodies of Commissioners . . . shall be paid at such time and by such instalments as the Joint Committee may direct into a fund, to be called the Medical Research Fund, under the control and management of the Joint Committee. . . ."

The remaining clauses formed the constitution of the Medical Research Committee and are quoted in full:

" 4. (1) A Committee shall be constituted for the purposes of research, called the Medical Research Committee, of which the persons whose names appear in the First Schedule to these Regulations shall be the first members.

(2) The first members of the Committee shall hold office for a period of not less than three years from the 20th day of August, 1913, and thereafter three members of the Committee, to be selected in such manner as the Committee may determine, shall retire at intervals of two years, but shall be eligible for re-appointment.

(3) Any vacancy whether casual or otherwise which may hereafter occur among members of the Committee shall be filled by appointment by the Chairman of the Joint Committee; but any person appointed to fill a casual vacancy shall only hold office for the remainder of the period of office of the member in whose place he is appointed.

5. (1) There shall also be constituted an Advisory Council for Research, of which the persons whose names appear in the Second Schedule to these Regulations shall be the first members.

(2) The first members of the Advisory Council shall hold office for a period of three years from the 20th day of August, 1913, and shall be eligible for re-appointment.

(3) All appointments to the Advisory Council whether in the event of any casual vacancy or otherwise shall hereafter be made by the Chairman of the Joint Committee in such manner and for such periods as he may determine from time to time.

6. (1) The Medical Research Committee shall appoint one of their members in writing to be Treasurer of the Committee, and it shall be the duty of the Treasurer to receive on behalf of the Committee all sums payable to the Committee out of the Medical Research Fund.

(2) The Committee may appoint such officers and servants and may expend such moneys for the administrative purposes of the Committee (including travelling expenses and subsistence allowances for members and staff) as it thinks fit, subject, as to the number of such officers and servants and their remuneration and as to the scale of travelling expenses and subsistence allowances, and as to the amount of such moneys, to the approval of the Chairman of the Joint Committee.

7. (1) The Medical Research Committee shall from time to time prepare schemes for research, including, if the Committee think fit, schemes for inquiries and the collection and publication of information and statistics, and shall submit such schemes to the Chairman of the Joint Committee for his approval.

(2) Every such scheme shall contain an estimate of the expenditure necessary for the carrying out of the scheme and shall specify the period within which such expenditure is to be incurred.

8. Subject to the provisions of these Regulations, the Medical Research Committee may, for the purposes of any scheme approved as aforesaid, apply any moneys received by the Treasurer of the Committee from the Medical Research Fund in the purchase or other acquisition of land or any interest therein, or any plant, furniture or other chattels, and in the erection, alteration or maintenance of any building or other works, and in the payment of any costs, charges and expenses of, or incidental to, the said scheme or any powers conferred by or pursuant to these Regulations.

9. (1) The Chairman of the Joint Committee may from time to time by writing appoint two or more members of the Medical Research Committee to be trustees of the Committee, and the provisions of the Trustee Act, 1893, shall apply accordingly.

(2) All property purchased out of moneys received by the Treasurer of the Medical Research Committee from the Medical Research Fund, or otherwise acquired for the purposes of the Committee, shall be vested in the trustees for the time being of the Committee, and in the case of land on trust for sale with full powers of management and disposition.

(3) No interest in land shall be acquired by the Medical Research Committee under these Regulations, or under any scheme made in pursuance thereof, without the consent in writing of the Chairman of the Joint Committee.

(4) The trustees shall execute a declaration of trust declaring such trusts and containing such powers and provisions relating to any property for the time being vested in them or the proceeds of sale thereof as the Chairman of the Joint Committee shall, subject to the provisions of these Regulations, approve.

10. Before approving any scheme so submitted to him by the Medical Research Committee, the Chairman of the Joint Committee shall consult the Advisory Council for Research.

11. There shall be paid from time to time out of the moneys standing to the credit of the Medical Research Fund:

> (a) to members of the Advisory Council for Research travelling expenses and subsistence allowances, upon a scale to be approved by the Chairman of the Joint Committee, incurred by them in attending meetings of the Council;

> (b) such sums as the Chairman of the Joint Committee may direct, as honoraria to members of the Medical Research Committee, not being the Chairman of the Committee or members of the Commons House of Parliament;

> (c) such sums as may be required for the administrative purposes of the Medical Research Committee;

> (d) such sums as the Chairman of the Joint Committee may from time to time direct to be paid to the Medical Research Committee for the purposes of any scheme or schemes approved as aforesaid.

12. (1) The accounts of the Medical Research Fund shall be made up for each financial year ending the 31st March, and shall be audited in such manner as the Treasury may direct. Any balance standing to the credit of the Fund as

at the end of any financial year shall, if the terms of the Parliamentary grant so provide, be carried forward to the next financial year.

(2) Any moneys from time to time standing to the credit of the Fund and not for the time being required for the purposes of these Regulations may, if the Joint Committee so direct, be invested in any securities for the time being authorised as investments for approved societies under subsection (2) of Section 56 of the Act.

13. The accounts of the Medical Research Committee shall be audited in such manner as the Treasury may direct.

14. Save as otherwise expressly provided in these Regulations, no moneys shall be paid by way of salary, fee or otherwise, out of the Medical Research Fund to any members of the Medical Research Committee or of the Advisory Council for Research."

First Schedule

The Right Hon. Lord Moulton of Bank, LLD, FRS (Chairman)

Christopher Addison, MD, MP

Waldorf Astor, MP

Sir T. Clifford Allbutt, KCB, MD, FRCP, FRS, Regius Professor of Physic, University of Cambridge

Charles John Bond, FRCS, Senior Honorary Surgeon, Leicester Infirmary

William Bulloch, MD, FRS, Bacteriologist to the London Hospital and Professor of Bacteriology in the University of London

Matthew Hay, MD, LLD Professor of Forensic Medicine and Public Health, Aberdeen University

Frederick Gowland Hopkins, MB, DSC, FRS, Reader in Chemical Physiology in the University of Cambridge

Brevet-Colonel Sir William Boog Leishman, MB, FRS, Professor of Pathology, Royal Army Medical College

Second Schedule

The Right Hon. Lord Moulton of Bank, LLD, FRS (Chairman)

Miss L. B. Aldrich-Blake, MD, MS

Sir W. Watson Cheyne, Bart., CB, FRCS, FRS

Sir William S. Church, Bart., KCB, MD

Sidney Coupland, MD

David Davies, MP

Sheridan Delépine, MB

Sir James Kingston Fowler, KCVO, MD

Sir Rickman J. Godlee, Bart., FRCS

Sir Alfred Pearce Gould, KCVO, FRCS

David Hepburn, MD

E. C. Hort, FRCP, Edin.

Arthur Latham, MD

Sir John McFadyean, MB

W. Leslie Mackenzie, MD

J. C. McVail, MD

W. J. Maguire, MD

S. H. C. Martin, MD, FRS

Robert Muir, MD

Alexander Napier, MD

Sir George Newman, MD

Arthur Newsholme, CB, MD

J. M. O'Connor, MB

Sir William Osler, Bart., MD, FRS

A. C. O'Sullivan, MB

Marcus S. Paterson, MD

Sir Robert W. Philip, MD

Sir William H. Power, KCB, FRCS, FRS

H. Meredith Richards, MD

Lauriston E. Shaw, MD

Albert Smith, MP

L. Lorrain Smith, MD, FRS

T. J. Stafford, CB, FRCSI

T. H. C. Stevenson, MD

Harold J. Stiles, FRCS, Edin

Sir Stewart Stockman, MRCVS

W. St. Clair Symmers, MB

Miss Jane Walker, MD

Norman Walker, MD

J. Smith Whitaker, MRCS, LRCP

Sir Arthur Whitelegge, KCB, MD

G. Sims Woodhead, MD

Appendix D

Orders in Council Relating to the Committee of Privy Council for Medical Research and the Medical Research Council

The following Orders were made, up to 1964, in pursuance of the Ministry of Health Act, 1919, and the remainder in pursuance of the Science and Technology Act 1965. Items 1, 9, 11 fix the dates of commencement of relevant parts of Acts. Items 2, 4, 6, 7, 8 and 10 relate to the constitution of the Committee of Privy Council, including its eventual dissolution (see also Appendix G). Items 3, 5, 12 approve drafts of the Royal Charters granted to the Council, and Item 12 allows amendments to the Charter of 1966 (Appendix E).

(Orders of the Committee of Privy Council for Medical Research (as distinct from Orders in Council) are regarded as internal documents and are not included in this Appendix. Such of them as were of more than a routine nature (e.g. allowing amendments to the Charter of 1920) are cited, by their dates, in Chapters 5 and 6 and their purport is sufficiently indicated in these references. Orders appointing new members of the Medical Research Council, annually or in casual vacancies, were a routine procedure.)

(1) **Order in Council of 9 February 1920:** Ministry of Health Act, 1919

(Date of Commencement) Order, 1920 (S.R. & O. 1920. No. 252)

It was ordered that 1 April 1920 be the date of commencement of the Act in respect of "Proviso (i) to subsection (1) of Section 3"; and "So much of subsection (2) of Section 11 and of the Second Schedule as repeals paragraph (*b*) of and the proviso to subsection (2) of Section 16 of the National Insurance Act, 1911".

(2) **Order in Council of 11 March 1920**

After recitals, the appointment of the Committee of Privy Council was ordered as follows:

"That the Lord President of the Council, the Minister of Health, the Secretary for Scotland and the Chief Secretary for Ireland, respectively, for the time being, be and they are hereby appointed a Committee for the purposes aforesaid.

And it is ordered that during His Majesty's pleasure the Minister of Health shall preside over the said Committee in the absence of the Lord President.

And it is further ordered that the said Committee may out of moneys provided by Parliament or otherwise available, and subject to such conditions as the Treasury may prescribe, furnish the Medical Research Council with such funds as may be necessary for the performance of their duties by the Council, and shall exercise and perform in relation to the Council such powers and duties as in the Charter aforesaid they shall be authorised and empowered to exercise and perform.

And it is further ordered that the Secretary of the Medical Research Council for the time being shall act as Secretary of the said Committee.

And it is ordered that the said Committee shall in every year cause to be laid before both Houses of Parliament a report of their proceedings and of the proceedings of the Medical Research Council during the preceding year."

(3) **Order in Council of 25 March 1920**

Promulgated the Draft of a Charter for creating the Members of the Medical Research Committee a Body Corporate, under the style and title of "The Medical Research Council"; and ordered that "one of His Majesty's Principal Secretaries of State do cause a Warrant to be prepared for His Majesty's Royal Signature, for passing under the Great Seal of the United Kingdom a Charter in conformity with the said Draft, which is hereunto annexed". (See Appendix E.)

(4) **Order in Council of 26 July 1926**

Ordered that the Committee of Privy Council "shall, as from the date of this Order, consist of the Lord President of the Council, the Secretary of State for Home Affairs, the Secretary of State for Dominion Affairs, the Secretary of State for the Colonies, the Minister of Health and the Secretary for Scotland, respectively, for the time being". ("for Home Affairs" should have read "for the Home Department"; the formal inaccuracy was copied for several years in the annual reports of the Medical Research Council.)

(5) **Order in Council of 30 June 1949**

Promulgated the Draft of a Supplemental Charter to be granted to the Medical Research Council; and ordered that it be prepared for Royal Signature. (Appendix E.)

(6) **Order in Council of 28 October 1955**

After recitals relating to the Committee of Privy Council, appointed "as Members of the said Committee the Lord President of the Council, the Secretary of State for the Home Department, the Secretary of State for Commonwealth Relations, the Secretary of State for the Colonies, the Secretary of State for Scotland, the Minister of Health and the Minister of Labour and National Service, respectively, for the time being". Also reaffirmed certain provisions of the Order of 11 March 1920.

(7) **Order in Council of 30 September 1959:** Minister for Science Order, 1959 (Statutory Instruments, 1959, No. 1826: Ministers of the Crown)

Ordered that the Minister for Science (newly appointed) be substituted for the Lord President of the Council as member and chairman of the Committees of the Privy Council for research, including the Committee for Medical Research. The Order came into operation on 3 November 1959.

(8) **Order in Council of 26 March 1964:** The Secretary of State for Education and Science Order 1964 (Statutory Instruments, 1964, No. 490: Ministers of the Crown)

Ordered that on 1 April 1964 there be transferred to the Secretary of State all functions of the Minister of Education and all functions of the Minister for Science; and that the Secretary of State be substituted for the Minister for Science as member and chairman of, *inter alia*, the Committee of Privy Council for Medical Research.

(9) **Order in Council of 24 March 1965:** Scientific Research: The Science and Technology Act 1965 (Commencement No. 1) Order 1965 (Statutory Instruments 1965, No. 597 (C. 3))

Fixed 1 April 1965 as the effective date of, *inter alia*, the amendment of the Income Tax Act 1952.

(10) **Order in Council of 14 April 1965:** Committees of the Privy Council (Medical, Agricultural, Scientific and Industrial Research) (Dissolution) Order 1965

Having regard to the Science and Technology Act 1965, formally dissolved the Committees named in the title.

(11) **Order in Council of 14 May 1965:** Scientific Research: The Science and Technology Act 1965 (Commencement No. 2) Order 1965. (Statutory Instruments 1965, No. 1127 (C. 6))

Fixed 1 June 1965 as the effective date of, *inter alia*, the repeal of a part of the Ministry of Health Act 1919 and a part of the Income Tax Act 1952.

(12) **Order in Council of 20 September 1966**

Approved the draft of a new Charter to be granted to the Medical Research Council. (Appendix E.)

(13) **Order in Council of 5 April 1971**

Approved amendments to the Charter of the Medical Research Council. (Appendix E.)

Appendix E
Royal Charters
of the Medical Research Council

Original Charter

This was granted on 1 April 1920 in accordance with an Order in Council of 25 March 1920 (Appendix D). It is here printed with the amendments subsequently allowed in accordance with Article 9 of the Charter, by the Committee of Privy Council for Medical Research, or made by the Supplemental Charter.

Words that were deleted are shown within heavy square brackets. Words that were added are printed in italic type. The dates in the margin are those of the respective amendments and refer to Orders of the Committee of Privy Council of 1 March 1926, 1 November 1943 and 15 May 1957; and to the Supplemental Charter granted on 27 July 1949.

The Charter was further amended in effect (not shown here) by clause 2 (4) of the Science and Technology Act 1965, which transferred the powers of the Committee of Privy Council to the Secretary of State for Education and Science, as from 23 March 1966.

Finally, the original Charter was revoked by the new Charter on 26 October 1966.

> GEORGE THE FIFTH, by the Grace of God of the United Kingdom of Great Britain and Ireland, and of the British Dominions beyond the Seas, King, Defender of the Faith:
>
> To all to whom these Presents shall come, Greeting.
>
> WHEREAS by proviso (i) to subsection (1) of Section 3 of the Ministry of Health Act, 1919, it is enacted that the duties heretofore performed by the body known as the Medical Research Committee shall after the date of the commencement of the Act be carried on by or under the direction of a Committee of Our Privy Council appointed by Us:
>
> And whereas by Our Order in Council, dated the ninth day of February, 1920, the first day of April, 1920, has been appointed as the date of the commencement of the Act for the purpose aforesaid and the Medical Research Committee as at present constituted will on and after that date cease to exist:
>
> And whereas We were pleased by Our Order in Council, dated the 11th day of March, 1920, to appoint the Lord President of

Our Privy Council, the Minister of Health, the Secretary for Scotland, and the Chief Secretary for Ireland, respectively, for the time being, to be the Committee of Our Privy Council for the purposes aforesaid:

And whereas the said Lord President, the said Minister of Health, the said Secretary for Scotland, and the said Chief Secretary for Ireland, have represented to Us that for the purpose of securing the continued performance of the duties heretofore performed by the Medical Research Committee and with a view to facilitating the holding of, and dealing with, any money provided by Parliament for medical research, and any other property, real or personal, otherwise available for that object, and with a view to encouraging the making of gifts and bequests in aid of the said object, it is expedient that the members of the Medical Research Committee should be created a Body Corporate:

NOW, THEREFORE, know ye that We, by virtue of Our Royal Prerogative and of all other powers enabling Us in that behalf, do, of our special grace, certain knowledge, and mere motion, by these Presents, for Us, Our Heirs and Successors, grant, will, direct, and ordain that:—

1. George Joachim, Viscount Goschen, CBE,

   William Graham, MP,

   The Hon. Edward Frederick Lindley Wood, MP,

   Charles John Bond, CMG, FRCS (Honorary Consultant Surgeon, Leicester Royal Infirmary),

   William Bulloch, MD, FRS (Professor of Bacteriology in the University of London),

   Thomas Renton Elliott, CBE, DSO, MD, FRS (Physician to University College Hospital),

   Henry Head, MD, FRS (formerly Physician to the London Hospital).

   Frederick Gowland Hopkins, DSC, FRS (Professor of Biochemistry in the University of Cambridge),

   Major-General Sir William Boog Leishman, KCMG, CB, FRS (Director of Pathology, Army Medical Service),

   Diarmid Noël Paton, MD, FRS (Regius Professor of Physiology in the University of Glasgow),

Added 1926 *and all other the persons who shall for the time being in pursuance of and in accordance with this Our Charter be Members of the Medical Research Council,* shall be one Body Corporate under the name of "The Medical Research Council", having a perpetual succession and a Common Seal, with full power by and in such name—

   (*a*) To sue and be sued;

   (*b*) To enter into such contracts or agreements in furtherance of the objects of the said Committee of Our Privy Council as the said Committee may direct;

   (*c*) To accept, hold, and dispose of, money or other personal property in furtherance of the said objects including sums voted by Parliament to that end;

   (*d*) To accept any trusts, whether subject to special conditions or not, in furtherance of the said Objects; and

(e) Generally to do all other lawful acts whatsoever that may be conducive or incidental to the attainment of the objects for which the said Committee of Our Privy Council has been appointed, and the said Medical Research Council is hereby established.

Amended 1949

We do hereby for Us, our Heirs and Successors, license, authorize and for ever hereafter enable the Medical Research Council to purchase take on lease or otherwise acquire any lands tenements or hereditaments within Our United Kingdom of Great Britain and *Northern* Ireland not exceeding in the whole the annual value of [£50,000] £*100,000* to be determined according to the value thereof at the time when the same are respectively acquired and to hold all or any lands tenements or hereditaments or interest therein, in perpetuity or on lease or otherwise and from time to time to grant demise alienate or otherwise dispose of the same or any part thereof.

Amended 1949

And We do hereby also for Ourselves, Our Heirs and Successors give and grant Our licence to any person or persons and any Body politic or corporate to assure in perpetuity or otherwise or to demise to or for the benefit of the Medical Research Council any lands tenements or hereditaments whatsoever within Our United Kingdom of Great Britain and *Northern* Ireland within the limits of value aforesaid.

Deleted 1926

[2. The said members of the Medical Research Council shall, subject as hereinafter provided, continue in office until the 30th day of September, 1921, when three members of the Council, to be selected in such manner as the said Committee of Our Privy Council may determine, shall retire, and thereafter three members shall retire at intervals of two years, but any member so retiring shall be eligible for reappointment.

3. Any vacancy, whether casual or otherwise, which may hereafter occur among members of the Medical Research Council shall be filled by appointment by the said Committee of Our Privy Council, but any person appointed to fill a casual vacancy shall only hold office for the remainder of the period of office of the member in whose place he is appointed.

4. Two members of the Medical Research Council shall at all times be members of the House of Lords and of the House of Commons respectively and shall vacate their membership of the Council on ceasing to be so qualified, and the other members of the Council shall be appointed after consultation with the President for the time being of the Royal Society and with the Medical Research Council:

Provided that nothing herein shall be construed as requiring any member of the Council being a Member of Parliament who is appointed after such consultation as aforesaid to vacate his membership of the Council on ceasing to be a Member of Parliament.]

Substituted 1926; deleted 1943

[2. (i) *After the 31st day of January, 1926, the Medical Research Council shall consist of so many members as shall, inclusive of those persons who are members of the Medical Research Council on that date, make up the number of eleven members.*

(ii) *The members of the Medical Research Council shall be appointed by the said Committee of Our Privy Council; eight members shall be appointed in respect of their scientific qualification, after consultation with the President for the time being of the Royal Society and with the Medical Research Council, and of the three remaining members, one shall be a member of the House of Lords and one of the House of Commons and either of these shall vacate his membership of the Council on ceasing to be so qualified.*

Provided that nothing in this Article shall require any member of the Medical Research Council who, being a member of the House of Lords or of the House of Commons, is appointed a member of the Medical Research Council otherwise than in respect of his membership of either House of Parliament, to retire from the Council by reason only of the fact that he has ceased to be a member of Parliament.

3. (i) *On the 30th day of September, 1926, two of the members of the Medical Research Council appointed in respect of their scientific qualifications, to be selected in such manner as the said Committee of Our Privy Council may determine, shall retire, and thereafter two members, to be selected in like manner, shall retire at intervals of one year, and no member retiring as aforesaid shall be eligible for reappointment until a period of at least one year has elapsed since the date of his last retirement.*

(ii) *On the 30th day of September, 1926, one of the other three members of the Medical Research Council, to be selected in such manner as the said Committee of Our Privy Council may determine, shall retire and hereafter one of the said three members, to be selected in like manner, shall retire at intervals of two years, but any of the said members retiring as aforesaid shall be eligible for immediate reappointment.*

4. *Any appointment to fill a casual vacancy which may occur among members of the Medical Research Council by reason of death, resignation or otherwise shall be made in like manner as the appointment of the member in whose place the appointment is made, but any person appointed to fill a casual vacancy shall continue to be a member only for the remainder of the period of office of the member in whose place he is appointed:*

Provided that any member appointed to fill a casual vacancy, who at the time of his retirement shall have been a member of the Council for less than three years shall, notwithstanding any of the provisions of this and the preceding Article, not be ineligible for immediate reappointment.]

Substituted
1943

2. *After the 30th day of September, 1942, the Medical Research Council shall consist of so many members as shall, inclusive of those persons who are members of the Medical Research Council on that date, make up the number of twelve members.*

3. *The members of the Medical Research Council shall be appointed by the said Committee of Our Privy Council; nine members shall be appointed in respect of their scientific qualifications, after consultation with the President for the time being of the Royal Society and with the Medical Research Council, and of the three remaining members, one shall be a member of the House of Lords and one of the House of Commons and either of these shall vacate his membership of the Council on ceasing to be so qualified.*

Provided that nothing in this Article shall require any member of the Medical Research Council who, being a member of the House of Lords or of the House of Commons, is appointed a member of the Medical Research Council otherwise than in respect of his membership of either House of Parliament, to retire from the Council by reason only of the fact that he has ceased to be a member of Parliament.

4. *On the 30th day of September, 1944, and thereafter at intervals of one year every member of the Medical Research Council who has served for four years or longer since the date of his last appointment as such shall retire, and no member appointed in respect of his scientific qualifications retiring as aforesaid shall be eligible for reappointment until a period of at least one year has elapsed since the date of his last retirement.*

5. The Medical Research Council shall with the approval of the said Committee of Our Privy Council appoint one of their members to be Chairman of the Council.

6. The Medical Research Council shall, with the approval of the said Committee of Our Privy Council, appoint one of their members to be Treasurer of the Council, and it shall be the duty of the Treasurer to receive on behalf of the Council all sums payable to the Council for the purposes of medical research.

7. The Medical Research Council shall appoint a Secretary of the Council and may appoint such other officers and servants and may expend such moneys for the administrative purposes of the Council (including travelling expenses and subsistence allowances for members and staff) as they think fit, subject, as to the number of such officers and servants and their remuneration and as to the scale of travelling expenses and subsistence allowances, and as to the amount of such moneys, to the approval of the said Committee of Our Privy Council.

8. The Medical Research Council shall so far as relates to the use and expenditure of any moneys provided by Parliament act in accordance with such directions as may from time to time be given to them by the said Committee of Our Privy Council.

9. The Medical Research Council may, by Special Resolution in that behalf, passed at any meeting by a majority of not less than two-thirds of the Members present and voting (being an absolute majority of the whole number of the Council), and confirmed at a meeting held not less than one month nor more than three months afterwards by a like majority, alter, amend or add to this Our Charter, and such alteration, amendment or addition shall, when allowed by the said Committee of Our Privy Council, become effectual so that this Our Charter shall thenceforward continue and operate as though it had been originally granted and made accordingly. This provision shall apply to this Our Charter, as altered, amended or added to in manner aforesaid.

10. All property for the time being vested in the Medical Research Council or the proceeds of sale thereof shall be held by them for the purposes of the Council in such manner as the said Committee of Our Privy Council, subject to the provision of this Charter or of any trust affecting such property, may approve.

Amended
1957

11. There may be paid as honoraria to Members of the Medical Research Council, not being Members of [either] *the Commons* House of Parliament, such sums as the said Committee of Our Privy Council may from time to time direct.

12. The accounts of the Medical Research Council shall be made up for each financial year ending the 31st day of March, and shall be audited in such manner as the Treasury may direct.

IN WITNESS whereof We have caused these Our Letters to be made Patent.

WITNESS Ourself at Westminster, the First day of April, in the year of Our Lord 1920, and in the Tenth Year of Our Reign.

BY WARRANT under the King's Sign Manual.

SCHUSTER.

Supplemental Charter

This was granted on 27 July 1949 in accordance with a draft approved by an Order in Council of 30 June 1949 (Appendix D). The effect was to make one substantial and two verbal amendments to the Original Charter, and these are shown in the version printed above.

GEORGE THE SIXTH by the Grace of God of Great Britain, Ireland and the British Dominions beyond the Seas King, Defender of the Faith:

To all to whom these Presents shall come, Greeting:

WHEREAS Our Royal Predecessor King George the Fifth in the year of our Lord 1920 by Royal Charter (hereinafter referred to as "the Original Charter") dated the first day of April in the tenth year of his reign constituted the ten persons therein named and all other the persons who should for the time being in pursuance of and in accordance with the Original Charter be Members of the Medical Research Council one Body Corporate under the name of "The Medical Research Council" having a perpetual succession and a Common Seal:

And Whereas the Original Charter was amended in accordance with the provisions of Article 9 thereof by two Special Resolutions of the Medical Research Council in manner therein mentioned and such amendments were respectively allowed by the Committee of Our Privy Council on the first day of March 1926 and the first day of November 1943:

And Whereas by the Original Charter Our said Predecessor for Himself His Heirs and Successors did license authorise and for ever thereafter enable the Medical Research Council to purchase take on lease or otherwise acquire any lands tenements or hereditaments within Our United Kingdom of Great Britain and Ireland not exceeding in the whole the annual value of £50,000 to be determined according to the value thereof at the time when the same were respectively acquired:

And Whereas by the Original Charter Our said Predecessor for Himself His Heirs and Successors did give and grant His licence to any person or persons and any Body politic or corporate to assure in perpetuity or otherwise or to demise to or for the benefit of the Medical Research Council any lands tenements or hereditaments whatsoever within Our United Kingdom of Great Britain and Ireland within the limits of value aforesaid:

And Whereas it has been represented unto Us that the annual value of the whole of the lands tenements and hereditaments within Our United Kingdom which may be acquired by the Medical Research Council should be extended to an annual value of £100,000 (to be determined according to the value thereof at the time when the same are respectively acquired) and that the Medical Research Council should be licensed and authorised to hold the same to such extended value:

NOW THEREFORE know ye that We, by virtue of Our Royal Prerogative and of all other powers enabling Us in that behalf do, of Our special grace, certain knowledge, and mere motion, by these Presents, for Us, Our Heirs and Successors, grant, will, direct and ordain as follows:

1. The Original Charter (so amended as aforesaid) shall be altered and extended and shall henceforth be read, construed and take effect as if the alterations hereby made had originally been contained therein, but otherwise the Original Charter (so amended as aforesaid) shall remain in full force and effect.

2. In Article 1 of the Original Charter, for the figures "£50,000" there shall be substituted the figures "£100,000", and for the expression "Our United Kingdom of Great Britain and Ireland" in the two places where it occurs there shall be substituted the expression "Our United Kingdom of Great Britain and Northern Ireland".

IN WITNESS whereof We have caused these Our Letters to be made Patent.

WITNESS Ourself at Westminster the twenty-seventh day of July in the thirteenth year of Our Reign.

BY WARRANT under the King's Sign Manual.

NAPIER

New Charter

This was granted on 26 October 1966 in accordance with a draft approved by an Order in Council of 20 September 1966 (Appendix D; and see Chapter 6). It is here printed with the amendments allowed by the Order in Council of 5 April 1971 (Appendix D); words that were deleted are shown within heavy square brackets, and those that were added or substituted are printed in italic type.

ELIZABETH THE SECOND by the Grace of God of the United Kingdom of Great Britain and Northern Ireland and of Our other Realms and Territories Queen, Head of the Commonwealth, Defender of the Faith:

To all to whom these Presents shall come, Greeting:

WHEREAS His Majesty King George the Fifth in the year of our Lord One thousand nine hundred and twenty by Royal Charter (hereinafter called "the Original Charter") dated the first day of April in the tenth year of His Reign constituted a Body Corporate by the name of "The Medical Research Council" (hereinafter referred to as "the Council") with perpetual succession and with power to sue and be sued by the said name and to use a Common Seal:

AND WHEREAS the Original Charter was amended from time to time by Special Resolutions of the Council, duly allowed by Orders of a Committee of the Lords of Our Most Honourable Privy Council, and by a Supplemental Charter dated the twenty-seventh day of July, One thousand nine hundred and forty-nine (hereinafter called "the Supplemental Charter"):

AND WHEREAS the Original Charter as so amended was further amended by the Science and Technology Act 1965:

AND WHEREAS it has been represented unto Us that it is

expedient for the better execution of the purposes thereof that the provisions of the Original Charter as so amended should be further amended and that this may best be done by the grant of a new Charter replacing the Original Charter:

NOW THEREFORE Know Ye that We, by virtue of Our Prerogative Royal and of all other powers enabling Us so to do have of Our especial grace, certain knowledge and mere motion granted and declared and do by these Presents for Us, Our Heirs and Successors, grant and declare as follows:

1. The provisions of the Original Charter, except insofar as they incorporate the Medical Research Council and confer upon it perpetual succession, and the Supplemental Charter are hereby revoked, but nothing in this revocation shall affect the legality or validity of any act, deed or thing lawfully done or executed under the provisions of the Original Charter or the Supplemental Charter.

Renumbered
1971

2. (1) The Council shall have a Common Seal, with power to break, alter and make anew the said Seal from time to time at their will and pleasure and by their name shall and may sue and be sued in all courts and in all manner of actions and suits, and shall have power to enter into contracts, to acquire, hold and dispose of property of any kind, to accept trusts and generally to do all matters and things incidental or appertaining to a Body Corporate.

Added 1971

(2) *Any real or personal property (including money and things in action) for the time being vested in or held by the Council may be invested in such stocks, funds, fully paid shares or securities as the Council shall from time to time think fit, whether within or outside Our United Kingdom of Great Britain and Northern Ireland or in the purchase of any interests in leasehold or freehold hereditaments in Our said United Kingdom including rents, provided that in the case of moneys held by the Council as Trustees, the powers conferred by this paragraph shall be exercised subject to the provisions of the law relating to investment by Trustees.*

3. (1) The objects for which the Council are established and incorporated are the purposes for which a Committee of the Lords of Our Most Honourable Privy Council was appointed by Order in Council dated the eleventh day of March One thousand nine hundred and twenty and all such other things as are conducive or incidental to any of those purposes.

(2) The Council may pursue their objects in Our United Kingdom of Great Britain and Northern Ireland or elsewhere.

4. All moneys and property howsoever received by the Council, including any moneys voted by Parliament, shall be applied solely towards the promotion of the objects of the Council and no portion thereof (except as otherwise provided in this Our Charter) shall be paid or transferred directly or indirectly to the members thereof.

5. (1) The Council shall consist of a Chairman, a deputy Chairman and not less than ten or more than fourteen other members.

(2) The Chairman and the Deputy Chairman shall be appointed by Our Secretary of State after consultation with the Council, and the terms of their appointment shall be determined by Our Secretary of State.

(3) The other members shall be appointed, and the terms of

their appointment shall be determined, by Our Secretary of State.

(4) Our Secretary of State shall appoint not less than three-quarters of the total number of members for the time being on account of their qualifications in Science: provided that before appointing any such member he shall consult the Council and the President for the time being of the Royal Society.

(5) Every member shall hold and vacate his office in accordance with the terms of his appointment and shall, on ceasing to be a member, be eligible for reappointment but

(a) a member other than the Chairman and the Deputy Chairman shall not be appointed for a term of more than four years;

(b) a member other than the Chairman and the Deputy Chairman appointed on account of his qualifications in Science shall not be eligible for reappointment before the expiration of one year from the end of that period; and

(c) a member may at any time by notice in writing to Our Secretary of State resign his office.

(6) Except as provided in paragraph (8) of this Article, the Council shall, in the case of any such member as Our Secretary of State, with the approval of the Lords Commissioners of Our Treasury, may determine

(a) pay to him such remuneration and allowances as may be so determined in his case; and

(b) pay to or in respect of him such pension, allowance or gratuity on his retirement or death, or make such payments towards provision for such a pension, allowance or gratuity, as may be so determined in his case.

(7) If a person ceases to be a member of the Council otherwise than on the expiration of his term of office, and it appears to Our Secretary of State that there are special circumstances which make it right that that person should receive compensation, the Council shall make to that person a payment of such amount as Our Secretary of State may, with the approval of the Lords Commissioners of Our Treasury, determine.

(8) The Council shall not in any circumstances or at any time make to or in respect of any person in his capacity as a member of the Council any payment of any kind whatsoever for or in respect of any period when he is also a member of Our Commons House of Parliament, other than a payment by way of reimbursement to him of actual out of pocket expenses previously and necessarily incurred by him in the performance of his duties as such member of the Council.

6. (1) The Council may act notwithstanding a vacancy among the members thereof and the validity of any proceedings of the Council shall not be affected by any defect in the appointment of a member thereof.

(2) The quorum of the Council shall be six members personally present or such greater number as the Council may from time to time determine.

7. Subject to the provisions of this Our Charter, the Council may regulate their own procedure.

8. (1) The Council may appoint Committees to exercise, or advise them on the exercise of, any of their functions and may:

(a) appoint to any such Committee persons who are not members of the Council; and

(b) at any time revoke the appointment of any member of any such Committee.

(2) Where the Council appoint to any such Committee any person who is not a member of the Council they may, if they, with the approval of Our Secretary of State and the Lords Commissioners of Our Treasury, so determine, pay to that person such remuneration and allowances as may be so determined in his case, but Article 5(8) of this Our Charter shall apply to any such person as though he were a member of the Council.

9. (1) The Council shall, with the approval of Our Secretary of State, appoint a Secretary and may appoint such other officers and take into their employment such other persons as the Council may determine subject, as to the number of such officers and other persons, to the approval of Our Secretary of State and the Lords Commissioners of Our Treasury.

(2) The Council may:

(a) pay to their Secretary and to their other officers and to other persons employed by them such remuneration and allowances as the Council may, with the approval of Our Secretary of State and the Lords Commissioners of Our Treasury, from time to time determine; and

Deleted 1971

[(b) as regards any officers or other persons employed in whose case it may be determined by the Council, with the approval of Our Secretary of State and the Lords Commissioners of Our Treasury, so to do, pay to or in respect of them such pension (including gratuities), or provide and maintain for them such pension schemes (whether contributory or not) as may be so determined.

(3) Where the holder of an office or employment with the Council, being a participant in any pension scheme applicable to the office or employment, is or becomes a member of the Council, he may be treated for the purposes of the pension scheme as if his service as a member of the Council were service in an office or employment with the Council, and his rights under the scheme shall not be affected by any provision of this Our Charter which requires that pensions, allowances or gratuities or payments towards the provision of them payable in the case of members of the Council shall be determined by Our Secretary of State with the approval of the Lords Commissioners of Our Treasury.]

Substituted 1971

(b) *as regards any officers or other persons employed in whose case it may be determined by the Council, with the approval of Our Secretary of State and Our Minister for the Civil Service, so to do, pay to or in respect of them such pension and other benefits or compensation (including gratuities) or provide and maintain for them such pension, benefit or compensation schemes (whether contributory or not) as may be so determined.*

(3) *Where the holder of an office or employment with the Council, being a participant in any pension, benefit or compensation scheme applicable to the office or employment, is or becomes a member of the Council, he may be treated for the purposes of the pension, benefit or compensation scheme as if his service as a member of the Council were service in an office or employment with the Council, and his rights under the scheme shall not be affected by any provision of this Our Charter which requires that pensions, allowances, gratuities, benefits, compensation or payment towards the provision of them payable in the case of members of the Council shall be determined by Our Secretary of State with the approval of Our Minister for the Civil Service.*

Appendix F
Nominal Roll of Responsible Ministers

Chairmen of the National Health Insurance Joint Committee

1913–15   The Rt Hon. C. F. G. Masterman, MP (also Financial Secretary to the Treasury)

1915   The Rt Hon. E. S. Montagu, MP (also Financial Secretary to the Treasury)

1915–17   Charles H. Roberts, MP (also Comptroller of HM's Household)

1917–19   Sir Edward Cornwall, Bart, MP (also Comptroller of HM's Household)

1919   The Rt Hon. Waldorf Astor, MP (also Parliamentary Secretary to the Local Government Board)

Minister of Health
(In that capacity from 1 July 1919 to 31 March 1920)

1919–20   The Rt Hon. Christopher Addison, MD, MP (later the Viscount Addison)

Chairmen of the Committee of Privy Council for Medical Research
As Lord President of the Council

1920–22   The Rt Hon. Arthur James Balfour, OM, FRS, MP (later the Earl of Balfour, GCVO)

1922–24   The Most Hon. the Marquess of Salisbury, GCVO (4th Marquess)

1924   The Rt Hon. Lord Parmoor of Frieth, KC

1924–25   The Most Hon. the Marquess Curzon of Kedleston, KG, GCSI, GCIE, DCL, LLD

1925–29   The Rt Hon. the Earl of Balfour, OM, FRS

1929–31   The Rt Hon. Lord Parmoor, KC

1931–35   The Rt Hon. Stanley Baldwin, MP (later Lord Baldwin of Bewdley)

1935–37   The Rt Hon. James Ramsay MacDonald, MP

1937–38   The Rt Hon. Viscount Halifax, GCSI, GCIE (later the Earl of Halifax)

1938   The Rt Hon. Viscount Hailsham, KC, LLD (1st Viscount)

1938–39   The Rt Hon. Viscount Runciman of Doxford

1939–40   The Rt Hon. the Earl Stanhope, DSO, MC

1940   The Rt Hon. Arthur Neville Chamberlain, MP

1940–43   The Rt Hon. Sir John Anderson, GCB, OM, GCSI, GCIE, MP, FRS (later Viscount Waverley)

1943–45   The Rt Hon. Clement Richard Attlee, KG, OM, CH, MP (later Earl Attlee)

1945   The Rt Hon. Lord Woolton, CH

1945–51   The Rt Hon. Herbert Morrison, CH, MP (later Lord Morrison of Lambeth)

1951   The Rt Hon. Viscount Addison, KG, MD, FRCS, FRCP

1951–52   The Rt Hon. Lord Woolton, CH (later Earl of Woolton)

1952–57   The Most Hon. the Marquess of Salisbury, KG (5th Marquess)

1957   The Rt Hon. the Earl of Home

1957–59   The Rt Hon. Viscount Hailsham, QC (2nd Viscount)

1959   The Rt Hon. the Earl of Home

As Minister for Science

1959–64   The Rt Hon. Viscount Hailsham, QC (also Lord Privy Seal, 1959–60; and Lord President of the Council from 1960: renounced title 1963, becoming the Rt Hon. Quintin (McGarel) Hogg, QC)

As Secretary of State for Education and Science

1964   The Rt Hon. Quintin (McGarel) Hogg, QC, MP (became Rt Hon. The Lord Hailsham of St Marylebone (Life Baron), June 1970)

1964–65   The Rt Hon. (Robert Maitland) Michael Stewart, MP

1965   The Rt Hon. (Charles) Anthony (Raven) Crosland, MP

Secretaries of State for Education and Science
(In that capacity from 23 March 1965)

1965–68   The Rt Hon. (Charles) Anthony (Raven) Crosland, MP

1968–70   The Rt Hon. Edward (Watson) Short, MP

1970–   The Rt Hon. Mrs Margaret H. Thatcher, MP

Appendix G
Composition of the Committee of Privy Council for Medical Research

Members *ex officiis*

1920–26   The Lord President of the Council (*Chairman*)
        The Minister of Health
        The Secretary for Scotland
        The Chief Secretary for Ireland—until 1922, when office ceased to
           exist

1926–55   The Lord President of the Council (*Chairman*)
        The Secretary of State for the Home Department
        The Secretary of State for Dominion Affairs—from 1947, for
           Commonwealth Relations
        The Secretary of State for the Colonies
        The Secretary of State for Scotland
        The Minister of Health

1955–59   The Lord President of the Council (*Chairman*)
        The Secretary of State for the Home Department
        The Secretary of State for Commonwealth Relations
        The Secretary of State for the Colonies
        The Secretary of State for Scotland
        The Minister of Health
        The Minister of Labour and National Service

1959–65   The Minister for Science (*Chairman*)—until 1964, when replaced by
           the Secretary of State for Education and Science
        The Secretary of State for the Home Department
        The Secretary of State for Commonwealth Relations
        The Secretary of State for the Colonies
        The Secretary of State for Scotland
        The Minister of Health
        The Minister of Labour

The Minister of Health was designated throughout as the member to preside in the absence of the Chairman.

The Secretary of the Medical Research Council was, *ex officio*, Secretary of the Committee of the Privy Council throughout.

Appendix H
Chairmen and Members of the Medical Research Committee and Council

In the following chronological list of members, the names of chairmen are picked out in heavy type. The figures in parenthesis refer to the subject fields represented by members appointed in respect of their scientific qualifications:

(1) Clinical Medicine
(2) Surgery
(3) Obstetrics and Gynaecology
(4) Psychiatry
(5) Ophthalmology
(6) Radiology
(7) Public Health
(8) Tropical Medicine
(9) Pathology
(10) Bacteriology and Immunology
(11) Zoology
(12) Physiology
(13) Pharmacology
(14) Biochemistry
(15) Anatomy
(16) Psychology
(17) Statistics

(Beginning dates are May in 1913, April in 1920 and October in the other years, while ending dates are March in 1920 and September in other years apart from the filling of casual vacancies.)

Medical Research Committee

1913–16   **The Rt Hon. Lord Moulton,** KCB, FRS. Chairman

1913–20   Christopher Addison, MD, MP (also 1948–51)

1913–20   **Major The Hon. Waldorf Astor,** MP; from 1919 **The Viscount Astor.** Treasurer 1913–16; Chairman 1916–20

1913–16   Professor Sir T. Clifford Allbutt, KCB, MD, FRS (1)

1913–20   C. J. Bond, CMG, FRCS. (Also 1920–21) (2)

1913–20   Professor William Bulloch, MD, FRS (also 1920–21) (9)

1913–16   Professor Matthew Hay, MD (7)

1913–20   Professor F. Gowland Hopkins, DSC, FRCP (also 1920–23, 1926–30) (14)

1913–20   Colonel Sir William B. Leishman, KCMG, CB, FRCP, FRS (also 1920–23, April–June 1926) (10)

1916–20   **The Viscount Goschen,** CBE. Treasurer 1916–February 1920; Chairman February–March 1920 (also 1920–24)

1916–18   A. K. Chalmers, MD, DPH (7)

1916–18   Professor George R. Murray, MD, FRCP (1)

1918–20   Henry Head, MD, FRCP, FRS. (also 1920–25) (1)

1918–20	Professor D. Noel Paton, MD, FRS (also 1920–24) (12)
1920	William Graham, LL B, MP (also 1920–24, 1924–28)
1920	The Hon. Edward F. L. Wood, MP. Treasurer (also 1920–21, 1924)
1920	Colonel T. R. Elliott, CBE, DSO, MD, FRS (also 1920–26, 1927–31, 1939–43) (1)

Medical Research Council

1920–24	**The Viscount Goschen,** CBE. Chairman (reappointed 1924)
1920	The Hon Edward F. L. Wood, MP. Treasurer (also 1924)
1920–24	The Rt Hon. William Graham, LL B, MP (also 1924–28)
1920–21	C. J. Bond, CMG, FRCS (2)
1920–21	Professor William Bulloch, MD, FRS (9)
1920–26	Professor T. R. Elliott, CBE, DSO, MD, FRS (also 1939–43) (1)
1920–25	Henry Head, MD, FRCP, FRS (later Sir Henry Head) (1)
1920–23	Professor F. Gowland Hopkins, D SC, FRCP, FRS (also 1926–30) (14)
1920–23	Major General Sir William B. Leishman, KCMG, CB, FRS (also 1926) (10)
1920–24	Professor D. Noel Paton, MD, FRS (12)
1921–37	The Rt Hon. F. B. Mildmay, MP; from 1922 Lord Mildmay of Flete. Treasurer (reappointed 1923, 1926, 1930, 1934)
1921–27	Sir Frederick W. Andrewes, OBE, DM, FRCP, FRS (10)
1921–27	Sir Cuthbert S. Wallace, KCMG, CB, FRCS (2)
1923–27	Professor George Dreyer, CBE, MD, FRC (reappointed 1923) (9)
1923–28	Sir Archibald E. Garrod, KCMG, MD, FRS (1)
1924	Major A. G. Church, DSO, MC, MP (also 1929–31)
1924	**The Rt Hon. Edward F. L. Wood,** MP (later Lord Irwin, and afterwards the Earl of Halifax). Chairman
1924–29	Professor E. P. Cathcart, CBE, MD, D SC, FRS (reappointed 1925) (12)
1924–29	**The Rt Hon. the Earl of Balfour,** KG, OM, FRS. Chairman
1924–28	The Rt. Hon. William Graham, LL B, MP (reappointed 1925)
1925–29	Sir Charles S. Sherrington, OM, GBE, SC D, FRS (also 1930–34) (12)
1926	Lieutenant-General Sir William B. Leishman, KCB, KCMG, FRS (10)
1926–30	Sir Charles J. Martin, CMG, D SC, FRS (reappointed Oct. 1926) (9)
1926–30	Sir Frederick Gowland Hopkins, OM, D SC, FRCP, FRS (14)
1927–28	Sir Hugh K. Anderson, MD, FRS (12)
1927–31	Professor T. R. Elliott, CBE, DSO, MD, FRS (also 1939–43) (1)
1928–29	The Rt. Hon. Sir Charles P. Trevelyan, Bart., MP
1928–32	Professor Robert Muir, MD, SCD, FRS (later Sir Robert Muir) (9)
1928–32	Sir John H. Parsons, CBE, D SC, FRCS, FRS (5)
1928–31	Professor J. B. Leathes, BM, FRCS, FRS (14)
1929–41	**The Rt. Hon. Viscount D'Abernon,** GCB, GCMG, FRS. Chairman (reappointed 1932)
1929–31	A. G. Church, DSO, MC, MP
1929–33	Professor J. J. R. Macleod, MB, D SC, FRS (12)
1929–33	Wilfrid Trotter, MD, MS, FRCS, FRS (2)
1930–34	J. A. Arkwright, MD, FRS (later Sir Joseph Arkwright) (10)
1930–34	Sir Charles S. Sherrington, OM, GBE, MD, SCD, FRS (12)

1931–35   The Rt Hon. Lord (later Vicscount) Dawson of Penn, GCVO, KCB, MD, PRCP (1)

1931–33   Professor Edward Mellanby, MD, FRS (later Sir Edward Mellanby, GBE, KCB) (12)

1932–36   The Rt Hon. W. S. Morrison, MC, QC, MP (later Lord Dunrossil)

1932–36   Professor E. D. Adrian, MD, FRCP, FRS (also 1939–40, 1940–44) (12)

1932–35   Professor A. E. Boycott, DM, FRCP, FRS (9)

1933–37   Sir Thomas Lewis, CBE, MD, DSC, FRCP, FRS (reappointed Oct. 1933) (1)

1933–37   Sir David P. D. Wilkie, OBE, MD, CHM, FRCS (2)

1933–39   Professor H. S. Raper, CBE, D SC, MB, FRCP, FRS (12) (reappointed 1935)

1934–36   **The Most Hon. The Marquess of Linlithgow,** KT, GCIE. Chairman

1934–38   Professor A. J. Clark, MC, MD, FRCP, FRS (also 1939–41) (13)

1934–38   Sir John C. G. Ledingham, CMG, DSC, FRCP, FRS (10)

1935–39   Professor J. A. Ryle, MD, FRCP (1)

1935–40   Professor Matthew J. Stewart, MB, FRCP (9) (reappointed 1936)

1936–40   Richard K. Law, MP (later the Rt. Hon. Lord Coleraine) (reappointed 1938)

1936–39   Professor John Mellanby, MD, FRS (12)

1936–48   **Lord Balfour of Burleigh,** DL. Chairman (reappointed 1944)

1937–48   Sir William M. Goodenough, Bart., DL, Treasurer (reappointed 1944)

1937–41   Professor G. E. Gask, CMG, DSO, FRCS (2)

1937–42   Professor L. J. Witts, MD, FRCP (also 1943–47) (1)

1938–42   Professor C. R. Harington, PHD, FRS (later Sir Charles Harington) (14)

1938–41   Professor W. W. C. Topley, MD, FRCP, FRS (10)

1939–41   Professor A. J. Clark, MC, MD, FRCP, FRS (13)

1939–43   Professor T. R. Elliott, CBE, DSO, MD, FRCP, FRS (1)

1939–44   Professor E. D. Adrian, OM, MD, FRCP, FRS (later Lord Adrian) (reappointed 1940) (12)

1940–42   The Rt. Hon. J. G. Stuart, MVO, MC, MP (later Lord Stuart of Findhorn) (reappointed 1940)

1940–44   Sir W. Wilson Jameson, KCB, MD, FRCP (7)

1941–45   Sir Ernest Rock Carling, MB, FRCP, FRCS (2)

1941–45   Professor S. P. Bedson, MD, FRS (later Sir Samuel Bedson) (10)

1941–47   Professor Frederic C. Bartlett, CBE, FRS (also 1948–52) (reappointed 1943) (16)

1942–46   Professor D. Keilin, SCD, FRS (14)

1942–46   Sir Henry H. Dale, OM, GBE, MD, FRCP, FRS (12)

1942–46   Sir Charles Glen MacAndrew, MP (later the Rt Hon. Lord MacAndrew)

1943–47   Professor L. J. Witts, MD, FRCP (1)

1943–48   Professor J. R. Learmouth, CBE, CHM, FRCSE (later Sir James R. Learmouth, KCVO) (2)

1944–48   A. N. Drury, CBE, MD, FRS (later Sir Alan Drury) (9)

1944–48   Professor J. C. Spence, MC, MD, FRCP (also 1952–54) (1)

1945–49   Professor P. A. Buxton, CMG, MRCS, FRS (11)

1945–49   Sir Alexander Fleming, MB, FRCS, FRCP, FRS (10)

1946–50   Professor C. A. Lovatt Evans, DSC, FRCP, FRS (later Sir Charles Lovatt Evans) (12)

1946–50   Professor R. A. Peters MC, MD, FRS (later Sir Rudolph Peters) (14)

1946–54   Group-Captain C. A. B. Wilcock, OBE, AFC, MP (reappointed 1950)

1947–48   Professor N. Hamilton Fairley, CBE, MD, DSC, FRCP, FRS (also 1949–51) (8)

1947–51   Professor J. H. Gaddum, SCD, MRCS, FRS (13)

1948–49   Professor H. P. Himsworth, MD, FRCP (later Sir Harold Himsworth, KCB, FRS) (also 1966–68) (1)

1948–51   **The Rt Hon. Viscount Addison,** KG, MD, FRCS, FRCP. Chairman

1948–52   Sir Frederic C. Bartlett, CBE, MA, FRS (16)

1948–52   Sir George E. Schuster, KCSI, KCMG, CBE, MC. Treasurer

1948–52   Sir Howard W. Florey, OM, PHD, MD, FRCP, FRS (later Lord Florey) (9)

1948–52   Sir Geoffrey Jefferson, CBE, MS, FRCS, FRCP, FRS (2)

1949–51   Sir Neil Hamilton Fairley, KBE, DSC, MD, FRCP, FRS (8)

1949–53   Sir Percival Hartley, CBE, MC, DSC, FRS (10)

1949–53   Professor J. McMichael, MD, FRCP (later Sir John McMichael) (1)

1950–54   Professor W. E. le Gros Clark, DSC, FRCS, FRS (later Sir Wilfrid le Gros Clark (15)

1950–54   Professor F. G. Young, DSC, FRS (later Sir Frank Young) (14)

1951–55   Sir James R. Learmonth, KCVO, CBE, CHM, FRCS (2)

1951–55   Professor G. L. Brown, CBE, MSC, MB, FRS (later Sir Lindor Brown) (12)

1952–60   **The Earl of Limerick,** GBE, KCB, DSO. Chairman (reappointed 1956)

1952–56   Professor G. R. Cameron, MB, DSC, FRCP, FRS (later Sir Roy Cameron) (9)

1952–56   Professor A. J. Lewis, MD, FRCP (later Sir Aubrey Lewis) (4)

1952–60   Sir Geoffrey Vickers, VC, MA. Treasurer (reappointed 1956)

1952–54   Sir James C. Spence, MC, MD, FRCP (1)

1953–57   Professor R. Platt, MSC, MD, FRCP (later Sir Robert Platt, Bart, afterwards Lord Platt) (1)

1953–57   Professor E. T. C. Spooner, MD (10)

1954–58   Professor G. W. Pickering, MD, FRCP (later Sir George Pickering) (1)

1954–58   Professor A. Bradford Hill, CBE, DSC, FRS (later Sir Austin Bradford Hill) (17)

1954–58   Professor G. F. Marrian, DSC, FRS (14)

1954–55   The Hon. R. F. Wood, MP

1955–59   Richard Fort, MP

1955–59   Professor R. C. Garry, MB, CHB, DSC, FRFPSG (12)

1955–59   H. J. Seddon, CMG, DM, FRCS (later Sir Herbert Seddon) (12)

1956–60   Professor G. Payling Wright, DM, FRCP (9)

1956–60   J. D. N. Hill, MB, FRCP, DPM (later Sir Denis Hill) (4)

1957–61   Professor A. A. Miles, CBE, MD, FRCP, FRS (later Sir Ashley Miles) (10)

K*

1957–61	Professor C. H. Stuart-Harris, CBE, MD, FRCP (later Sir Charles Stuart-Harris) (1)
1958–62	Professor R. H. S. Thompson, BSC, DM (14)
1958–62	Professor E. J. Wayne, MD, PHD, FRCP (later Sir Edward Wayne) (1)
1958–62	Professor Sir Brian Windeyer, MB, MRCP, FRCS, FFR (also 1968–71) (6)
1959–64	Sir Hugh Linstead, OBE, FPS, MP (reappointed 1963)
1959–63	Professor A. L. Hodgkin, MA, FRS (later Sir Alan Hodgkin) (12)
1959–63	Professor R. Milnes Walker, MS, FRCS (2)
1960–68	Sir Edward Collingwood, CBE, SC D. Treasurer (reappointed 1964)
1960–64	Professor T. Crawford, MD, FRFPSG (9)
1960–64	Professor W. M. Millar, MD (4)
1960–61	**The Rt. Hon. the Viscount Amory.** Chairman
1961–65	Professor M. L. Rosenheim, CBE, MD, FRCP (later Sir Max Rosenheim, afterwards Lord Rosenheim) (1)
1961–65	Professor Wilson Smith, MD, FRS (10)
1961–65	**The Rt. Hon. Lord Shawcross,** QC. Chairman
1962–66	Professor G. M. Bull, MD, FRCP (1)
1962–66	Professor A. Neuberger, CBE, MD, PHD, FRS (14)
1962–65	Professor M. Swann, PHD, FRS (later Sir Michael Swann) (11)
1963–67	Professor H. J. B. Atkins, DM, MCH, FRCS (later Sir Hedley Atkins, KBE) (2)
1963–67	Professor W. D. M. Paton, DM, FRS (13)
1964–68	Professor A. R. Currie, BSC, MB, FRCPE, FRCPG (9)
1964–68	Professor Martin Roth, MD, FRCP, DPM (later Sir Martin Roth) (4)
1964–65	Austen Albu, B SC, MP
1965–67	Arthur Blenkinsop, FCIS, MP
1965–69	**The Rt. Hon. the Viscount Amory,** GCMG. Chairman
1965–69	Professor W. Melville Arnott, TD, B SC, MD, FRCP (later Sir Melville Arnott) (1)
1965–69	Professor D. G. Evans, DSC, FRS (10)
1965–69	Professor J. L. Gowans, DPHIL, MB, FRS (10)
1966–70	Professor D. A. K. Black, MD, FRCP (later Sir Douglas Black) (1)
1966–70	Professor W. T. J. Morgan, CBE, FRS (14)
1966–67	Lord Platt, MD, MSC, FRCP (1)
1966–68	Sir Harold Himsworth, KCB, MD, FRCP, FRS. Deputy Chairman and Secretary (1)
1967–71	Professor A. W. Kay, MD, CHM, FRCS, FRCSE, FRCSG (later Sir Andrew Kay) (2)
1967–71	Professor R. A. Gregory, DSC, MRCS, FRS (12)
1968–	Sir John Gray, MB, SCD FRS. Secretary (12)
1968–71	Professor Sir Brian Windeyer, DSC, FRCP, FRCS (6)
1968–69	Mr D. Marquand, MP
1969–	**His Grace the Duke of Northumberland,** KG, FRS. Chairman
1969–72	Professor D. A. Pond, MD, FRCP (4)
1969–72	Professor T. Symington, MD, FRCP, FRCPG (9)
1969–71	Professor A. S. V. Burgen, MD, FRS (13)
1969–	Professor R. E. O. Williams, MD, FRCP (10)

1969–   Laurence Pavitt, MP
1970–   Professor Sir Richard Doll, OBE, MD, DSC, FRCP, FRS (1)
1970–   Professor R. R. Porter, PHD, FRS (14)
1970–   Professor P. M. B. Walker, PHD (11)
1971–   Professor W. S. Peart, MD, FRCP, FRS (1)
1971–   J. P. Bull, MB, FRCP (1)
1971–   Professor R. B. Welbourn, MD, FRCS (2)
1971–   D. G. Davey, OBE, PHD (13)

Appendix J*

Senior Members of the Headquarters Staff of the Medical Research Committee and Council

(Names under highest rank attained; titles as at latest date)

Secretaries:

Sir Walter M. Fletcher, KBE, CB, MD, SCD, FRCP, FRS (1914–33)

Sir Edward Mellanby, GBE, KCB, MD, FRCP, FRS (1933–49)

Sir Harold P. Himsworth, KCB, MD, FRCP, FRS (1949–68; also Deputy Chairman 1967–68)

Sir John Gray, MB, SCD, FRS (from 1968; earlier Second Secretary 1966–68)

Second Officers (various titles):

Sir A. Landsborough Thomson, CB, OBE, DSC (1919–57; as Assistant Secretary 1913, Principal Assistant Secretary 1936, Under Secretary 1946 and Second Secretary 1949; later employed part-time for special duties 1957–70).

R. H. L. Cohen, CB, MRCS (1957–62, as Deputy Chief Medical Officer; earlier Principal Medical Officer 1955, Senior Medical Officer 1950, on staff from 1948; later seconded to Ministry of Health, and successor Department of Health and Social Security, where ranked as PMO 1962, DCMO 1967, Chief Scientist 1972–73)

C. Y. Carstairs, CMG (1963–65, as Deputy Secretary, while temporarily seconded from Civil Service)

Sir Charles R. Harington, KBE, SCD, FRS (1965–66, as Acting Second Secretary; and as Consultant Adviser 1962–65 and 1966–67, after retirement as Director, NIMR)

S. G. Owen, MD, FRCP (from 1968, as Second Secretary)

Administrative Secretaries (third officers, from 1965)

D. A. Smith, BSC (1965–67, while temporarily seconded from Civil Service)

J. G. Duncan, LLB (from 1967; earlier Assistant Secretary 1954, with supplementary grading as Principal Administrative Officer 1960; on staff from 1945)

Principal Medical Officers

F. H. K. Green, CBE, MD, FRCP (1949–55; earlier SMO 1947; on staff from 1929)

F. J. C. Herrald, CBE, MB, FRCPE (1955–70; earlier SMO 1949; on staff from 1938)

B. S. Lush, MD, FRCP (1961–73; earlier SMO 1957; on staff from 1951)

* Equivalent lists of senior scientific staff, at the National Institute for Medical Research and elsewhere, are given in appendices to Volume Two.

Joan Faulkner, MB, MRCP (Lady Doll) (1968–72; earlier SMO 1957, with supplementary grading as Principal SMO from 1964; on staff from 1943; seconded to DHSS 1972)

M. P. W. Godfrey, MB, MRCP (from 1970; earlier SMO 1964; on staff from 1960)

R. C. Norton, MB (from 1972; earlier SMO 1959; on staff from 1958)

Assistant Secretaries

D. V. T. Fairrie, CBE, FCA (1950–61, with supplementary grading as Principal Administrative Officer from 1957; on staff from 1934; seconded to PHLS Board 1961–68

J. D. Whittaker, MBE (1957–68; on staff from 1946; seconded to PHLS Board 1968)

C. A. Kirkman (from 1960, on transfer from Civil Service)

R. Wakefield (1964–70, while temporarily seconded from Civil Service)

A. E. Turner (from 1968; on staff from 1949)

F. Rushton (from 1969; on staff from 1948)

G. M. Levack, OBE (from 1968)

D. Noble (from 1971; on staff from 1962)

Senior Medical Officers

J. M. Rogan, MD, FRCPE (1948–51)

H. W. Bunjé, MD, FRCP (from 1964; on HQ staff from 1960)

P. J. Chapman, MB (from 1968; on staff from 1959)

Sheila Howarth, MB, MRCP (Lady McMichael) (from 1968; on staff from 1964)

M. Ashley-Miller, MB (from 1969; on staff from 1964)

Katherine Lévy, MB (from 1970; on staff from 1964)

Elizabeth Neale, BM, MRCP (from 1971; on staff from 1965)

A. M. Baker, MRCS (from 1971; on staff from 1967)

Other senior staff for ten or more years in or above grade of medical officer, principal or equivalent (dates show total service on staff)

D. J. Cawthron, MA (from 1950)

E. M. B. Clements, MB (1954–72)

Margaret Gorrill, MB (Lady Mallinson) (1955–69)

J. H. Dixon, MBE (1920–56)

R. F. Smart, OBE (1928–68)

J. C. R. Hudson (1954–68; seconded to Department of Education and Science 1968–71, later transferred)

J. M. Jeffs, AACCA (from 1947)

Secretaries, Industrial (Fatigue) Health Research Board

Sir Duncan R. Wilson, CBE, MA (1919–28, on secondment from duty as H.M. Inspector of Factories)

Air Vice-Marshal Sir David Munro, KCB, CIE, MB, FRCSE (1929–42)

R. S. F. Schilling, MD (1942–46)

Index of general subjects

T

U

Index of personal* names

---

* Peers who had that rank at date of first mention are entered under
titles; other peers and all knights are entered under surnames, with title
following within parenthesis. Where title and surname differ, cross-
references are given.

Printed in England for Her Majesty's Stationery Office
by The Campfield Press, St. Albans

Dmd. 505619.   K.11.   12/73.